Population Dynamics
and Infectious Diseases in Asia

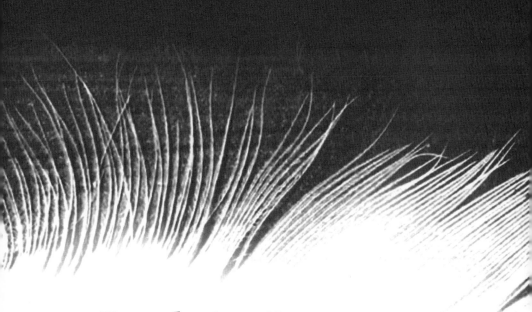

Population Dynamics
and Infectious Diseases in Asia

Editors

Adrian C Sleigh
NCEPH, Australian National University, Australia

Chee Heng Leng
Asia Research Institute, NUS, Singapore

Brenda SA Yeoh
Asian MetaCentre for Population and Sustainable Development Analysis,
Asia Research Institute, NUS Singapore

Phua Kai Hong
Lee Kuan Yew School of Public Policy, NUS, Singapore

Rachel Safman
Department of Sociology, NUS, Singapore

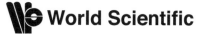 **World Scientific**

NEW JERSEY · LONDON · SINGAPORE · BEIJING · SHANGHAI · HONG KONG · TAIPEI · CHENNAI

Published by

World Scientific Publishing Co. Pte. Ltd.

5 Toh Tuck Link, Singapore 596224

USA office: 27 Warren Street, Suite 401-402, Hackensack, NJ 07601

UK office: 57 Shelton Street, Covent Garden, London WC2H 9HE

British Library Cataloguing-in-Publication Data
A catalogue record for this book is available from the British Library.

ISBN 981-256-833-6

Typeset by Stallion Press
Email: enquiries@stallionpress.com

Printed in Singapore by World Scientific Printers (S) Pte Ltd

Contributors

Niels G BECKER is Professor of Biostatistics at the National Centre for Epidemiology and Population Health. ANU College of Medicine and Health Sciences, The Australian National University. He is also a member of the National Centre for Biosecurity at ANU. His research has focused on developing new statistical methods for health studies, with recent work concerned with the association between deep vein thrombosis and air travel. He also has a longstanding interest in the use of modeling to inform infectious disease control, including vaccine preventable infections and outbreaks of emerged infections such as SARS.

David J BRADLEY is Ross Professor of Tropical Hygiene Emeritus at the London School of Hygiene and Tropical Medicine and Leverhulme Emeritus Fellow in the Department of Zoology, Oxford University. He has worked on the epidemiology and control of vector-borne and infectious diseases, water in relation to health, and concepts in international health since 1961, living in East Africa for ten years and working in many countries worldwide.

CHAN Chee Khoon is Professor (Health & Development) at the School of Social Sciences, Universiti Sains Malaysia. He was a founding executive board member of the International Society for Equity in Health (www.iseqh.org) and has served on the editorial advisory boards of the *International Journal for Equity in Health* and *Global Social Policy*. He contributed a chapter on genomics and population health (co-written with Gilles de Wildt and Helen Wallace) for *Global Health Watch*, 2005–2006 (Zed Books, 2005). His recently published work, on the political economy of health care reforms and the social ecology of emergent infectious outbreaks, is addressed to public interest, international agency and academic constituencies.

CHEE Heng Leng is Senior Research Fellow at the Asia Research Institute, National University of Singapore. Before coming to the NUS, she was an Associate Professor at Universiti Putra Malaysia. She has researched and written widely on community health and health care issues, and was one of the writers of the 2002 WHO report *Genomics and World Health*.

Suok Kai CHEW is Deputy Director of Medical Services, Epidemiology and Disease Control Division, Ministry of Health, Singapore. He is also Adjunct Associate Professor, Department of Community, Occupational and Family Medicine, National University of Singapore. He has published extensively in the field of communicable and non-communicable diseases.

Vincent J DEL CASINO, Jr. is Associate Professor, Department of Geography, California State University, Long Beach. He has published on the geographies of health, healthcare, and HIV/AIDS in a number of journals, including *Health and Place, The Professional Geographer*, and *Disability Studies Quarterly*. His broader co-authored work on the politics of space, representation and identity has also appeared in *Progress in Human Geography* and *Social and Cultural Geography*. He has co-published research on organisational geographies in *Geoforum* and in a forthcoming title from SUNY Press titled *Who Gets What Where? Advancing the Sociology of Spatial Inequality*. He has also been Principal Investigator on a University-Wide AIDS Research Program grant that examined the intersections of drug use, HIV risk, and identity politics among men who have sex with men in Long Beach, California.

Kathryn GLASS is Research Fellow at the National Centre for Epidemiology and Population Health, ANU College of Medicine and Health Sciences, The Australian National University. Her research interests are in developing mathematical models to describe transmission of childhood infectious diseases such as measles, and emerging infectious diseases such as SARS.

Kee Tai GOH is Senior Consultant, Communicable Diseases, and Director, WHO Collaborating Centre for Environmental Epidemiology, Ministry of Health, Singapore. He is also Clinical Associate Professor, Department of Community, Occupational and Family Medicine, National University of Singapore. He has published extensively in the fields of infectious diseases and environmental epidemiology.

Mei–Ling HSU is Professor of Journalism at the National Chengchi University in Taiwan. She is also an Adjunct Professor of the Graduate Institute of Public Health at the Taipei Medical University. She has researched and published widely in the field of health communication. Her current research interests include topics such as social construction of health in the media, health campaign design and evaluation, lay discourse of medicine, and ethics in health information dissemination.

Sukhan JACKSON is Senior Lecturer at the School of Economics, The University of Queensland, Brisbane, Australia. She has published extensively on health economics including the economics of disease control and health financing in China, and on the economics of ageing in Australia.

David KELLY worked in academic positions focused on China's economic and political reforms (Contemporary China Centre, The Australian National University, and School of Politics, Australian Defence Force Academy) after completing a PhD in Chinese studies at Sydney University and holding a Fulbright Fellowship in the United States (University of Chicago). He lived and worked professionally in Beijing from 2000 through the SARS crisis of 2003, and is currently Senior Research Fellow in the East Asian Institute, National University of Singapore.

Vernon JM LEE is a public health physician with the Communicable Disease Centre at Tan Tock Seng Hospital. A graduate of the NUS Medical School and Johns Hopkins Bloomberg School of Public Health, his areas of interest are healthcare economics, management and infectious disease epidemiology. He has conducted research on national pandemic preparedness strategies, and on the impact and prevention of infectious diseases such as influenza, dengue, HIV/AIDS, and hospital acquired infections.

Yuguo LI is Associate Professor (Senior Lecturer) at the Department of Mechanical Engineering, the University of Hong Kong. He has worked for 15 years at the interface areas between fluid dynamics, indoor environment and health in Sweden, Australia and Hong Kong. He has published widely on natural ventilation, bioaerosols, engineering control of infectious diseases including SARS and computational fluid dynamics.

LIEW Kai Khiun is currently pursuing his PhD at the Wellcome Trust Centre for the History of Medicine at University College London. His field of research concerns the role of civil society in the provision of public health in British Malaya. He has published articles and book reviews relating to historical subjects on occupational health, mental asylums, venereal diseases and influenza.

Ching-I LIU is currently a Research Assistant at the National Applied Research Laboratories in Taiwan. She has a Master of Arts degree in Journalism from the National Chengchi University in Taiwan. Her thesis deals with news coverage of SARS in the Taiwanese media.

Xi-Li LIU is Doctor-in-Chief at Henan Centre for Disease Control and Prevention (Henan CDC), China. He has been Principal Investigator for several TDR/WHO Projects since 1990. The research outcome of "Economics of malaria control in China: cost, performance and effectiveness of Henan's consolidation programme" was judged as an outstanding advance in scientific knowledge in an international context by the SEB Steering Committee of WHO/TDR. He has published on malaria, TB, community health and health economics.

Chris LYTTLETON is Head of the Anthropology Department, Macquarie University, Sydney, Australia. His primary research work focuses on the social impact of HIV/AIDS in Thailand and Laos; changing patterns of drug abuse in mainland SE Asia; and mobility, social change and cross-border disease vulnerability in the Upper Mekong. He has published widely on these topics including the monograph. *Watermelons, Bars and Trucks: Dangerous Intersections in Northwest Laos* (Institute for Cultural Research, Vientiane, 2004) and book *Endangered Relations: Negotiating Sex and AIDS in Thailand* (Routledge/Martin Dunitz, and White Lotus Press, 2000).

Xiaopeng LUO is Director, Center for Poverty Alleviation Stuides, University of Guizhou. He holds a doctorate in agricultural economics from the Unitersity of Minnesota. He was formerly a senior staffer in the Economic Reform Institute under the State Council, which directly advised Premier Zhao Ziyang and oversaw the early rounds of agricultural modernisation. Formerly China Representative of International Development Enterprises, an American NGO, and Dean of the Oxbridge Business School, Beijing, he has numerous publications in rural reform and public policy.

Anthony J McMICHAEL is Director of the National Centre for Epidemiology and Population Health, ANU College of Medicine and Health Sciences, The Australian National University. He has taken a special interest in studies of how large-scale environmental, social and technological changes influence patterns of infectious disease occurrence. A particular interest is the role of climate change in facilitating the spread of various climate-sensitive infectious diseases, including the study of environmental and climatic influences on mosquito-borne infectious diseases in Australia. He has written widely on the evolutionary, historical and cultural contexts to the ever-changing relationship between humans and the microbial world.

Tran Lam NGUYEN studied medical anthropology at the University of Amsterdam. His PhD project is about indigenous people in Vietnam and emerging epidemics. He edited a book about the HIV/AIDS program in Vietnam and has written various articles about indigenous people, infectious disease, migration, and development. One of his articles will be published in *Indigenous People: Development Process or Domestication?* (All India Press, 2006).

Shir Nee ONG is a Geography lecturer at Hwa Chong Institution (College), Singapore. She has completed a Master degree with a Thesis on SARS in Singapore and co-published a journal article on SARS in *Health Policy* (June 2005). Her current research interests are geographies of health and ill-health, including AIDS and SARS.

PHUA Kai Hong is Joint Associate Professor at the Lee Kuan Yew School of Public Policy and the Yong Loo Lin School of Medicine, National University of Singapore. Dr Phua has published widely in the field of health care management and related areas including the history of health services, health and population ageing, health economics and financing. His current research interests are comparative health policy, especially organisational and financing systems, and health sector reforms in the Asia-Pacific region. He is active as Chairman, Executive Board of the Asia-Pacific Health Economics Network (APHEN), Founding Member of the Asian Health Systems Reform Network (DRAGONET), and had served previously as Associate Editor of the *Asia-Pacific Journal of Public Health*. He has undertaken health-care consulting assignments for numerous governments and organisations throughout the Asia-Pacific region, including the World Bank and World Health Organization.

Hua QIAN is a doctoral student at the Department of Mechanical Engineering, the University of Hong Kong. His research interest lies in indoor environment engineering and sciences. He has published several papers on natural ventilation and the ventilation of hospital wards.

Rachel SAFMAN is Assistant Professor in the Department of Sociology at the National University of Singapore. Her research focuses on the impact of and responses to infectious disease outbreaks in mainland Southeast Asia.

Adrian C SLEIGH is Professor of Epidemiology at the National Centre for Epidemiology and Population Health, ANU College of Medicine and Health Sciences, The Australian National University. He is also a member of the National Centre for Biosecurity at ANU. He has worked for many years with resource-poor communities on health, development and disease control, and has published research on health effects of dams, parasitic infections, tuberculosis and viral diseases, including SARS.

Guixiang SONG is Professor of Health Statistics and Director for Department of Health Statistics at Shanghai Municipal Center for Diseases Prevention and Control. She has published research papers on Shanghai mortality.

Guo-Jie WANG is Associate Doctor-in-Chief at Henan Centre for Disease Control and Prevention, China. He has worked for many years with tuberculosis control and has published research in the field of tuberculosis.

Annelies WILDER-SMITH is Head of the Travellers' Health and Vaccination Centre at the Tan Tock Seng Hospital, Singapore. She is also concurrently Adjunct Associate Professor at the Department of Community,

Occupational and Family Medicine, National University of Singapore. She researches on meningococcal disease related to the Hajj pilgrimage.

Tze Wai WONG is Professor of the Department of Community and Family Medicine, the Chinese University of Hong Kong. He has been practicing public health and occupational medicine for 28 years, with 20 years of research experience in air pollution, infectious diseases and public health. He has published more than 130 journal papers on public health and infectious diseases including SARS and hantaviruses.

Xiushi YANG is Professor, Department of Sociology and Criminal Justice, Old Dominion University. He has worked and published extensively in the field of internal migration. His recent and ongoing research focuses on migrants' reproductive and HIV risk behaviours and the interplay of migration and gender in influencing female migrants' health behaviour in China. His most recent publications include research on HIV risk and sexual behaviours among female entertainment workers and on links between migration and spread of HIV risk behaviours at both individual and community level.

Brenda SA YEOH is Professor, Department of Geography, National University of Singapore as well as Research Leader of the Asian Migration Research Cluster and Principal Investigator of the Asian MetaCentre at the University's Asia Research Institute. She recently published an edited volume on *Migration and Health in Asia* (Routledge, 2005, with Santosh Jatrana and Mika Toyota).

Ignatius TS YU is Professor at the Department of Community and Family Medicine, the Chinese University of Hong Kong. He has worked for 25 years in occupational medicine and public health. He has published widely on occupational medicine, environmental health and epidemiology.

Shengnian ZHANG is Professor of Toxicology and Epidemiology and the Director for Shanghai Municipal Center for Diseases Prevention and Control. He has published more than 30 research papers in epidemiology and toxicology.

Zhongwei ZHAO is Senior Fellow at Demography and Sociology Program, The Australian National University, and Bye Fellow at Pembroke College, University of Cambridge. He has been working in the following areas: simulating changes in kinship structure and household composition, fertility behaviour in the past, using genealogies for demographic research, and health and mortality transition in China. He has published widely in major demography journals.

Feng ZHOU is Professor of Epidemiology at Department of Health Statistics at Shanghai Municipal Center for Diseases Prevention and Control. He has published research papers on mortality.

Tingkui ZHOU is Professor of Epidemiology and Director for Shanghai Preventive Medicine Association. He has conducted many field studies and published research papers on infectious diseases.

Preface

We are pleased to bring together theoretical and applied research under-way on population dynamics and infectious diseases in Asia. This volume is based on a wide range of selected papers first presented at an international workshop entitled "*Population Dynamics and Infectious Diseases in Asia*", held in Singapore in October 2004. The workshop was organised by the Asian MetaCentre for Population and Sustainable Development Analysis at the National University of Singapore, and was supported by the Wellcome Trust, UK. From the conception of the workshop to selecting, editing and putting together the papers into a book, our work was facilitated by many individuals who gave generously of their time and assistance. First, we are grateful for the support we received from the Asia Research Institute of the National University of Singapore, and the National Centre for Epidemi-ology and Population Health of The Australian National University. We are also indebted to the Senior Administrative Officer, Verene Koh at the Asian MetaCentre for her unstinting help in receiving and organising the papers both for the workshop and this volume. Ludovic Francois, Kelly Fu, Theodora Lam provided us with timely research assistance and invalu-able help with the myriad tasks associated with copy-editing this volume of papers. To all the contributors of the volume, we would like to express our gratitude for collaborating with us in bringing this book project to fruition.

The Editors

Contents

Contributors   v

Preface   xiii

INTRODUCTION

1. Transdisciplinary Approaches to Population Dynamics and
    Infectious Diseases in Asia   3
    *Adrian C Sleigh, Chee Heng Leng, Brenda SA Yeoh, Phua Kai Hong
    and Rachel Safman*

FRAMEWORKS FOR UNDERSTANDING
POPULATION DYNAMICS AND INFECTIOUS
DISEASES IN ASIA

2. Ecological and Social Influences on Emergence and
    Resurgence of Infectious Diseases   23
    Anthony J McMichael

3. Landscape Epidemiology and Migration: Insights and Problems
    at Several Scales for Transmissible Diseases   39
    David J Bradley

4. Water, Dams and Infection: Asian Challenges   57
    Adrian C Sleigh

5. The Impact of Imported Infection   73
    Niels G Becker and Kathryn Glass

6. Demographic and Epidemiological Transitions in Asia:
    Comparative Health Policies for Emerging Infectious Diseases   97
    Phua Kai Hong and Vernon JM Lee

DEVELOPMENT AND INFECTIOUS DISEASES IN ASIA

7. Control of Infectious Diseases and Rising Life Expectancy in
    Shanghai: 1950–2003   113
    *Zhongwei Zhao, Feng Zhou, Guixiang Song, Shengnian Zhang
    and Tingkui Zhou*

8. Social Change and Infectious Diseases in Northern Mountain
    Vietnam   133
    Tran Lam Nguyen

9. NGOs and the Re-Organisation of "Community
    Development" in Northern Thailand: Mediating the Flows of
    People Living with HIV and AIDS   159
    Vincent J Del Casino Jr

10. HIV/AIDS in Singapore: State Policies, Social Norms and Civil
    Society Action   187
    Shir Nee Ong and Brenda SA Yeoh

POPULATION MOBILITY AND INFECTIOUS DISEASES IN ASIA

11. Cultivating the Market: Mobility, Labour and Sexual Exchange
    in Northwest Laos   207
    Chris Lyttleton

12. Household Poverty, Off-farm Migration and Pulmonary
    Tuberculosis in Rural Henan, China   231
    Sukhan Jackson, Adrian C Sleigh, Guo-Jie Wang and Xi-Li Liu

13. Migration, Gender, and STD Risk: A Case Study of Female
    Temporary Migrants in Southwestern China   245
    Xiushi Yang

14. The Hajj Pilgrimage: Public Health Consequences of the
    Largest People Mass Movement   271
    Annelies Wilder-Smith

COMPARATIVE PERSPECTIVES ON SARS IN ASIA

15. Epidemiology of Emerging Infectious Diseases in Singapore,
    with Special Reference to SARS   287
    Kee Tai Goh and Suok Kai Chew

16. Probable Roles of Bio-Aerosol Dispersion in the SARS
    Outbreak in Amoy Gardens, Hong Kong   305
    Yuguo Li, Hua Qian, Ignatius Tak Sun Yu and Tze Wai Wong

17. Discourse of "Othering" During the SARS Outbreak in
    Taiwan: A News Analysis   329
    Mei-Ling Hsu and Ching-I Liu

18. Risk Perception and Coping Responses in a SARS Outbreak
    in Malaysia   351
    Chan Chee Khoon

19. A Defining Moment, Defining a Moment: Making SARS
    History in Singapore   369
    Liew Kai Khiun

20. SARS and China's Rural Migrant Labour: Roots of a
    Governance Crisis   389
    David Kelly and Xiaopeng Luo

DRAWING LESSONS FROM THE PAST TO
RESPOND TO FUTURE CHALLENGES

21. Avian Flu: One More Infection Challenge from Asia   411
    Adrian C Sleigh, Rachel Safman and Phua Kai Hong

Index   431

SECTION 1
INTRODUCTION

1

Transdisciplinary Approaches to Population Dynamics and Infectious Diseases in Asia

Adrian C Sleigh, Chee Heng Leng, Brenda SA Yeoh, Phua Kai Hong and Rachel Safman

Introduction

The population determinants and the outcomes of infectious diseases persisting or emerging in Asia are rarely considered together. Yet, both the causal factors and the outcomes are intricately intertwined with regional population dynamics. If better understanding and management of infectious diseases in Asia is the goal, then knowledge must be shared at many levels across multiple academic disciplines. This challenge is addressed here.

Exchange of information, concepts and analyses across disciplines is always difficult and has not been attempted for infectious diseases in Asia. Accordingly, the Asian MetaCentre for Population and Sustainable Development Analysis (National University of Singapore), together with the National Centre for Epidemiology and Population Health (Australian National University), invited over 40 scholars from Asia, Europe, Australia and North America to Singapore for an International Workshop on the *Population Dynamics of Infectious Disease in Asia* (October 27–29, 2004).

Papers presented covered diverse aspects of medicine, epidemiology, public health, history, demography, sociology, anthropology, geography, economics, politics, journalism, engineering, and mathematical modeling — all in relation to various infectious disease problems in many parts of Asia. The dialogue among participants before and at the conference, and over the following year as we prepared this book, promoted our understanding of the many possible perspectives on the infectious disease problems.

We found ourselves developing new integrative thoughts that crossed the disciplines, and taking the first steps towards transdisciplinary understanding (Parkes *et al.*, 2005). We hope the readers of this book will also be drawn to such an analysis, an integrated approach that goes beyond a simple exchange of views across disciplines, as we present some of the complex issues arising from persistence, resurgence or emergence of infectious diseases in Asia.

Population Dynamics in Asia

Asia's 3.6 billion people account for about three fifths of the world's population (United Nations, 2005). China, the most populous nation in the world, has a current population of more than 1.2 billion people. Following closely behind is India, the world's second most populous country with a population that is slightly over a billion (United Nations, 2005; U.S. Census Bureau, 2002). Although world population growth is now generally declining, and in Asia it is likely to fall even further below the global rate, nonetheless, the developing countries of Asia will still be major contributors to world population growth for many decades to come (U.S. Census Bureau, 2005b).

Considering Asia as one geographical entity, however, belies the diversity in cultures and populations, as well as a wide range of economies and differences in demographic change. On the one hand, there is Japan with a developed economy and an aged population. There are also the rapidly growing economies of China and India, within each of which are found extensive variations, and which together with Pakistan, Bangladesh, Indonesia and Malaysia, have populations that are still relatively young. There are also places such as Hong Kong and Singapore, metropolitan centres with rapidly ageing populations, and finally, countries such as Cambodia, Laos, and Myanmar with developing economies and high fertility and mortality rates (UNESCAP, 2005; Population Reference Bureau, 2001).

Against this backdrop of wide variations, two distinct trends which have relevance to infectious diseases may be identified. They are increased population mobility and large-scale migratory flows within and between countries, and a very rapid rate of urbanisation. These trends in urbanisation and migration have particularly profound implications for the ecology of infectious diseases, interacting in complex ways with other biological and social factors, and opening multiple pathways for the emergence of new infections and the resurgence of existing ones.

Migration and mobility

Asia has witnessed large movements of people both within and between countries in recent decades. The migration of labour in Asia, whether legal or illegal, is largely voluntary, essentially motivated by economic necessity or opportunity. However, there are also migrants who are refugees, driven out by political reasons or by conflict. And large numbers of Asian women are trafficked around the world, contributing to an increasing global problem. More recently, migration from Asia to other developed regions such as Europe, United States and Australia has also been growing.

Human mobility affects the population size and composition of both the host and receiving communities, and may also alter prevailing mortality and fertility trends (Lentzner *et al.*, 2002). Within Asia, Japan, Singapore and South Korea are predominantly the recipients of large numbers of migrants, while Malaysia and Thailand both send and receive significant numbers of migrants (see Table 1 for the number of migrants in the labour-importing countries). Malaysia and Thailand also have the highest number of unauthorised or illegal migrants in their countries, with numbers estimated to be about 500,000 (IOM, 2005). At the sending end, The Philippines, India, Bangladesh, Pakistan, Indonesia, China, Sri Lanka and Myanmar are among the largest exporters of migrants. Altogether, they contribute around one-half to two-thirds of all legal immigrants entering the international migration stream (IOM, 2005).

A large proportion of Asian migrants are unskilled workers, seeking employment in plantations, construction sites or in homes as domestic workers. Women made up about 47% of the total in 2001 (Zlotnik, 2003). However, Asian migration is becoming increasingly feminised, with women accounting for a growing proportion of labour migrants. For countries such as The Philippines, Indonesia, Thailand and Sri Lanka, women already constitute the majority — approximately 60% to 80% — of all labour

Table 1. Migrants in labour-importing countries in Asia, 2000.

	National labour force (thousands)	Foreign population (thousands)	Total migrant workers* (thousands)	Legal migrant workers* (thousands)	Migrant workers share of labour force (per cent)	Migrant workers with Legal Status (per cent)
Malaysia	9,600	1,500	1,239	789	13	64
Thailand	34,000	1,250	1,000	700	3	70
Singapore	2,190	1,000	960	940	44	98
Japan	68,000	1,700	670	420	1	63
Province of Taiwan	10,000	350	345	329	3	96
South Korea	22,000	350	310	95	1	31
Hong Kong, SAR	3,380	400	300	235	9	78
Total	149,170	6,550	4,824	3,508	3	73

*Note: Total migrant workers are legal migrants plus students and trainees and unauthorised workers. Legal migrant workers are foreign workers (1) with work permits and (2) considered to be workers under labour law.
Source: Martin and Widgren, 2002.

migrants (Asis, 2003). By the late 1990s, some one million Filipina, 500,000 Indonesian and 40,000 Thai female migrants had worked overseas (Wille and Passl, 2001). Approximately 250,000 of the foreign permanent residents in Japan are also women working in either skilled or unskilled jobs (IOM, 2005); most are second, third and fourth generation Koreans and Chinese.

Urbanisation

The second distinctive and significant trend in our consideration of infectious diseases is the increasing urbanisation in Asian countries, as larger proportions of the population shift from rural to urban settings. In 1975, only 25% of Asians lived in urban areas. However, the percentage has risen to 37% in 2000 and is expected to rise further to 53% by 2030 (Lentzner *et al.,* 2002). The changes in urban populations are reflected in Table 2. As part

Table 2. Percent urban: 1975, 2000 and 2030.

	1975	2000	2030
Asia	24.7	36.7	53.4
Republic of Korea	48.0	81.9	90.5
Japan	75.7	78.8	84.8
The Philippines	35.6	58.6	73.8
Malaysia	37.7	57.4	72.7
Indonesia	19.4	40.9	63.5
Pakistan	26.4	37.0	55.9
China	17.4	32.1	50.3
India	21.3	28.4	45.8
Bangladesh	9.8	24.5	43.8
Myanmar	23.9	27.7	46.6
Sri Lanka	22.0	27.5	39.3
Lao PDR	11.4	23.5	42.6
Thailand	15.1	21.6	39.1
Viet Nam	18.8	19.7	33.7
Cambodia	10.3	15.9	31.9

Source: United Nations Population Division, 2001.

of urbanisation, mega-cities have sprouted in Asia, with "12 of the world's 20 largest urban agglomerations" being found there (Lentzner *et al.,* 2002: 11). In addition, secondary cities have also been growing in Asia. At least 170 urban areas with over 750,000 inhabitants can be found in India and China alone (United Nations Population Division, 2001).

Urbanisation impacts on many aspects of life, including living conditions, behaviours and values, and political, social and economic processes (Lentzner *et al.,* 2002: 11). It is thus expected to have a considerable impact on population dynamics, especially mortality. From the data gathered from both developed and developing nations, mortality rates are generally lower in cities due to their health advantage over rural areas. This has been reflected in many Asian countries, with cities generally having better overall health outcomes than rural areas (Lentzner *et al.,* 2002). However, this advantage may not last as mega-cities and urban populations continue to grow at an uncontrollable rate. Moreover, numerous hazards such as pollution exist within urban areas. These hazards should not be ignored, as they may have critical influences on mortality in the near future (Mutatkar, 1995).

Urbanisation also affects fertility rates. Asians living in urban areas tend to marry later, with the mean marriage age increasing to >22 years for women and >25 years for men. This is true for all Asian countries except Nepal, India and Bangladesh (Lentzner *et al.*, 2005). Nonetheless, even India's mean age at marriage in both urban and rural areas has risen by 3.6 years during the period from 1961 to early 1990s (Das and Dey, 1998). The increasing age at marriage has resulted in dramatic declines in fertility. Changes in lifestyles, namely sexual activity outside of marriage, may also lead to unwanted and terminated pregnancies, as well as increasing the spread of sexually-transmitted diseases. Finally, it is interesting to note that most such demographic changes arise first in major cities before moving to smaller cities and rural areas.

Infectious Diseases in Asia

Infectious diseases are still important public health problems in Asia today. Previous optimism in the 1960s and 1970s that almost all serious infections would be controlled was misplaced (Morens *et al.*, 2004). Many old infections have persisted and several lethal new human infections like SARS, avian influenza and Nipah virus have emerged (from animal populations) in Asia in the last decade. In 2003, SARS spread around the world and paralysed trade, travel and some health systems for 6 months; it reappeared as dangerous laboratory outbreaks in Singapore, Taiwan and China in 2004. SARS could revisit at any time.

Avian influenza is now causing worldwide concern as it repeatedly appears in East Asia and spreads south and west, with the ever-present risk of becoming a lethal airborne human influenza pandemic. HIV had entered the region and spread exponentially for the last 20–30 years, currently infecting nearly 9 million people in Asia, 21% of the global total (UNAIDS, 2004). As more people are infected with HIV, the Asian population becomes more vulnerable to other infections, especially TB, because the HIV virus disables the natural ability to fight off infection. Other infections, including hookworm, other intestinal parasites, dengue, Japanese B encephalitis, sexual infections and meningococcal meningitis, have persisted or re-emerged. Dengue has become more severe and spread to other continents, while still affecting most of Asia.

Age-old infections such as TB and malaria have become more resistant to control techniques that worked well in the past, while plague, human influenza and cholera still threaten the world with the possibility of escalating into global epidemics. Although large areas of Asia have been freed from previously endemic malaria and schistosomiasis that used to kill many people and debilitate surviving populations, transmission of these vector-borne diseases persists in less fortunate areas, usually intimately associated with ongoing poverty and rural subsistence occupations.

These worrisome infection trends occur in parallel with many other socio-economic and environmental developments which are themselves rapidly changing. We have already identified the two distinct trends i.e., migration and urbanisation that will have significant effects on infection risks. Furthermore, there are the ecological consequences of rapidly increasing trade, travel and transport of goods and animals, certain human behaviour linked to both transitional and traditional societies and their economies and cultures, intensified agriculture and animal food production and associated misuse of pesticides and antibiotics. We also cannot neglect the effects of progressive climate and ecological change. Microbial evolution, in dynamic interplay with these factors, and with the intrinsic properties of organisms transacting their existence in complex and changing environments, is also part of the causal web of infection trends in Asia. It is in the context of such a multitude of factors and players, and their complex inter-relationships, that we will have to understand the current unfolding situation of infectious diseases in Asia today.

Outline of Sections

The book is divided into six sections, starting with this *Introduction* (Chap. 1), highlighting our transdisciplinary approach and summarising the material presented. The next section sets up *Frameworks for Understanding Population Dynamics and Infectious Diseases in Asia* (Chaps. 2-6), overarching concepts or problems that are of general relevance to any analysis of infectious disease patterns in Asia or beyond. We consider the forces driving infectious diseases, introduce novel approaches to analysis with special reference to unstable landscapes and migration, and consider the impact of large dams. We also explore the biomathematics of infection outbreaks and the implications for infection control, and analyse diverse health system responses manifested across Asia.

Section 3 considers *Development and Infectious Disease in Asia* (Chaps. 7–10). This section covers the extraordinary historical successes in Shanghai, the adverse impact of social change in mountain Vietnam, the tensions surrounding NGO services for mobile HIV-infected persons in Thailand, and the complex interactions of the state and civil society in relation to HIV/AIDS in Singapore. Section 4 covers *Population Mobility and Infectious Diseases in Asia* (Chaps. 11–14). This is where we examine a new road in Laos as a risk for sexually transmitted diseases (STD), rural work migration in China as a risk for TB, urban migration of females in Southwest China and the risk of STD, and the many infections associated with the largest annual human movement, the Hajj.

Section 5 deals with *Comparative Perspectives of SARS in Asia* (Chaps. 15–20). The SARS experience of Singapore is first noted in the context of the many infections that have been introduced to that central Asian city. This is followed by an analysis of the risks exposed by a notorious SARS outbreak in a high rise building in Hong Kong. Diverse reports followed from Taiwan (stigma and SARS), Malaysia (SARS and risk perception) and China (SARS and governance). In the final section, *Drawing Lessons from the Past to Respond to Future Challenges* (Chap. 21), the recent and ongoing problem of avian influenza is analysed and connected back to the many themes running through the book.

Outline of Following Chapters

Chapter 2 is Anthony J McMichael's account of *Ecological and Social Influences on Emergence and Resurgence of Infectious Disease*. He examines, broadly, the ways in which the emergence and resurgence of infectious diseases in the Asia-Pacific region reflect dynamic and rapid changes that have been brought about by the processes of 'globalisation'. Historic transitions include the appearance of zoonotic diseases with the advent of agriculture and animal husbandry 10,000 years ago, subsequent east-west microbial exchange between the Chinese and Roman empires, then the spread of infections (smallpox, measles) to vulnerable populations by European navigators several hundred years ago, and now global warming and destabilisation of ecosystems and biophysical processes needed for the world's life-support system. McMichael notes three ongoing socio-ecological phenomena that promote emerging infections: (i) increasingly intense modification of natural environments; (ii) the disturbance of natural ecosystems; (iii) poverty, crowding, social disorder and political instability. He points out that we live non-negotiably in a microbially-dominated world. Thus, we must think more in ecological terms and less in military terms about our relations with microbes. Indeed, we should aim to improve at coexisting.

Chapter 3 is David Bradley's approach to transmissible diseases at several scales incorporating *Landscape Epidemiology and Migration*. He relates space-time to infection at ecological 'edges' or zones of change known as 'tones'. These include spatial 'ecotones' (such as the canopy-floor zone within a forest, or a forest fringe) and temporal 'chronotones' (unstable landscape interposed in time between two stable states, such as a recently dammed valley). Both ecotones and chronotones are rich sources of human infection and are often in flux due to human activity. He notes that the landscape is structured ecologically into patches, corridors and matrices which determine the existence and transmissibility of infection. People create and adapt to landscapes. Migrants entering landscapes contact new infections, especially when crossing ecotones or chronotones. They also carry cultural adaptations from their former landscapes, and these may become maladaptations and pose new risks in new landscapes.

Adrian Sleigh (Chap. 4) analyses *Water, Dams and Infection*, an important and emerging feature of the Asian landscape with a direct impact on infectious diseases. Growing problems of water stress, food production, desertification and urbanisation are driving Asian countries to build large dams. These were a 2 trillion dollar investment in the 20th century, as the global inventory grew to 45,000 such dams, mostly in China and India. That investment was often imprudent and of exaggerated benefit. When located in Asia's heavily populated river valleys, the dams cause massive human displacement, much more so than in Western countries. As many as 50 million people have been displaced by large dams in India and China since 1950. Infections result, notably schistosomiasis and malaria, but other endemic infections of poverty such as pneumonia and diarrhoea are also exacerbated due to the prolonged adverse socioeconomic effects of dams.

In Chap. 5, Niels Becker and Katie Glass consider the biomathematics underlying *The Impact of Imported Infection*. They use mathematical transmission models to assess the impact of imported infections in two settings, that of vaccine-preventable disease such as measles, and that of a newly-emerged infection such as SARS. The results indicate that the appropriate public health response is rather different in these settings. When controlling an infection by a routine vaccination schedule, there is no need for a response to an imported infection if the immunity coverage achieved is below the threshold required for sustained elimination. The number of extra cases resulting from importation is generally so small that more cases are prevented by focusing the effort on improving the immunity coverage. In contrast, to prevent a major outbreak from an emerged infection for which there is no vaccine, the public health response should focus on prompt traditional interventions; the models demonstrate that early isolation of new cases in the early days of such an outbreak can avert an epidemic.

Phua Kai Hong and Vernon Lee (Chap. 6) examine the role of Asian health systems in responding to newly emerging infectious diseases. The health systems now affected by emerging infections such as SARS and avian influenza are quite diverse in their capacity and finance. At issue is an accurate account of the costs of such infections and the determination of the appropriate threshold for public investment in national and regional preparedness and capacity to respond. The recent Asian fiscal crisis, as well as growing trends of privatisation and cost containment, provides many challenges to those responsible for planning health systems that are responsive to the infectious diseases of the future.

In Chap. 7, Zhongwei Zhao, Feng Zhou, Guixiang Song, Shengnian Zhang and Tingkui Zhou report on the *Control of Infectious Diseases and Rising Life Expectancy in Shanghai: 1950–2003*. Infectious diseases were the major killer in Shanghai before 1950. Since then, the Shanghai municipal government has taken effective measures to combat infectious diseases. They examine the huge impact of infectious diseases prior to the 1950s, the methods adopted for their control in the last half of the century, and the great impact on life expectancy. They also note recent patterns of resurging or emerging infections (TB, gonorrhoea, HIV) and problems with reappearance of old infections such as measles among poor migrant groups in Shanghai.

In Chap. 8, Nguyen Tran Lam reports on the *Social Change and Infectious Diseases in Northern Mountain Vietnam*. Changing social conditions affect the lives and livelihoods of particular minority people in ways that significantly influence the spread of infectious diseases and condition the shape of epidemics. Primary drivers are contextually varied, including among others, contaminated water, poor sanitation and hygiene awareness, under-nutrition and hunger, material and seasonal deprivation, poor housing conditions, migration, drug resistance, and uneven distribution of health services. Major health problems arising from the socio-political conditions in this area are diarrhoea, pneumonia, influenza, TB, AIDS, malaria, reproductive tract infections and hepatitis. There is a resurgence of TB, Japanese encephalitis and dengue fever.

In Chap. 9, Vincent Del Casino traces the rising tensions regarding questions of mobility and local development in the wake of the growing impact of HIV/AIDS in Northern Thailand. In so doing, he investigates the ways in which healthcare management and development programmes affect mobility patterns and how those mobility patterns impact NGO goals of sustaining local development initiatives. The dynamic relationship between mobility and local needs raises the question of how to provide economic opportunities for people living with HIV and AIDS (PLWHA), as well as those affected by HIV/AIDS locally, such as children and grandparents. Non-governmental organisations (NGOs) have intervened to provide both care programmes and community development support and organisation as a way of enhancing local development, in attempts to "keep people local" and focused on community development. Many of these projects have also found favour with the Thai government, which since the "1997 crash" has promoted "local development" more vigorously. The long-term goals of many NGO initiatives is to develop sustainable local economic development that will also enhance the growing drive to promote participation and local governance initiatives in Northern Thai communities. Yet, there is a tension between the growing interest of NGOs to promote local economic development and the desire of PLWHA and others to participate in the growing globalised national economy.

Focusing on HIV/AIDS but in the context of the globalising city of Singapore, Shir Nee Ong and Brenda Yeoh in Chap. 10 consider the dominant state and socio-cultural discourses that surround HIV/AIDS and PLWHA in the city-state, and how these discourses attempt to discipline Singaporean bodies by encouraging 'safer sex' practices. Some discourses also (re)present HIV-positive bodies as 'deviant' bodies creating 'dis-ease' and therefore requiring regulation. The chapter also examines the extent of civil society activism and response through a consideration of how individuals and organisations help PLWHA in a number of ways, i.e., by providing 'space' for PLWHA to interact, by integrating them socio-spatially into the workplace, and through advocacy work in protecting their rights.

In Chap. 11, Chris Lyttleton explores the impact of *Cultivating the Market: Mobility, Labour and Sexual Exchange in Northwest Laos*. In the late 1990s, a million dollars from the World Bank upgraded a haphazard trail into an all-weather highway through Northwest Laos, linking China with the Mekong and Thailand. Although only 74 km long, Route 17B offers a microcosm of the multiple impacts that follow rapid social change for both itinerant and host communities in areas where infrastructure developments introduce transnational flows of ideas, people and goods. Numerous trucks now move through from China ferrying goods to and from the river connection with Thailand. The complex mix of ethnicity, economy, migration and politics has increased vulnerability to HIV and other sexually transmitted diseases in roadside communities in Northwest Laos. Rapid commoditisation of daily life for resettled Akha and other ethnic minority groups is fostering diverse sexual networks among internal and cross-border populations. Notions of ethnic customs and cultural difference are frequently cited by health professionals as a catalyst for the spread of sexually transmitted infections in this region, but simplistic ideas of ethnic difference pose a serious obstacle to effective health promotion.

In Chap. 12, Sukhan Jackson, Adrian Sleigh, Wang Guo-Jie and Liu Xi-Li consider *Household Poverty, Off-Farm Migration and Pulmonary Tuberculosis in Rural Henan, China*. They compare new TB cases and their controls for association with poverty (as measured by household economic status) and off-farm migration. They also calculated the economic costs of TB and its huge impact on the household. In China's poverty reduction programme, it is critical that financial support be offered to TB sufferers impoverished by lost income and capital due to the economic burden of this disease. The poorest farmers migrate for work and these migrants are then at high risk for TB, impoverishing them further. Thus, in rural China today, poverty and TB form a vicious cycle, each inducing the other.

In Chap. 13, Xiushi Yang reports on *Migration, Gender, and STD Risk: A Case Study of Female Temporary Migrants in Southwestern China.* He examines the interplay of migration and gender power relations that render female migrants vulnerable to sexual infections. Rural female migrants in urban centres, particularly those in the personal service and entertainment industry, have disproportionate increases in dangerous sexual behavior and are at a high risk of STDs and HIV. Economic hardship and competition leave female migrants with little control of casual or commercial sex encounters and unable to resist the pressure for unprotected sex. Gendered moral and social values further subject them to a subordinate position, limiting their power in negotiating protective measures, and putting them at a high risk of acquiring and subsequently transmitting STDs/HIV which has dire implications. At any point in time in China there are several million female migrant workers in this industry, and the cumulative number could be many times larger since many typically work for only a few years, returning to home villages subsequently to get married. The possibility of them becoming the unwitting source in the spread of STDs/HIV in China is therefore real and serious.

Annelies Wilder-Smith (Chap. 14) then introduces another regional issue influencing infectious disease patterns in Asia and across the World, that of the annual Hajj pilgrimage. More than 2 million Moslems migrate for the Hajj every year, the largest mass movement of people on earth. The over-crowded conditions and convergence of populations carries a high risk of person-to person infections such as influenza, tuberculosis and meningococcal disease, and worldwide spread of these diseases after the pilgrims return. She examines the information available on the many infections that result and reviews strategies that can reduce these risks.

Goh Kee Tai and Chew Suok Kai (Chap. 15) give a comprehensive account of the *Epidemiology of Emerging Infectious Diseases in Singapore, with Special Reference to SARS.* This chapter reveals the constant pressure placed on Singapore to detect and control many food–borne infections, encephalitis and dengue, as well as unexpected intrusions. The stress reached new levels with the outbreak of SARS and they give us a detailed account of how it spread and of its severe impact on the Singapore health system. The final outcome was a laboratory incident with lessons for the whole region for the prevention and management of infection.

In Chap. 16, Yuguo Li, Hua Qian, Ignatius Yu and Tze Wai Wong examine the *Probable Roles of Bio-Aerosol Dispersion in the SARS Outbreak in Amoy Gardens, Hong Kong.* They use an engineering approach to evaluate and model the probable mode of transmission in this notorious community outbreak affecting 321 residents and causing 42 deaths in a high–rise apartment complex in that densely populated city. They conclude that the virus became externally airborne from a source case in one flat, enabling faeco-respiratory transmission between flats and buildings at different levels in the apartment complex, with transmission affected by prevailing weather conditions and the wind. This analysis raises the issue of high rise building safety, as urbanisation proceeds elsewhere in Asia and the need for better building design and more research on the topic.

In Chap. 17, Mei-Ling Hsu and Ching-I Liu examine how various groups have been stigmatised in the public discourse about SARS in Taiwan's society. Adopting a conceptual framework of stigma formation, they performed a textual analysis of the news content in three mainstream newspapers — namely, *China Times, United Daily News,* and *Min Seng Daily,* in Taiwan. The time frame of news selection ranges from the first reported local SARS case on 1 March 2003 to 5 July 2003, the date when Taiwan was removed from the World Health Organization's SARS list. They noted that 'others' were frequently constructed in the news texts informing the public about the epidemic and prevention of the infectious disease. The 'others' were distinguished from 'us' and were blamed and denigrated for putting the population at risk. Only healthcare workers had the power to escape from their initial 'other' status, but blue collar workers, the homeless and the foreigners were unable to do the same and bore the blame for SARS.

In Chap. 18, *Risk Perception and Coping Responses in a SARS Outbreak in Malaysia,* Chan Chee Khoon explores the theme of *risk perception* and what influences it may have had in the SARS outbreak which swept through East and Southeast Asia in 2003. He points out that while much credit has been given to institutional responses such as isolation, contact tracing, and quarantines for rapidly bringing the epidemic under control, less mentioned were the individual–coping responses and risk avoidance behaviors (reduced travel, avoidance of crowded locations, avoidance of hospitals). In fact, because of the economic and financial stakes involved, official sources in Malaysia tried to avert "overreaction" in the risk avoidance responses to the outbreak (at the same time, and in obvious contradiction, urging caution upon those who contemplated travel to SARS-affected destinations such as China, Hong Kong, Taiwan, Singapore, and Toronto). In conclusion, he argues that the perception of risk associated with the SARS infectious outbreak was disproportionate to the threat it posed to global population health, and that this inflated perception of risk was driven more by economic rather than epidemiological considerations.

In Chap. 19, Liew Kai Khiun examines the response to the framing of the SARS epidemic in Singapore, looking at the role which the epidemic played in reinforcing government legitimacy and reifying themes which have been central to the nation-building project since independence. As such, his study demonstrates the ways in which public health and disease control efforts are nested within broader political and social concerns and may serve to either contravene or reinforce these other agendas.

In Chap. 20, David Kelly and Luo Xiaopeng examine the roots of a crisis in governance that were exposed by the SARS epidemic in 2003. Not only was the public health system extremely weak, particularly in the rural areas, but there was a large floating population of migrant labour that commuted between urban and rural areas, serving as a potential reservoir as well as a vector for the emergent infection. Kelly and Luo explain the characteristics of China's economy and polity which gave rise to this large migrant pool, and point out that the difficulties in changing the system are essentially due to weaknesses in the governance structure of the country.

In the final chapter, we address the latest infectious disease threat to emerge from Asia. Not only is avian influenza considered a danger to the whole world, it has forced us to re-examine the often forgotten experience with previous influenza pandemics, especially the catastrophic 1918 and 1919 pandemic. The many lessons arising from the preceding chapters in the book are considered as we appraise the risks now posed by H5N1 infection. We may be better prepared for the next pandemic of influenza, but must make decisions to share the risks and burdens of necessary invest-ments regionally in our Asian health systems. Retreat to national solutions will make any prospects of control more difficult, and will not be in the best interests of anyone. This matter has now become a global concern, but Asia has a vital interest in the outcome of preparations for the next pandemic of influenza, as it will probably be the source and the first region to be affected.

Conclusion

This book covers an array of problems from many perspectives, but certain topics are of outstanding importance when considering population dynamics and infectious diseases in Asia. Firstly, the volume emphasises the importance of *place*, expressed through *landscape and culture*. Location determines the risk of infection and also modifies the response. Secondly, of significance too is the *alteration of the landscape* for economic development with local, national, regional and global effects. A third crucial element relates to *human mobility across the landscape*, driven by spiritual faith, involuntary displacement, and the forces of economic development, including both poverty and affluence. Fourthly, it is important to consider the *cumulated legacy of previous changes in place*, with human movement reflecting ties from the past, and resulting in infections being introduced. Finally, the all important effects of *poverty* cannot be ignored. This is driving millions of people to change where they reside, exposing them to risks they cannot resist and for which the local place- and culture-based health systems are currently inadequate.

As the chapters of this book unfold, it becomes apparent that understand-ing and responding to the challenges posed by infectious diseases takes us beyond a traditional epidemiological or biomedical framework towards a transdisciplinary analysis. We hope that this book will encourage readers to begin that intellectual journey on Asia.

References

Asis M. (2003) *Asian Women Migrants: Going the Distance, but Not Far Enough.* Migra-tion Information Source, Washington DC, 1 March.
Das NP, Dey D. (1998) Age at marriage in India: Trends and determinants. *Demog India* **27**(1): 91–115.

IOM. (2005) *World Migration 2005: Costs and Benefits of International Migration*. International Organization for Migration, Switzerland.

Kinsella K, Gist YJ. (1998) *International Brief: Gender and Aging, Mortality and Health*. US Census Bureau, IB98-2, US Government Printing Office, Washington DC.

Lentzner H *et al.* (2002) *Health Consequences of Population Changes in Asia: What are the Issues?* Asian MetaCentre Research Paper Series No. 6, Asian MetaCentre for Population and Sustainable Development Analysis, Singapore.

Martin P, Widgren J. (2002) International migration: Facing the challenge. *Pop Bull* **57**(1).

Morens DM, Folkers GK, Fauci AS. (2004) The challenge of emerging and re-emerging infectious diseases. *Nature* **430**: 242–8

Mutatkar RK. (1995) Public health problems of urbanisation. *Soc Sci Med* **41**(7): 977–981.

Parkes MW, Bienen L, Breilh J, Hsu L-N, McDonald M, Patz JA, Rosenthal JP, Sahani M, Sleigh A, Waltner-Toews D, Yassi A. (2005) All hands on deck: Transdisciplinary approaches to emerging infectious disease. *Ecohealth* **2**: 258–272.

Population Reference Bureau (2001) *2001 World Population Data Sheet*. PRB, Washington DC.

UNAIDS (2004) AIDS Epidemic Update. UNAIDS/WHO, Geneva, December.

United Nations (2005) *Global Trends: Asia*. Available at http://www.unhabitat.org/habrdd/asia.html, Accessed 11 October 2005.

UNESCAP (2005) *Dynamics of Population Ageing: How can Asia and the Pacific Respond?* Available at http://www.unescap.org/pdd/publications/survey2005/9_Survey05_Ch-III.pdf, Accessed 30 September 2005.

United Nations Population Division (2001) *World Urbanisation Prospects: The 2001 Revision*. United Nations, New York.

United Nations Population Division (2002) *World Population Ageing 1950–2050*. United Nations publication, Sales No. E.02.XIII.3, United Nations Population Division, New York.

U.S. Census Bureau (2002) *Global Population Profile: 2002*. Available at http://www.census.gov/ipc/www/wp02.html, Accessed 11 October 2005.

U.S. Census Bureau (2005a) *World Population Information*. Available at http://www.census.gov/ipc/www/world.html, Accessed 11 October 2005.

U.S. Census Bureau (2005b) *Population Size and Growth*. Available at http://www.census.gov/ipc/ prod/wp96/wp96005.pdf, Accessed 11 October 2005.

Wille C, Passl B. (2001) *Change and Continuity: Female Labour Migration in South East Asia*. Asia Research Centre for Migration, Bangkok.

World Bank (2005) *World Bank Atlas*. Available at http://siteresources.worldbank.org/INTPRH/Resources/population.pdf, Accessed 11 October 2005.

Zlotnik H. (2003) *The Global Dimensions of Female Migration*. Migration Information Source, Washington DC, 1 March.

SECTION 2

FRAMEWORKS FOR UNDERSTANDING POPULATION DYNAMICS AND INFECTIOUS DISEASES IN ASIA

2

Ecological and Social Influences on Emergence and Resurgence of Infectious Diseases

Anthony J McMichael

Introduction

During the third quarter of the 20th century, the age-old scourge of infectious disease, the biblical 'Fourth Horseman of the Apocalypse; was widely assumed to be receding in the developed world. The antibiotic era had begun with great success in the 1940s; vaccine know how was accelerating, pesticides were available for controlling mosquito populations, and surveillance and control measures (border controls, quarantine, other social controls, public education) were becoming internationally coordinated. Not surprisingly, by the early 1970s, various eminent scientists and government authorities proclaimed the imminent end of the infectious disease era.

In retrospect, this proclamation was premature. By late 20th century, it had become evident that the world faced a generalised upturn in emerging and resurgent infectious diseases (Weiss and McMichael, 2004). Over 30 new infectious diseases were identified in the last quarter of last century, including HIV/AIDS, 'mad cow disease' as a source of human variant Creutzfeldt Jakob Disease (CJD), hepatitis C, Nipah virus and many viral haemorrhagic fevers. Since 2000, this narrative has continued worldwide, and particularly in the Asia-Pacific region, with severe acute respiratory syndrome (SARS) and the avian flu virus. Meanwhile, many of the long-established infectious diseases such as tuberculosis, malaria and dengue fever have increased.

On the whole, this return and revival of new and old infectious diseases is a reflection of the distinctive conditions in a modern globalising world, i.e. persistent poverty (especially in urban slums), rapid increases in population size and density, urbanisation, mobility (air-travel, refugees, rural–urban migration, etc.), long-distance trade, conflict and warfare. There are also contributions from human–induced global environmental changes, i.e. the disturbance and destabilisation of ecosystems and biophysical processes such as the climate system. Political ignorance, denial and obduracy (as with HIV/AIDS) often compound the problem. Meanwhile, diarrhoeal disease and acute respiratory infections, especially in conditions of poverty and squalor, continue to kill millions of infants and children every year.

Cholera — the seventh pandemic

Cholera well illustrates how large-scale changes in social, economic and environmental conditions can affect the pattern of infectious disease occurrence. This disease is currently seeing its largest-ever and longest-ever pandemic — the seventh. Meanwhile, a new eighth cholera pandemic (entailing a new strain of the cholera bacterium) is currently emerging in South Asia.

Epidemics of a cholera-like disease have been described in the Ganges delta in India over the past four centuries (Lee and Dodgson, 2000). Cholera (its genotype apparently reinforced with a newly acquired toxin-producing gene) first extended its range beyond South Asia in 1817. This initial extension followed the Great Kumbh annual religious festival in the Upper Ganges, in which Hindu pilgrims from all over India came to bathe in the sacred waters. Their subsequent dispersal and contacts with British troops mobilising in the northwest frontier region sparked a cholera pandemic that spread from India to the Arabian peninsula and along the trade routes to Africa and the Mediterranean coast. In the early 1830s, the faster-travelling steamboats enabled cholera to cross the Atlantic. The disease reached North America in 1832, and spread rapidly around the United States coastline and inland via major rivers.

This current seventh pandemic has extended further than ever before, affecting Asia, Europe, Africa, North America and Latin America. It began in 1961 and is by far the longest lasting cholera pandemic to date (Lee and Dodgson, 2003; WHO, 2003a). The pandemic entails the El Tor strain, which, in mid-twentieth century, replaced the more lethal classical biotype of the nineteenth-century pandemics. The extraordinary scale of this pandemic seems particularly to reflect the great increase in human movement between continents, the greater rapidity and distance of modern shipping-based trade, the growth of urban slums with unsafe drinking water, and the increased nutrient enrichment of coastal and estuarine waters by phosphates and nitrates in agricultural and domestic run-off water (and which enhance proliferation of vibrio-harbouring phytoplankton and zooplankton) (McMichael, 2001).

Infectious disease in populations: an ecological perspective

Our understanding of the changing patterns of infectious diseases in populations can be much enriched by both an ecological and an historical perspective. The worldwide dispersal of the human species over the past 50,000–100,000 years, accompanied by cultural evolution and inter-population contacts, has profoundly transformed the relationship between *Homo sapiens* and the microbiological world. During this grand odyssey, there have been several major transitions at the key historical junctures, each entailing the emergence of various new or unfamiliar infectious diseases (McNeill, 1976).

The coevolution of humans and infectious agents of course has a long history. In human prehistory, two profound transitions in this relationship occurred: the first when early humans became serious meat-eaters, thereby exposing themselves to various animal parasites, and the second, when our *Homo sapiens* ancestors spread out of Africa into new environments and climates where they encountered unfamiliar microbes. Since the advent of agriculture and animal husbandry, three other great transitions have occurred in the human-microbe relationship (Weiss and McMichael, 2004). First, early agrarian-based settlements enabled enzootic microbes to cross the species barrier and make contact with *Homo sapiens*. Hence, the early city-states of the Middle East, Egypt, South Asia, East Asia and

Central and South America each acquired their own distinct repertoire of locally evolving 'crowd' infectious diseases. Second, over the course of a thousand years or so, the ancient civilisations of greater Eurasia (Egypt, India, Rome, China) made contact, swapped their dominant microbes and painfully equilibrated. Third, from the 15th century onwards, expansionist sea-faring Europe, pre-eminent technologically, inadvertently exported its lethal, empire-winning, germs to the Americas and later to the South Pacific, Australia and Africa.

We seem now to be living through the fourth great historical transition, one that extends globally for the first time. Today's apparent increased lability in the occurrence, spread and biological behaviour of infectious diseases reflects the impact of widespread demographic, commercial, environmental, behavioural, technological and other rapid changes in human ecology. Modern clinical medicine, via blood transfusion and hypodermic syringes, has created new opportunities for microbes that have contributed to the rises in hepatitis C, HIV/AIDS and several other viral infections.

Perhaps a new equilibration will occur as the post-genome era of molecular biotechnologies yields new ways to constrain the natural biological impulses of microbes. However, the future will certainly not entail a world free of infectious disease. We must recognise and accommodate the existence of the myriad of microbial species that are part of the interdependent system of Life on Earth. A tiny proportion of those microbes now, as will others in future, causes infectious diseases in humans. Human ecology is now characterised by rapid changes around the world and it is important to sharpen our understanding of the social, economic, technological and environmental influences on infectious disease occurrence.

Social, Economic and Associated Influences

Infectious diseases remain the world's leading cause of death, accounting for one in three of all deaths. Each year, 17 million people, mostly young children, die from infectious diseases, with acute respiratory infections killing almost 4 million people, diarrhoeal diseases killing 3 million, HIV/AIDS killing 2.5 million, tuberculosis killing 2 million, and malaria killing 1.5 million people annually (WHO, 2003b). The discrepancy in mortality profiles between the rich and the very poor countries is huge; infections cause 1 to 2% of all deaths in the former, but >50% in the latter. Indeed, among the world's poorest sub-populations, infectious disease causes almost two-thirds of deaths.

Diseases such as tuberculosis, leprosy, cholera, typhoid and diphtheria are known to be pre-eminently diseases of poverty. As happened historically with tuberculosis, HIV infection now seems to be entrenching itself among the world's poor and disempowered, especially in sub-Saharan Africa and South Asia. Much of the spread of HIV has been along international 'fault lines', tracking the inequality and vulnerability that accompany migrant labour, educational deprivation and sexual commerce (Farmer, 1999). The health ramifications of economic disadvantage that occur under free trade agreements are well illustrated by hepatitis A and cyclosporiasis (a protozoal infection) that occurred in the United States in the 1990s. Outbreaks of these diseases were caused by faecally contaminated strawberries and raspberries imported from Central America. The North American Free Trade Agreement had degraded environmental and labour standards (such as providing toilet facilities for workers) in response to the demands of open competition and profitability. With modern air-transport, diners in New York were able to consume these berries two days after they were picked and were quickly exposed to these faecally transmitted infections.

Socially disordered populations living in circumstances of privation, unhygienic conditions and close contact are susceptible to infectious diseases. History abounds with examples. The severity of the bubonic plague (Black Death) in mid 14th century Europe appears to have partly reflected, the nutritional consequences and attendant impoverishment caused by several preceding decades of unusually cold and wet weather with crop failures (McMichael, 2001). This adverse experience, occurring in conjunction with the incipient destabilisation of the hierarchical feudal system, would have heightened the vulnerability of the European populations to epidemic disease.

The urban environment has recently become the dominant human habitat; approximately half of the world's population now lives in cities or large towns, compared with an estimated 5% about two centuries ago. Cities have been referred to as highways for 'microbial traffic' (Morse, 1992). Urbanism typically entails a breakdown in traditional family and social structures, and brings greater personal mobility along with extended and labile social networks. These features, accompanied by access to modern contraception, have facilitated a diversity of sexual contacts, and hence the spread of STDs. The growth in sex tourism in today's internationally mobile world, which capitalises in exploitative fashion on the desperation of poverty, amplifies the risk of STD transmission in many of today's developing countries.

Rapid urbanisation, boosted by the urge to enter the cash economy in a globalising marketplace, boosts the risk of old infectious diseases such as childhood pneumonia, diarrhoea, tuberculosis and dengue. It also facilitates the spread of various 'emerging' diseases. For example, high-rise housing can create new infectious disease risks, as was recently observed for SARS in Hong Kong. Such housing also typically increases the risks of infection via the processes of family breakdown and social instability, leading to intra-venous drug abuse, and sexual transmission of infections (Cohen, 2003).

Food sources and production

The spectacular outbreak of 'mad cow disease' (bovine spongiform encephalopathy, BSE) in the UK in the mid 1980s underscores the infec-tious disease risks inherent in changes in food sources and food production methods. In that particular case, the source of the problem lay with the intensification of meat production, entailing the cost-cutting use of recycled bovine offal (including parts of the nervous system). This unnatural practice of feeding animal protein to herbivores inadvertently exposed the artificially 'carnivorous' cattle to a surprising quasi-infectious agent, the prion protein.

Across cultures, there is a widespread predilection for eating meat from various exotic species of animals. This exacerbates the risk of exposure to unfamiliar infectious agents. Indeed, such exposure probably triggered the 2003 epidemic of Severe Acute Respiratory Syndrome, SARS, in the Guangzhou region of Southern China (Peiris and Guan, 2004). The nat-ural reservoir species for the SARS coronavirus remains uncertain. How-ever, infection of Civet cats with SARS-related viruses has been reported, although it is not yet known if this is the original source species. Surveys have shown that the live markets and restaurants in Guangzhou sold vari-ous species of small carnivores (e.g. civet cat, racoon dog and ferret badger) that were captured in China, Laos, Vietnam and Thailand, transported to markets (often across national borders), and that were thereby brought into close proximity (Bell *et al.*, 2004). Thus, infectious agents have much opportunity to move between edible species. Indeed, the recent regionalisation and high-volume intensification of what was previously a local practice, in order to meet the burgeoning urban demand in Southern China, has greatly amplified the health risks of what were previously localised cultural practices in rural settings.

In Africa, consumption of bush-meat (much of it from hunted primates, which are now under increasing threat of extinction) entails a serious risk of acquiring new infectious diseases from zoonotic sources. As an ominous example, molecular genetic studies have shown that the HIV virus has crossed from chimpanzees into humans at least three times (Hahn *et al.*, 2000).

On the international economic front, globalisation of the food market has amplified the movement of pathogens from one region to another. For example, the commercial movement of fruits and vegetables facilitates the redistribution of anti-microbial resistance genes between strains and types of organisms. In the 1990s, alfalfa sprouts grown from a contaminated seed sent to a Dutch shipper caused outbreaks of infections with *Salmonella* species in both the USA and Finland (Mahon *et al.*, 1997).

Travel and trade

Microbes do not respect political and administrative borders. The mobility of humans, animals and birds is a constant stimulus to changes in the pattern of infectious disease occurrence. Vector mosquito species can travel with trade and transport (as apparently did the bubonic plague-infected black rat, travelling westwards across the Silk Road, towards the Black Sea and Europe, in the 14th century). HIV/AIDS has spread quickly around the world in the past twenty years. SARS spread readily from Hong Kong to Vietnam, across to Germany and Toronto. In the case of SARS, infected travellers are often not easy to identify; a prominent carrier was a doctor attending a conference who displayed no signs of illness at all (McLean *et al.*, 2005).

Dengue fever, numerically the most important vector-borne viral disease of humans, provides a good example of how patterns of trade, travel and settlement can influence various infectious diseases. Although dengue is primarily a tropical disease, its extension in recent decades into various temperate countries reflects both the introduction of the disease's main mosquito vector species, *Aedes aegypti* (which is behaviourally adaptable to a cold climate), and the increase in imported cases resulting from increased air travel (Kuno, 1995). It also reflects the rapid evolutionary adjustment of this mosquito species to coexistence with urban-dwelling humans, having originated in forest Africa. Indeed, *Aedes aegypti* has followed human kind on its travels and migrations around the world (Monath *et al.*, 1994). A major alternate mosquito vector for the dengue virus, *Aedes albopictus* (the 'Asian tiger mosquito'), has been disseminated widely in recent years via the unwitting intercontinental exportation of mosquito eggs in used car tyres from Asia into Africa and the Americas (Reiter and Sprenger, 1987).

Neisseria meningitidis, a global pathogen, causes seasonal epidemics of meningitis in the 'meningitis belt' of Sahelian Africa. Studies with molecular markers have shown that in recent decades, Muslim pilgrims brought an epidemic strain of *N. meningitidis* from Southern Asia to Mecca, where they passed it on to pilgrims from sub-Saharan Africa, who after returning home, initiated strain-specific epidemic outbreaks in several locations (Moore *et al.*, 1989).

The West Nile virus, newly emergent in North America as a human infection, further illustrates the impact of long-distance trade and travel. The disease originated in Africa, and it occurs sporadically in the Middle East and in parts of Europe. It was unknown in North America until it arrived in New York in 1999, perhaps via an infected mosquito on an aeroplane. Birds were affected first and later humans. The apparently favourable environmental conditions for the virus to survive and spread within New York City were these:

(i) Early season rain and summer drought provided ideal conditions for *Culex* mosquitoes.
(ii) July 1999 was the hottest July on record for New York City.
(iii) Suburban/urban ecosystems support high numbers of select avian host and mosquito vector species adapted to those conditions, enabling close interaction of mosquitoes, birds and humans.
(iv) High populations of susceptible bird species existed, especially crows.

West Nile virus subsequently spread widely across the United States, and by early 2004, it had established itself as an endemic virus, harboured by animals including birds and horses, and transmitted via mosquitoes. In July 2003, Mexico declared a state of emergency when West Nile virus arrived in that country. There is concern that the disease could spread more rapidly in Central and South America than in North America, because the warmer Latin American countries nurture large bird populations and year-round mosquito populations (Mackenzie *et al.*, 2004).

On another front, the escalating international trade in exotic pets also yields unexpected infectious disease outbreaks. For example, the monkey pox virus was recently introduced into the USA in imported African rodents, with subsequent transmission to pet prairie dogs and from them to the other pets and the pet owners (Di Giulio and Eckburg, 2004).

Land use and environmental change

Humans have always changed their environments. With population growth and the intensification of economic activities, such changes are rapidly increasing in magnitude, reflected in tropical deforestation, irrigation, dam building, urban sprawl, road building, intensified crop and animal production systems, and pollution of coastal zones. The increasing scale of this encroachment on, and the disturbance of the natural environment accelerates the emergence of new infectious diseases.

The Nipah virus provides a good recent example. Human contact with this bat-borne virus followed the establishment of pig farms close to the tropical forest in Northern Malaysia, where the Nipah virus first crossed over from fruit bats to pigs and thence to pig farmers in 1999 (Chua *et al.*, 1999). Thousands of pigs and several hundred infected farmers and their family members died from the infection. The destruction of natural forest in many other locations has also encouraged fruit bats to relocate nearer human habitation. Indeed in 1997, the Hendra virus, deriving from Australian fruit bats, fatally infected a veterinarian examining a sick horse in Queensland, Australia (Halpin, 1999).

Rodents are a prominent source of new and re-emerging infections, as occurred in the 1990s with Hanta viruses in the USA. Rodent-borne hantavirus is widespread in agricultural systems in South America and

East Asia, in arid grasslands in North America and elsewhere. In mid 1993, an unexpected outbreak of acute, sometimes fatal, respiratory disease occurred in humans in Southwest USA (Parmenter *et al.*, 1993). This 'hantavirus pulmonary syndrome' was caused by a previously unrecognised virus that is maintained in the natural environment, primarily within the native deer-mouse, and which is transmitted via rodent excreta. The 1991–1992 El Niño event, causing unseasonally heavy summer rains and a proliferation of piñon nuts within Southwest USA, hugely amplified local rodent populations, leading to the 1993 outbreak of 'hantavirus pulmonary syndrome' (Parmenter *et al.*, 1993; Engelthaler *et al.*, 1999).

Various other environmental changes also influence the occurrence of human infection. In the USA, nature conservation and increased contact with woodland in the Eastern states has led to the emergence of Lyme disease (borreliosis). The ixodic ticks that transmit the spirochaete *Borrelia burgdorferi* normally feed on deer and white-footed mice, with the latter being the more competent viral host species. However, forest fragmentation has led to changes in biodiversity. This includes the loss of various predator species such as wolves, foxes, raptors and others, and a resultant shift of ticks from the less competent to the more competent host species (white-footed mice). These changes, along with middle-class suburban sprawl into woodlands, have interacted in the emergence of this disease (Glass *et al.*, 1995; Schmidt *et al.*, 2001).

Global Environmental Changes and Anticipating the Future

Many of the large-scale environmental changes that humankind is now imposing on the biosphere have profound implications for the future pattern of infectious disease occurrence and transmission. Much of the recent formal research in this emerging topic area has been done in relation to global climate change. However, it is important to recognise that many of these environmental changes will affect infectious diseases, and that they will often do so in concert, including via interactive effects. Further more, the disease impact of changing environmental conditions will usually be modulated by the level of susceptibility of the human population, a function of population density, immune status, the nutritional status, the extent of mobility, the level of social organisation/disorganisation, flexibility of political systems and of governance, and various other such social-environmental factors.

Global climate change

The now-certain prospect of human-induced global climate change raises long-term questions about how infectious diseases will respond in the coming century and beyond. Many infectious agents, their vector organisms and their reservoir non-human species, are sensitive to climatic conditions and to resultant environmental changes.

In the Asia-Pacific region, El Niño fluctuations appear to affect the occurrence of dengue fever, the world's most prevalent vector-borne viral disease spreads primarily by the *Aedes aegypti* mosquito. (Dengue causes an estimated 100 million cases annually in tropical and sub-tropical countries.) Similarly, inter-annual variations in climatic conditions in Australia, especially those due to the El Niño cycle, influence the pattern of outbreaks of Ross River virus disease (Tong *et al.*, 2002; Woodruff *et al.*, 2002).

Climate change, via both a shift in background climate conditions and changes in regional climatic variability, will affect the potential (spatial and seasonal) transmission of various vector-borne infectious diseases. These would include malaria, dengue fever, various types of viral encephalitis, schistosomiasis (spread by water-snails), leishmaniasis (spread by sand-flies in South America and around the Mediterranean coast), onchocerciasis (West African 'river blindness', spread by black flies) and yellow fever (also spread by the *Aedes aegypti* mosquito).

The key phrase here is *potential transmission*. It is perfectly relevant to estimate how the world's intrinsic infectious disease transmission properties would alter in response to climate change. Indeed, such research is in the classic tradition of experimental science, which seeks to hold all other factors constant, while estimating the effect induced by varying just one key factor. Nevertheless, we know that the *actual* transmission of diseases such as malaria, is and will be much affected by economic and social conditions, and by the robustness of public health defences. Hence, we must strive to develop methods of modelling that incorporate other reasonably foreseeable contextual changes.

Both statistical and biologically-based ('process-based') models have been used to assess how shifts in ranges of temperature and patterns of rainfall would affect the transmission potential of various vector-borne diseases (Martens, 1999; Hales *et al.,* 2002). However, this genre of future scenario-based modelling has not yet been able to address all aspects of the topic. For example, how will domestic and urban water use (particularly relevant to dengue fever occurrence) change in a warmer world with altered patterns of precipitation? How would an increase in the tempo of extreme weather events and natural disasters affect infectious disease occurrence? There are still many things to learn about how the impending shift into unfamiliar climatic conditions will affect the complex processes of infectious disease transmission, especially the vector-borne diseases.

In the meantime, there is suggestive evidence that the climate change observed over the past 30 years has influenced cholera outbreaks in Bangladesh (Rodo *et al.*, 2002), the extension of tick-borne encephalitis in Sweden (Lindgren and Gustafson, 2001), and more debatable, the range and seasonality of malaria in some parts of Eastern Africa (Patz *et al.*, 2002).

Anticipating future infectious disease risks

A tantalising question is whether we can estimate the future probabilities of infectious disease emergence and resurgence. This is obviously extremely difficult given that we could not have foreseen the emergence of HIV/ AIDS, Mad Cow Disease or SARS. High-precision deterministic models are not achievable since the world is inherently stochastic, and hence microbial mutation occurs in random fashion (as it is intrinsic to Darwinian biological evolution), and the evolution of human culture and behaviour is unpredictable. Nevertheless, there are techniques for modelling the approximate likely range and form of future infectious disease epidemics (Brockman *et al.*, 2005).

However, we do know that the following situations create auspicious conditions for (new) microbes to become human infections:

(i) Increasingly intense modification/exploitation of natural environments, often entailing new human–microbe contacts.

(ii) The disturbance of natural ecosystems and their various internal biotic controls. This results in the disruption of the natural constraints on infectious pathogens and on their host species and vector organisms.

(iii) Poverty, crowding, social disorder and political instability.

Consider influenza where the molecular-biological and clinical aspects are well understood. However, the underlying ecological dimensions (e.g. the poultry-pig-human interactions) remain less definitive (Weiss and McMichael, 2004). A typical scenario is where wild fowl infected with avian flu come in contact with intensely-farmed poultry, with pigs acting as a mediating (and perhaps genetically recombining) host; this is followed by the co-infection of a farm-worker who already carries the preceding strain of human flu, leading to a highly infectious genetically-recombinant form which spreads to the other people, some of whom board an airplane bound for a major population centre.

We can better approach the anticipation of future risks if we have both ecological and historical insights. Much can be learnt from past experience about the sorts of composite situations that increase the probability of either new microbes entering human populations or known infectious agents extending their range, their seasonality or their virulence (particularly the salutary experience, over recent decades, of having induced widespread antimicrobial resistance among many infectious pathogens).

Conclusion

As ever, the world is replete with microbes striving for supplies of nutrients, energy and molecular building blocks. The right microbe fortuitously in the right place can extend, re-start or found a dynasty. It has happened many times before and it will continue to do so.

We can better engage with the topic if we apply both ecological and historical perspectives to it. Since we live non-negotiably in a microbially-dominated world, we must think more in ecological terms about our relations with microbes. The lesson of recent times is that we cannot conquer the microbial world. However, we could (and must) get better at coexisting.

As the scale of human impact on the biosphere escalates, and as the structures and fluidity of human societies change along with the levels of susceptibility of local human populations, so these large-scale changes create various opportunities for infectious agents, both new and resurgent. Today, this process appears to be occurring at an accelerated rate, and on a global scale. We are undergoing a fourth and larger-than-ever transition in the overall relationship between the human species and the microbial world.

References

Bell D, Roberton S, Hunter PR. (2004) Animal origins of SARS coronavirus: Possible links with the international trade in small carnivores. *Philos Trans R Soc Lond B Biol Sci* 2 **359**: 1107–1114.

Brockmann D, Hufnagel L, Geisel T. (2005) Dynamics of modern epidemics, in McLean A, *et al.* (eds.), *SARS: A Case Study in Emerging Infections*. Oxford University Press, Oxford.

Chua KB, Goh KJ, Wong KT, *et al.* (1999) Fatal encephalitis due to nipah virus among pig-farmers in Malaysia. *Lancet* **354**: 1257–1259.

Cohen A. (2003) Urban unfinished business. *Int J Environ Health Res* **13**: S29–S36.

Di Giulio D, Eckburg P. (2004) Human monkeypox: An emerging zoonosis. *Lancet Infect Dis* **4**: 15–25.

Engelthaler DM, Mosley DG, Cheek JE, *et al.* (1999) Climatic and environmental patterns associated with hantavirus pulmonary syndrome, four corners region, United States. *Emerg Infect Dis* **5**: 87–94.

Farmer P. (1999) *Infections and Inequalities. The Modern Plagues*. University of California Press, Berkeley.

Glass G, Schwartz B, Morgan JI, Johnson D, Noy P, Israel E. (1995) Environmental risk factors for Lyme disease identified with geographical information systems. *Am J Public Health* **85**: 944–948.

Hahn BH, Shaw GM, De Cock KM, Sharp PM. (2000). AIDS as a zoonosis: scientific and public health implications. *Science* **287**: 607–614.

Hales S, de Wet N, Maindonald J, Woodward A. (2002) Potential effect of population and climate changes on global distribution of dengue fever: An empirical model. *The Lancet* **360**: 830–834.

Halpin K, Young P, Field H, Mackenzie J. (1999) Newly discovered viruses of flying foxes. *Vet Microbiol* **68**: 83–87.

Kuno G. (1995) Review of the factors modulating dengue transmission. *Epidemiol Rev* **17**: 321–335.

Lee K, Dodgson R. (2000) Globalisation and cholera: Implications for global governance. *Global Govern* **6**: 213–236.

Lindgren E, Gustafson R. (2001) Tick-borne encephalitis in Sweden and climate change. *Lancet* **358**: 16–18.

MacKenzie J, Gubler D, Petersen L. (2004) Emerging flaviviruses: The spread and resurgence of Japanese encephalitis, West Nile and dengue viruses. *Nat Med* **10**: S98–S109.

Mahon BE, Ponka A, Hall WN, *et al.* (1997) An international outbreak of Salmonella infections caused by alfalfa sprouts grown from contaminated seeds. *J Infect Dis* **175**: 876–882.

Martens P. (1999) How will climate change affect human health? *Am Scientist* **87**: 534–541.

McLean A, May R, Pattison J, Weiss R. (2005) SARS: *A Case Study in Emerging Infections*. Oxford University Press, Oxford.

McMichael AJ. (2001) *Human Frontiers, Environments and Disease: Past Patterns, Uncertain Futures*. Cambridge University Press, Cambridge.

McNeill W. (1976) *Plagues and People*. Penguin, Middlesex.

Monath T. (1994) Dengue: The risk to developed and developing countries. *Proc Natl Acad Sci USA* **91**: 2395–2400.

Moore P, Reeves M, Schwartz B, Gellin B, Broome C. (1989) Intercontinental spread of an epidemic group. A neisseria meningitidis strain. *Lancet* **2**: 260–263.

Morse SS. (1992) Global microbial traffic and the interchange of disease. *Am J Public Health* **82**: 1326–1327.

Parmenter R, Brunt J, Moore D, Ernest S. (1993) The hantavirus epidemic in the southwest: Rodent population dynamics and the implications for transmission of hantavirus-associated adult respiratory distress syndrome (HARDS) in the four corners region. *Sevilleta LTER Publication* **41**: 324–328.

Patz J, Hulme M, Rosenzweig C, *et al.* (2002) Climate change — regional warming and malaria resurgence. *Nature* **420**: 627–628.

Peiris JS, Guan Y. (2004) Confronting SARS: A view from Hong Kong. *Philos Trans R Soc Lond B Biol Sci* **359**: 1075–1079.

Reiter P, Sprenger D. (1987) The used tire trade: A mechanism for the world-wide dispersal of container-breeding mosquitoes. *J Am Mos of Control Assoc* **3**: 494–501.

Rodo X, Pascual M, Fuchs G, Faruque A. (2002) ENSO and Cholera: A non-stationary link related to climate change? *Proc Nat Acad Sci* **99**: 12901–12906.

Schmidt K, Ostfeld R. (2001) Biodiversity and the dilution effect in disease ecology. *Ecology* **82**: 609–619.

Tong S, Bi P, Donald K, McMichael A. (2002) Climate variability and ross river virus transmission. *Epidemiology* **13**: 2.

Weiss RA, McMichael AJ. (2004) Social and environmental risk factors in the emergence of infectious diseases. *Nat Med* **10**: S70–S76.

WHO. (2003a) *Global Defence against the Infectious Disease Threat*. Geneva: WHO: 74–79.

WHO. (2003b) *World Health Report 2002*. Geneva: WHO: 86–87.

Woodruff RE, Guest C, Garner M, *et al.* (2002) Predicting ross river virus epidemics from regional weather data. *Epidemiology* **13**: 384–393.

3

Landscape Epidemiology and Migration: Insights and Problems at Several Scales for Transmissible Diseases

David J Bradley

(In Memoriam: Sir Richard Southwood)

Introduction

This chapter addresses two large themes in the population dynamics of disease.[1] The first is the spatial structure of disease and its contexts, where technical innovations have transformed the scene, but have tended to substitute for a theoretical basis for such spatial thinking. I shall argue that there is a useful subject, best named landscape epidemiology, which is more than just applied geographical information systems (GIS). The recent history of public health thinking about different scales for communicable disease epidemiology will also be considered.

---

[1] In preparing a draft version of this chapter for a meeting devoted largely to epidemic contagious diseases in urban Asia, I had to ask what someone whose expertise and thinking is primarily on endemic vector-borne diseases in rural Africa has to offer. This has driven me back to what interests me most: how we conceptualise issues in public health, what ideas from other aspects of science have to offer us, and the strategic consequences of technical advances. I trust the ideas here may help give an overall and rounded picture of the field, which is both intellectually challenging and poses huge practical problems for medicine and the public health.

There will be some elaboration of two related special topics in relation to space and scales of change. One is well established and will always be particularly associated with the Malay Peninsula: the role of *ecotones* in epidemiology of emergent infections (Audy, 1968). The other is an analogous concept but rooted in time rather than space: *chronotones* and their importance in human development of space (Bradley, 2004). These two concepts are linked together in space-time clustering of both disease problems and health opportunities.

From my earlier years in research, it seemed clear that two factors in life generally, and in disease specifically, were greatly under estimated: one was genetics and the other migration. Thirty years from then, the importance of genetics has been fully appreciated, first with vectors (insecticide resistance) and species complexes, closely followed by pathogens because of drug resistance, and much more slowly in human and other mammalian hosts, in relation to susceptibility and resistance to disease. Although Sabin (1952) and Bang (1960) had done beautiful work showing that resistance of mice to group B arboviruses (such as yellow fever) and mouse hepatitis respectively is under single gene control, I learned it from visceral leishmaniasis in mice later (Bradley, 1974, 1977), finding the *Lsh* (later *Nramp1* and now *SLC11A1*) gene that 30 years later was shown to affect human susceptibility to tuberculosis (Li *et al.*, 2002). However, our understanding of the genetics of mammalian host resistance to infection still lags behind our understanding of the genetics of drug resistance by pathogens and of resistance to insecticides by vectors. The great implication for pathogen dynamics is that we should now look at population genetic models of disease more thoroughly and not simply follow the fixed genetic species epidemiological models of the past when we think about such diseases as malaria (Bradley, 1999). The present issues with bird influenza that worry farmers and scientists in Asia and worldwide only serve to underline this conclusion.

However, systematic treatment of the role of migration has remained neglected in spite of some attempts long ago (for example, Prothero, 1965). The way we conceptualise migration will be my second main theme. In many ways, it is the antithesis of the first. Migration can completely confuse the results of a spatially constructed analysis of disease and my example is malaria in South China. Yet, the significance of migration is only clearly visible if we have a spatially structured model of disease dynamics. Were diseases transmitted by vectors flying randomly among equally randomly distributed hosts, as in most epidemiological models for vector-borne disease, we could continue to ignore the importance of movement and migration.

For a holistic perception of migration, we may turn to particular models of landscape epidemiology to make sense of changing epidemiological determinants, human life patterns and emerging diseases. Our models need to be not only population genetic models, but also models embracing a geographically structured view of the environment and of metapopulations (Hanski, 1999) linked by intensive migration.

The expansion of what is tractable epidemiologically

The last few decades have seen remarkable changes in the descriptive epidemiology of communicable disease. It would not be a caricature to describe field epidemiology of endemic infections in the 1960s as annual cycles of infections in villages. This was partly because the scales of funding and of available time (often constrained to the maximum of 15 months that is feasible during a PhD study) meant that to gain real understanding, one focused only on a small community over an annual cycle of transmission. The process was felt to be orderly and repeated and sometimes rudely disrupted by a drought or flood, but essentially predictable with those exceptions. Epidemic investigation, by contrast, was viewed as a more disorderly *ad hoc* process with a limited theoretical basis that needed much practical skill. The other important limitation was that in rigorous epidemiology, space was largely ignored or reduced to a one-dimensional variable such as "distance from the index case" or source.

This has changed in several respects, not always consciously acknowledged, as a result of research in other areas of science and of technical innovations in gathering and processing information. The most obvious advances are in information technology: the development of geographical information systems (GIS) of such power and capacity that it is possible to handle spatial data on a large scale (in the cartographic sense of detailed representation and also in the more general sense of covering large areas). These have been fed by devising global positioning apparatus to rapidly define the places of interest on the earth and by satellite imagery, which can acquire vast amounts of information from large areas rapidly.

There is also a growing awareness that large-scale (I shall hereafter use this to mean big areas, in the general, and not cartographical, sense) events may be explicable in scientific terms. The demonstration that continental drift was explicable in terms of plate tectonics, and was not a form of vague historical metaphysics, was for me a crucial event. It was reinforced by similar changes in our perception of how far events were explicable over long time periods, for example, our increasing awareness of the El Niño Southern Oscillation phenomenon and its pervasive effects (Kovats *et al.*, 2003). Those working on village level epidemiological problems, who had been comfortable with the annual cycles of temperature and rainfall and the agricultural cycles linked to them, realised that one could be rational over the longer term and larger scale determinants of disease.

When we look at the intermediate scales of human activity and diseases, the district, county or other population unit between 5,000 and 500,000, it is important to realise that different "populations" are involved. There are clearly human populations; almost as clear are populations of pathogens: both the populations within an individual host and the metapopulations of all the populations in a given locality. For vector-borne diseases, insect vector population dynamics are crucial to our understanding and to the approaches to control. For zoonoses, the populations of other host species will be relevant. However, for some cycles, the 'habitat population' dynamics may be of importance, comparable to patch dynamics in landscape epidemiology terminology (Forman and Godron, 1986; Forman, 1995). An example is seen in the analysis of the large increases in malaria transmission detected in the grazing areas of Southwest Uganda (Okello-Onen and colleagues, work in progress). One variable to be investigated is the increase in small water bodies: valley tanks of various sizes for general access in drought and individual household on-farm ponds that have proliferated since the settlement of primarily nomadic pastoralists. Years ago, conscious of the complexity of populations of snails as intermediate hosts of *Schistosoma haematobium* and of our ignorance of human behaviour in relation to them, the use of the population of ponds that formed the snail habitats as units for modelling was suggested, regardless of their detailed content (Bradley, 1965). However, this consideration of populations needs to extend further in some cases. In the absence of predation and culling, African elephant populations have greatly multiplied, destroying the trees in their habitat, and effecting changes in vegetation cover and greatly affecting insect vector and snail intermediate host populations. At the other extreme of scale, and especially if we are considering migration, the key elements in drug resistance of microbes are the resistance genes.

Landscape Epidemiology

There are difficulties if we seek to handle spatial knowledge in general public health terms, whether to measure concerns about disease emergence and spread or to define risk areas for several types of disease or where the detailed life cycles are unclear. The detailed three or more component models will prove too complex if spatial structure is added, due more to the limitations of data than to model complexity or demands for computing power.

There are many ways to classify and categorise space, but two approaches seem fruitful. The first is the metapopulations approach, for which pathogens are particularly suited. Those old enough to have learned their ecology from Andrewartha and Birch (1954) will have encountered their diagrams of local habitats. The medical microbiologist may feel that each little circle is too similar to the others to represent a wood or lake, but if we are considering people infected with a pathogen, then the model becomes more convincing (Bradley, 1972).

Not only are pathogens by nature presented as "metapopulations = infected people", but many have stages in their transmission where either they or their vectors are inhabitants of small water bodies, comprising another level of metapopulations. Moreover, there is an extensive theoretical literature on island biogeography (MacArthur and Wilson, 1967). If we view the ponds as islands and the land between as analogous to sea; or even if we view people as the islands, some of the island biogeographical theory has relevance.

More immediately relevant is the body of work carried out in what was then the USSR by Pavlovsky and his many followers, on what Western and Southeast Asian workers termed the epidemiology of the zoonoses, but which Pavlovsky (1963, 1966) named "Landscape Epidemiology". His work was carried out in the 1920s and 1930s when new communities were being established in Siberia and in the then Soviet Central Asia. He observed that the settlers contracted several diseases that were associated with the particular ecosystem of settlement. In the forest or taiga, spring-summer encephalitis tended to occur, and was shown to be tick-borne; in the semi-desert steppe cutaneous leishmaniasis and plague were problems, with a reservoir in the huge populations of burrowing gerbils and transmitted by sandflies and by rodent fleas respectively. Pavlovsky's emphasis was on the relation between landscape type and its typical disease pattern.

The third and most immediate source of spatial theory relevant to the epidemiology is the subject known as "Landscape Ecology". It arose, as does this chapter in part, from dissatisfaction with an ecology that stayed within particular habitat types and treated them as homogeneous. Such workers as Forman and Godron (1986), building on much work by geographers, conservation workers, and the metapopulation ecologists such as Hanski (1999), sought to emphasise the discontinuities in the landscape, viewing it as being made up of patches and corridors of landscape elements set in a matrix of the predominant element. This is not the place for a critique of an evolving theory with both strengths and weaknesses, but its picture of regions made up of landscapes comprising a series of recurring landscape elements is of real use in considering the patterns of endemic, epidemic and emerging diseases, especially those which are vector-borne or zoonotic, as are so many emerging diseases.

For our purposes, we may take a simplified view of landscape, as a struc-tured environment. It is something we can look at; indeed one meaning of "landscape" is a view or painting of a view, of scenery. As such, it can be recognised; it assembles a range of environmental variables that may affect pathogens and health, and it can also be made accessible to non-specialists and used as a means of communication of health risks, an aspect to which I shall return at the conclusion of this chapter.

With this tentative definition, it is clearer that landscape epidemiology will be much influenced by geo-referenced data, but it should not be equated with GIS, in the same manner that electron microscopy was essential for cell biology, but is a technique and not a subject in itself.

Landscapes typical for various disease risks such as sleeping sickness/ trypanosomiasis (Robertson, 1963), tick-borne relapsing fever (Walton, 1962), and onchocerciasis are easily shown. Cultural landscapes of a rural type have particular disease risks. Urban and peri-urban sites have more complex assemblages of risks; moreover, peri–urban areas vary between the major continents in the type and degree of interpenetration of agricultural elements into the poor urban landscape, with different disease implications.

Ecotones and Chronotones

In a Southeast Asian context, the importance of ecotones in disease emergence and epidemiology needs no belabouring, when the archetypal example of this is scrub typhus in Malaysia, beautifully described by Audy (1968) in his book *Red Mites and Typhus*. An ecotone is the boundary between two ecosystems (Hansen *et al.*, 1988); in the Malaysian case, it is a clearing in the jungle. It had the consequence of bringing the trombiculid mites of the jungle into contact with the human beings, and the transfer of *Rickettsia tsutsugamushi* from its endemic jungle hosts to people with dire consequences. Ecotone theory suggests that such edges between environments with different fauna allow contact between species that otherwise do not meet, and also that the ecotones may have a rich fauna from both ecosystems, plus a group of species peculiar to the ecotone itself (Lachavanne and Juge, 1997).

The other classical example concerns transmission of yellow fever, that is endemic in jungle canopy monkeys, from them to human beings. In East Africa, this may occur via the traditional vector responsible for spread between monkeys, *Aedes africanus*, which lives in the canopy but which briefly descends to the floor of the forest from the canopy, just before dark. People entering the forest to gather wood at that time may be bitten and contract yellow fever. In other sites, there is a species of mosquito that lives at the forest edge ecotone, *Aedes simpsoni*, and may bite both monkeys and people. Once people are infected, the peridomestic and urban yellow fever vector, *Aedes aegypti*, takes over and epidemic outbreaks occur (Haddow *et al.*, 1948; Lumsden, 1951).

In human development (or, more neutrally, human alteration) of the environment, there is much confusion over the health effects of the changes that are taking place. The comment, often seen, that "deforestation increases malaria" is less than half true in many parts of the world. It is true in several areas that those who cut down the forests and live by the forest edge may have an increased risk of malaria, but when all the trees have gone, the risk of malaria may fall. The *process* of deforestation increased malaria and the *state* of deforestation reduced it (Walsh *et al.*, 1993).

When a great dam is erected, a reservoir created and the water used for power generation or irrigation, there is a complex period from the beginning of the works to some years after their completion, when many disease risks rise, as do opportunities to cope with them (Stanley and Alpers, 1975). In the case of Volta Lake in Ghana (Bradley, 2004) where inundation took place without tree clearance, a sequence of events involving schistosomiasis epidemics took place (Scott *et al.*, 1982) and it took about 15 years for the fluxes of disease to settle to a new set of steady states.

Forest or arid countryside may have persisted for centuries, and the deforested agricultural land or the reservoir may continue for many decades. However, the crucial intermediate processes of deforestation or of reservoir construction, filling and stabilisation may occupy from a year to more than a decade during which all things are in flux. This boundary in time between two steady states of the landscape I have called a chronotone, by analogy with the ecotone (Bradley, 2004).

Chronotones are times of high risk for disease emergence and proliferation. They are often times of great in and out migration of people. Old threats to health may meet a non-immune population of temporary workers on the dam, and they may bring new diseases with them. Chronotones are also periods of great opportunity to establish healthcare facilities as well as to take preventive measures. They usually require substantially higher health inputs than times before or after (these should be charged to the project), but such expenditure may have substantial long-term pay-offs. Usually, the chronotone period is massively under budgeted.

Migration

The limitations of spatial knowledge

To move on to the limitations of spatial knowledge in epidemiology, I consider attempts to use GIS as a guide to the operations of malaria control. Three studies of this type have been done by our group in the Brazilian Amazon (Breitas, personal communication, 1990), the Pacific coastal plain of Colombia (Osorio *et al.*, 2004) and in rural Yunnan, China (Luo, 2001).

All point in the same direction but the Yunnan work by Luo Dapeng is both the clearest and most likely to be of most interest to readers of this volume.

Luo (2001) carried out a detailed GIS characterisation of an area near the Red River, using many variables to describe the environment in relation to likely malaria transmission, and then compared predicted with observed malaria in very careful studies. From the original cases of falciparum malaria recorded in his survey, many were excluded because they had travelled to other malarious areas during the usual incubation period of malaria. Among those apparently not travelling, it was found that those with a travel history outside the usually recognised incubation period still had a very much elevated relative risk of malaria. When these were taken into consideration, even in this part of rural Yunnan over two thirds of cases had contracted their malaria outside their home villages and therefore the detailed GIS was not of use in directing the Malaria Control Programme's case finding activities.

We have shown that for the recent malaria studies in spatially structured human populations, migration is a huge confounding variable to the simple use of GIS as a guide to what is happening to the human and parasite populations. From a practical viewpoint, it means that environmental information, such as is obtainable from satellite imagery, is a very poor guide to the control of malaria in people, however good it may be for defining the sites of malaria transmission. The spatial noise from migration exceeds in volume the signal from local transmission. This does not mean that we can safely regress to the panmictic populations of people and mosquitoes of the simple transmission models. We need to know much more about detailed patterns of migration, and some further examples of superficially very different types of migration and malaria can drive the discussion on.

In the UK, I have looked after the UK Malaria Reference Laboratory's (MRL) epidemiology for 30 yrs. Imported into the UK annually, and for the 17 years from 1987–2003 inclusive, we maintained a standard protocol and the same epidemiological staff. Currently, this unique data set is being analysed from various viewpoints. Over time, there has been a shift, most noticeably in London, from predominantly vivax malaria contracted in South Asia to overwhelmingly falciparum malaria contracted in Africa (Phillips-Howard *et al.*, 1988, 1990). There are several reasons for this and till now, some mysteries still remain. Today, malaria imported into London is primarily a disease of ethnic minorities, with 90% of London's falciparum malaria burden falling on its African ethnic population, and almost half of imported malaria being the result of "visiting friends and relations" (VFR) back in Africa. The vivax malaria that predominated two decades ago also resulted from VFR by South Asians who had settled in the UK earlier than the African population (Bradley, 1989a; Bradley *et al.*, 1998).

For many years, our focus was on getting better epidemiological data on the place and time of infection, and we are able to say in which countries most of our imported cases contracted their malaria infections. More recently, we have mapped the homes in the UK of imported cases, using postcodes (a topic to which I shall return). There is a high degree of concentration of cases so that some 90% of imported falciparum cases in ethnic Africans are reported from under 20% of the 600 electoral wards into which London is divided (Dos Santos, 2002). Vivax malaria is still more focal, with 90% of the cases in only 10% of the wards. In other words, there is a high degree of focality of imported malaria at the site of illness as well as at the source of infection. This has substantial implications for the strategy of prevention, especially as rates of compliance with chemoprophylaxis in ethnic minority travellers are less than in travellers in general. The aggregation of cases in certain wards is of course more a matter of co-location of ethnic groups who travel to the same malarious regions than of any forces driving cases themselves together. However, since cases are an unequivocal indicator of risk, the malaria case distribution maps provide a good aid to targeting prophylactic interventions (and one less open to misinterpretation politically); focusing on sites of maximal risk of malaria is somewhat easier to explain than selecting minority groups for special attention per se.

Africans in Britain overwhelmingly live in London, but South Asians who have settled in the Midlands and North of England show comparable focality of *Plasmodium vivax* malaria. Moreover, it is possible to map parts of South Asia onto the UK map, e.g. immigrants from the Sylhet region of NE Bangladesh have particularly settled in Leicester. In this example, migration and landscape epidemiology come together. The variations in endemicity of malaria in the places from which particular ethnic groups have come, and to which they return when visiting friends and relations, is reflected in the frequency and drug resistance patterns of malaria shown by these people in the UK.

However, people on the move are not only responsible for transporting pathogens from their endemic area to a new region where it will be of clinical importance (made worse because the diagnosis is more likely to be missed there) and of possible public health importance, if in the case of vector-borne disease, the home destination is receptive, or if it be endemic for the infection but lacks drug resistance present in the imported parasite. Migrants also transport their beliefs about diseases and their views on severity, appropriate health-seeking behaviour and the like. This is clearly seen in malaria in the UK and in some highland areas of Kenya.

Movement of disease 'culture'

In the UK, African immigrants who were exposed to high levels of malaria transmission during childhood in Africa hold the view that malaria is merely a mild nuisance illness, as it is for many adults in holoendemic areas, and may be unaware that immunity decays rapidly in the absence of continual re-infection. More seriously, they may be unaware that their children born in the UK are essentially non-immune and liable to life-threatening falciparum malaria during visits to friends and relations in Africa.

In Kenya, Doi (2001) showed how three groups of migrant workers on tea estates at an altitude liable to epidemic malaria had three very different views of malaria and the appropriate action to take, views more suitable to the home environments that each group had left many years or decades earlier. In her words, each group had a "malaria culture" appropriate to their location many years ago.

These two examples illustrate the general concept that migrants may not only carry and suffer from communicable disease from their earlier homes, but also carry a "disease culture", often acquired much earlier still, which will affect their responses to perceived illness, sometimes in a maladaptive way. This "disease culture" may also determine the care that their children receive should they fall ill, or the nature of any preventive action during visits to their original homeland.

Movement, travel and migration

The complexity and rapidity of movement is far greater than in the past, as is its total extent for many people. As those who have investigated outbreaks of highly contagious disease will know, as the carrying capacity of aeroplanes rises from 7 to 330, the number of secondary contacts of an index case, where 30% of travellers take a further journey, will increase three thousand fold.

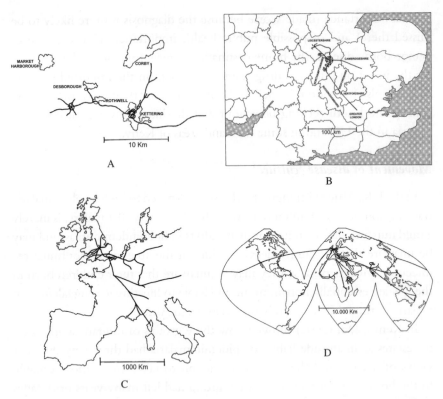

Fig. 1. Maps of the life-time track of four generations of the same English family. The linear scale increases by a factor of 10 and the map area by a factor of 100 between each pair of adjacent figures. Figure 1A represented the track of the great-grandparental generation, 1B grandparents, 1C parents and 1D the author's generation. Reproduced from Bradley (1989b) with permission from the publishers.

The range increases too. Figure 1 shows the range of movements of four generations of a UK family. The linear extremes of range rose 10-fold per generation and the area over which they roamed increased by a figure of the order of 100-fold per generation.

Even the daily and weekly migrations of people in many countries are both diverse and complex. In studies of persistent (asymptomatic) imported malaria infections in the UK from the MRL database, undertaken as a basis for policy advice to the blood transfusion service, a number of very long intervals between travel abroad and detection of *P. falciparum*, of the order of four years, were observed. In cases where it was possible to undertake local investigations, it emerged that some people were travelling to the tropics with a high but unadmitted frequency.

The lifetime track

These observations, and the complicated routes taken by backpackers during long overseas visits, all point to the inadequacy of travel and migration histories as generally taken and recorded. Similar inadequacies have been remarked by Baker (1978) in his exhaustive documentation of animal migration. Until patterns of migration are more fully described, we suggest a similar research approach, of investigating from an epidemiological viewpoint the lifetime track of people, that is, the complete movement pattern from birth to death. Groups for whom this approach may be specially revealing are those with highly migratory lives, such as migrants who have largely settled in a new country, but may be visiting relatives or doing business in their countries of origin with a high frequency. Another group comprises those that are living in areas undergoing rapid and complex environmental change, such as settlers in the Amazon forest clearings in Brazil, populations affected by dam construction, nomads being heavily encouraged to settle, some homeless urban dwellers and the like, as well as the many populations who are forcibly internally displaced or war refugees. Studies of this type by those interested in the movement of people may form a good basis for subsequent selection of high risk migration patterns in relation to disease emergence or spread at the public health level, as well as those at a high risk of suffering.

A particular tool known as the postcode has emerged as being of great help in recording locations, and changing locations in the UK, although it certainly may not solve the problems of the highest risk movements. In the UK, the postcode identifies an address with a high degree of accuracy as less than 15 houses usually share a postcode. Moreover, there are computer programmes that give the precise spatial location of the centroid of any UK postcode. This has proved to be a highly useful epidemiological tool in determining risk in populations living in the plume of factory smoke suspected of containing radioactivity, and it could be used to record complex movement patterns over time with precision and in a concise way. For the majority of the world's population with no such easy identifiers of location, GPS apparatus provides a rapid and reliable means of mapping sites visited in the field.

It is obvious that complete lifetime track histories of people are not going to be collected for large populations. However, even a few samples are likely to be illuminating in relation to sites of high risk for disease emergence, the use of ecotones and other places of complex environmental interaction, and routes of epidemic propagation. To give a simple livestock example, had veterinary public health workers been more aware of the movement patterns and rates of stock bought from UK markets, they would perhaps have been more aware of epidemic risk and better motivated to ban the market events that led to the huge UK foot and mouth disease outbreak and the public might have been more accepting of strong action.

When lifetime track type information is combined with the landscape epidemiological way of looking at places and habitats, we begin to have the type of knowledge system that can help us analyse and predict disease emergence, problems of disease control and of the role of human beings in changing the face of the earth.

I have addressed several vast themes too rapidly, with the aim of creating not an entire theory, since the data and issues are far too complex, but a framework of some generality that may help us to accommodate those key variables of spatial structure and of migration that are often omitted from classical epidemiological theory. This is needed for communicable disease epidemiology in the present era where environmental changes and genetic variation in complex situations are the basis of many disease problems.

Practical Application

As we consider what should be done, we are faced with several difficult problems for society and political economy. Success in combating infectious diseases in the past was achieved by the firm imposition of general public health measures, in ways that have broken down in many affluent countries, and were not implemented in the poor countries.

Even today, violation of basic public health rules has underlain some of the most devastating of our recent epidemics, e.g. the foot and mouth disease outbreak in the UK in 2002, and many other infections that arise or spread because of large scale profitable activities. The drive for cheap food, market share, new products and exotic novelties will all tend to favour the entrepreneur who sails close to the wind, and the greater the competitive pressure, the more incentive there is to bypass sound regulations, both for the tycoon and the peasant. The very poor will lack both the information and the means to comply. The diminution of state control and the increase of individualism, in the absence of strong cultural constraints will tend to increase the risks of disease emergence and outbreak frequency. How will the increase of liberty without licence be achieved? Will the development of transdisciplinary approaches and "sustainability science", which at least seek to grapple with the problems, lead to implementable solutions? Will society be able to combine democracy with a long-term perspective?

To conclude, I would like to descend from these levels of general theory to practical public health. A landscape is not only the aggregation of land-forms in a particular place, but also the portion of land or scenery as seen by the eye in a single view or a picture of a view of scenery, both in English usage and in that of several other European languages. In other words, it is a way of visually communicating a structured environment. Landscape lends itself to communication and to the type of transdisciplinary activity needed to involve the public in its own health. If the historic directive approach to public health action has been weakened, the approach of landscape epidemi-ology lends itself to the participatory public health needed at this moment and in the future, in the same way that consciousness of lifetime tracks can assist people generally and their health advisers in understanding risks and preventive measures, and to help bridge the rather artificial boundaries between environmental and "lifestyle" explanations of disease risk.

References

Andrewartha HG, Birch LC. (1954) *The Distribution and Abundance of Animals.* University of Chicago Press, Chicago.

Audy JR. (1968) *Red Mites and Typhus.* Athlone Press, London.

Baker, RR. (1978) *The Evolutionary Ecology of Animal Migration*, Hodder & Stoughton, London.

Bang FB, Warwick A. (1960) Mouse macrophages as host cells for the mouse hepatitis virus, and the genetic basis of their susceptibility. *Proc Natl Acad Sci US* **46**: 1065–1075.

Bradley DJ. (1965) Consequences of pond transmission for theory of bilharzial epidemiology. *J Appl Ecol* **2**: 413–414.

Bradley DJ. (1972) Regulation of parasite populations. A general theory of the epidemiology and control of parasitic infection. *Trans Roy Soc Trop Med Hyg* **66**: 697–708.

Bradley DJ. (1974) Genetic control of natural resistance to *Leishmania donovani*. *Nature* **250**: 353.

Bradley DJ. (1977) Regulation of leishmania populations within the host. II. Genetic control of acute susceptibility of mice to *L. donovani* infection. *Clin Exp Immunol* **30**: 119–129.

Bradley DJ. (1989a) Current trends in malaria in britain. *J Roy Soc Med* **82** (Suppl) **17**: 8–13.

Bradley DJ. (1989b) The scope of travel medicine, in Steffen R *et al.* (eds.) *Travel Medicine*. Springer-Verlag, Britain.

Bradley DJ. (1998) The influence of local changes in the rise of infectious disease, in Greenwood B & De Cock K (eds.) *London School of Hygiene and Tropical Medicine Seventh Annual Public Health Forum. New and Resurgent Infections. Prediction, Detection and Management of Tomorrow's Epidemics*, pp. 1–12, John Wiley & Sons, UK.

Bradley DJ. (1999) The last and the next hundred years of malariology. *Parassitologia* **41**: 11–18.

Bradley DJ. (2004) An exploration of chronotones: A concept for understanding the health processes of changing ecosystems. *Ecohealth* **1**: 165–171.

Bradley DJ, Warhurst DC, Blaze M, Smith V, Williams J. (1998) Malaria imported into the united kingdom in 1996. *Euro Surveillance* **3**: 40–42.

Doi Y. (2001) *Communities, Malaria Culture and the Resurgence of Highland Malaria in Western Kenya: A KAP Study*. PhD Thesis, University of Liverpool.

Dos Santos MP. (2002) *Microdistribution of Imported Malaria Cases in London*. MSc Thesis, London School of Hygiene and Tropical Medicine.

Forman RTT. (1995) *Land Mosaics: The Ecology of Landscapes and Regions*. Cambridge University Press, Cambridge.

Forman RTT, Godron M. (1986) *Landscape Ecology*. Wiley, Chichester.

Haddow AJ, *et al.* (1948) Implication of the mosquito *Aedes africanus* in the forest cycle of yellow fever in Uganda. *Annals Trop Med Parsitol* **42**: 218–223.

Hansen AJ, Di Castri F, Naiman RJ. (1988) Ecotones: What and Why? in Di Castri F, Hansen AJ & Holland MM (eds.), *A New Look at Ecotones: Emerging International Projects on Landscape Boundaries. Biology International* **17**: 9–46.

Hanski I. (1999) *Metapopulation Ecology*. Oxford University Press, Oxford.

Kovats RS, Bouma MJ, Hajat S, Worrall E, Haines A. (2003) El Niño and health. *Lancet* **362**: 1481–1489.

Lachavanne JB, Juge R (eds.) (1997) *Biodiversity in Land-Inland Water Ecotones*. Paris: UNESCO, Parthenon, New York.

Li CM, Campbell SJ, Kumararatne DS, Bellamy R, Ruwende C, McAdam KP, Hill AV, Lammas DA. (2002) Association of a polymorphism in the p2x7 gene with tuberculosis in a Gambian population. *J Infect Dis* **186**:1458–1462.

Lumsden WHR. (1951) Probable insect vectors of yellow fever virus from monkeys to man in Bwamba county, Uganda. *Bull Entomol Res* **42**: 317–330.

Luo D-P. (2001) *Spatial Prediction of Malaria in the Red River Basin, Yunnan, China Using Geographical Information Systems and Remote Sensing*. PhD Thesis, London School of Hygiene and Tropical Medicine, University of London.

MacArthur RH, Wilson EO. (1967) *The Theory of Island Biogeography*. Princeton University Press, Princeton.

Osorio L, Todd J, Bradley DJ. (2004) Travel histories as risk factors in the analysis of urban malaria in Colombia. *Am J Trop Med Hyg* **71**: 380–6.

Pavlovsky EN. (1963) *Human Diseases with Natural Foci*, YN Pavlovsky (ed.) [transl. from Russian by D Rottenberg], Foreign Languages Pub House, Moscow.

Pavlovsky EN. (1966) *Natural Nidality of Transmissible Diseases: With Special Reference to the Landscape Epidemiology of Zooanthroponoses* (English translation edited by Norman D. Levine, translated by Frederick K. Plous, Jr.), University of Illinois Press, Urbana.

Phillips-Howard PA, Bradley DJ, Blaze M, Hurn M. (1988) Malaria in Britain 1977–1986. *Br Med J* **296**: 245–248.

Phillips-Howard PA, Radalowicz A, Mitchell J, Bradley DJ. (1990) Risk of malaria in British residents returning from malarious areas. *Br Med J* **300**: 499–503.

Prothero RM. (1965) *Migrants and Malaria*. Longmans, London.

Robertson DHH. (1963) Human trypanosomiasis in southeast Uganda. *Bull Wld Hlth Org* **28**: 627–643.

Sabin AB. (1952) Nature of inherited resistance to viruses affecting the nervous system. *Proc Natl Acad Sci US* **38**: 540–546

Scott D, Senker K, England EC. (1982) Epidemiology of human schistosoma haematobium infection around Volta Lake, Ghana, 1973–75. *Bull World Health Org* **60**: 89–100.

Stanley NF, Alpers MP (eds.) (1975). *Man-made Lakes and Human Health*, Academic Press, London.

Walsh JF, Molyneux DH, Birley MH. (1993). Deforestation: Effects on vector-borne disease. *Parasitology* **106** (Suppl): S55–S75.

Walton GA. (1962) The *ornithodorus moubata* superspecies problem in relation to human relapsing fever epidemiology, in Arthur DR (ed.) *Aspects of Disease Transmission by Ticks. Symposia of the Zoological Society of London No. 6*, pp. 83–156.

4

Water, Dams and Infection: Asian Challenges

Adrian C Sleigh

Introduction

Throughout Asia, the growing needs and aspirations of the huge population now engaged in very rapid economic development are placing great strains on the ecosystem. Hydrological resources are under particular stress (Pearce, 1992; World Commission on Dams, 2000). For example, the Yangtze and Ganges river valleys, with 224 and 375 persons per square km, respectively, support many more people than comparable river valleys in the Americas. Throughout most of Asia, the surface and underground water is increasingly polluted by animal and human excreta, poisoned by factory and agricultural effluents, withdrawn for agriculture, industry and households, and manipulated for navigation, flood control and power generation. National goals for economic development, safe water supplies, food security and good health are competing, even colliding. Central to meeting many of the above demands, especially those relating to food, water and economic development, are large dams and irrigation systems. Thousands have already been built in Asia. Indeed, China and India together now have over half the global total of large dams. It seems certain that thousands more large dams will be commissioned over the next two to three decades. Once

again, China and India will account for most of them. The dams themselves
will pose additional risks to already stressed ecosystems, but the water and
the energy that they provide will also enhance many lives. Unfortunately,
millions will be adversely affected and dam-associated infectious diseases will
play a significant role in generating such negative effects. Given the large
proportion of the dams that will be located in Asia, this topic is of special
importance in that region.

Dams and their reservoirs transform the environment. A set of river-
related resources such as water, fauna, flora and landscape are converted
into another set of natural resources. The fauna and flora are changed, often
completely, and even the climate can alter with rising humidity and temperature. The water table rises, fish no longer migrate, people and animals
cannot traverse the landscape, farmland is submerged, people are displaced
and livelihoods are destroyed. A large lake appears, but its level fluctuates in
unnatural ways and it often becomes polluted. Downstream flows are altered
as well, with great changes forced upon the agricultural system, alteration
of fisheries and estuaries, erosion of flood dykes due to lack of silt below
the dam, and decreased river flow due to upstream extraction for irrigation.
Ancestral graves and archaeological sites are flooded. Another group of people and animals, often remote from the dam site, benefits from these changes,
with generation of power and water supplies for domestic and industrial use.
There are always winners and losers. When the losers are indigenous people,
with traditional lives and lands lost, they cannot recover as their culture is
place-based and unique. With increasing construction of very large dams
(more than 150 metres in height) Asian river valleys are being affected at an
alarming rate, with dense population areas now considered for dam developments. This means that displaced populations are also increasing, with the
Three Gorges Dam in China as a good example with nearly two million
people displaced from the reservoir area, and hundreds of millions affected
downstream.

In this chapter, I review the general attributes of large dams, consider their
documented impacts on infections, and suggest ways that the development
community can integrate resources to mitigate these unwanted health effects.
My interest in this topic first arose when I studied water-related diseases in
Brazil many years ago. This made me consider the link between agriculture, water and infection. I worked in some areas that were irrigated, visited

several large dams and encountered many people displaced and marginalised by one large dam. Later, I had the opportunity to join the impact mitigation teams working on large dams in China, including the two biggest, Three Gorges Dam on the Yangtze river and the World Bank-financed Ertan Dam on the Yalong river, 1,000 km further upstream (Sleigh and Jackson, 1998, 2001; Jackson and Sleigh, 2000, 2001). I worked with experienced Chinese and international colleagues and learned much from them about big dams, their ecological and social impacts, and the furious debate then (and now) raging about the role of dams in development (Alvares and Billorey, 1988; Morse and Berger, 1992; Fearnside, 1994; Dorcey *et al.*, 1997; Cernea, 1988, 1999; McCully, 2001). However, I was usually the sole health person on the team, so under-resourcing health assessments and constraining mitigation of health impacts even when the social and ecological impacts were being seriously considered by the dam builders. But this was better than previous practice, as most earlier dams were built without giving the health sector any voice at all (Hunter *et al.*, 1993; World Health Organization, 1999).

Dams, Population and Development

Human societies have constructed dams for most of recorded history. As far as we know, hydraulic works began with civilisation itself. We know that Mesopotamians built dams and irrigation canals 8,000 years ago and town water supply systems have been used in the Middle East since 3,000 BC. Ancient water systems and dams were also built in Asia and South America and the capture of energy from flowing water was practised in ancient Egypt and Sumeria, using wheels and buckets.

Taking a long view of history, one could argue that the most successful agricultural development arose in China. Dams and water played a major role, but the environmental toll has been great and the next 100 years will be the most challenging that China has ever faced. A huge population, associated pollution, progressive northern desertification, sinking aquifers and rivers that no longer reach the sea are the legacy of this past success. The economic historian David Landes attributes China's precocious and (until now) long-lasting agricultural success to its early focus on hydraulic works and irrigation (Landes, 1998). In this much praised book, he examines and attempts to explain the wealth and poverty of nations. Landes notes that the 2,500 year-old Chinese strategy of ensuring political survival and economic development of the Han by stimulating and enabling their rapid demographic growth. The population growth required a commensurate increase in the food supply, achieved by adopting labour-intensive agriculture. Intensive agriculture was in turn enabled by the demographic growth, requiring more agricultural production and creating a treadmill effect and more population growth. Underpinning this development strategy in China was the invention, construction and the firm central control of dams and irrigation at that time. The process began in the rich loess soils of the Upper Yellow river, a veritable school for water control, irrigation technology and adaptation of water buffalo as draft animals. The population then expanded further down that same river basin where floods and droughts were later to affect large settled populations, becoming China's "Sorrow". Eventually, after 2,500 years of human manipulation of the river water for storage, irrigation, flood control and finally power generation, the Yellow river began to run dry before reaching the sea. Currently, the lower reaches of the river are dry on most days of the year and the surrounding region, including Beijing, has a severe water shortage.

Eventually, beginning about 1,300 years ago, the Han expanded south into the warmer and wetter Yangtze and Pearl river basins, embracing irrigated rice and double or triple annual cropping, substantially boosting caloric yields and population growth. This water-based development of labour-intensive agriculture led to Wittfogel's political theory that the required 'hydraulic centralism' inevitably produced an autocratic form of government, which he injudiciously named Oriental Despotism (Wittfogel, 1957). Landes concurs that the intensive Chinese system of irrigated agriculture led to the need for absolute central power over a critical and ever-growing system of big dikes, dams, canals, flood control, repair and relief. It is not hard to link such historical descriptions to the situation prevailing in China today, with the obvious preoccupation with maintaining the water-based food supply for its now huge population. This is a direct result of 2,500 years of hitherto successful and always inventive hydraulic manipulation of the national ecosystem, and its central engineer-focused decision making for matters dealing with large dams, flood control, irrigation and water supply.

It remains to be seen whether such central control can now rescue China from its looming environmental fate, with widespread soil erosion, severe water pollution, and a population that is almost too large for the available water supplies.

While China developed technologically, Europe did not do so well in the field of dam development, at least for the first 2,000 years. The Romans ground their corn with watermills 2,100 years ago, but these were not adopted widely until 500 years later in medieval England. Finally, in the 19th century, Britain began to develop dams more than 15 metres in height to supply water to its new industrial cities. Dams of this size are now defined as 'large dams' (World Commission on Dams, 2000). In 1832, Benoit Fourneyron invented a water turbine to capture the energy of falling water, and advance on the ancient flow-dependent waterwheels. Eventually, turbines were connected to generators and the first hydroelectric plant began producing electricity in Wisconsin in 1882. Hydropower is a combination of four complex technologies, i.e. dams, turbines, generators, and electricity transmission. At last, energy from water in one location could reach another location for flexible use in multiple productive and comforting tasks (Smith, 1971).

Dams and power stations quickly grew from 30 metre heads (in 1900) to 200 metre heads (1930s) and spread rapidly in Europe and North America. In 1902, the British built the Low Aswan Dam to regulate the Nile and irrigate cotton fields, but the uptake of large dam technology remained limited in the developing world for another 50 years. After World War II, big dams began to spread to the developing world, and both India and China started to invest heavily in them. From 1950 to 1980, China built around 600 such dams per year, but quality was poor. Many dams burst, some catastrophically. For example, it has been reported that 250,000 people were killed in Henan in 1975 when 62 dams burst after an extraordinary rainfall (McCully, 2001). Dam failure rates in China appear to have been higher than elsewhere during this period.

The World Bank, other development banks, the Food and Agriculture Organization (FAO) and the UN Development Programme (UNDP) played an important role in promoting large dams and irrigation schemes in developing countries after 1970. The US Agency for International Development (USAID) and the British Overseas Development

Administration (ODA) also helped to plan and fund dams. Such aid-supported construction companies based themselves in rich countries once the work at home had declined. The most definitive statistics on the global situation are those given by the World Commission on Dams (2000). It reported that around $20 billion is spent every year on large dams and 100–200 are commissioned. Over the last 100 years, two trillion US dollars has been invested in 45,000 large dams worldwide. Unfortunately, few have been evaluated economically, environmentally or socially; even fewer have been systematically studied for health effects.

Health and Social Effects of Dams

Dams are built to enable socio–economic development and thus by definition, they should not make people worse off, or produce disease. However, disease caused by dams has been well documented, especially infections. Although published information on the impacts of large dams comes mostly from studies conducted in Africa and the Caribbean, there are parallel problems with dams in Asia (Hunter *et al.*, 1993; Jobin, 1999; World Health Organization, 1999).

Many disease problems are an indirect result of the adverse social impact of large dams, especially the decapitalisation that results from the loss of land, home and livelihood. Previous capital invested is lost and for many years before the dam is built, new investment is withheld. These socio-economic effects have been studied more extensively than health effects (Morse and Cernea, 1988, 1999; Berger, 1992; Scudder, 1997; Cernea and McDowell, 2000). However, the economic drivers needed to reconstruct shattered lives have been relatively neglected due to the short-term follow-up of most assessments. Dams are an important component of the ongoing global problem of human displacement, with dams accounting for millions of people affected every year. Michael Cernea, the World Bank sociologist who has done much to sensitise that institution to this problem, estimates that development programs over the last 20 years forced 200 million people from homes and livelihoods. This exceeds the number of refugees displaced by conflict over the same period (Cernea, 2000). A large part of the development and displacement problem arises from large dams and the World Commission on Dams (2000) recently released informative estimates. In China alone, the official figure for the period 1950–1990 is 10.2 million, but unofficial estimates point to this number just for the Yangtze basin. In India, the number of dam-displaced persons for that same period is estimated at 16 to 38 million, and the global figure is 40 to 80 million. For World Bank development projects, large dams account for 63% of all resulting human displacement. The numbers displaced by ancillary works are not included in estimates, nor are hundreds of millions whose livelihoods were displaced by downstream effects of altered flows and other ecological changes.

Overall, dam-related vector-borne diseases have been reported frequently, especially epidemics erupting around large or small reservoirs and the associated irrigation works. These problems arise after reservoirs form and river basins change their character, creating conditions that are suitable for certain infections. The most notorious dam-associated infection and one quintessentially linked to agriculture and irrigation is schistosomiasis. This disease is variously known as bilharzia in Africa, snail fever in Asia or water belly in South America. Schistosomiasis is caused by blood flukes (schistosomes) residing in pairs inside the venous system surrounding the gastrointestinal or urinary tracts. The female constantly lays eggs that digest their way through the tissues to the faecal or urinary stream, reach fresh water and hatch into "miracidia" that infect snails present in the water bodies. They multiply inside the snails and emerge as numerous free swimming larvae ("cercariae") that infect human hosts by passing through the skin of people who enter the water. Several species of schistosome infect humans, including *S. japonicum*, which is endemic to a large part of central and Southern China where it also infects many domestic mammals. Schistosomiasis is present in 73 countries including much of Africa, parts of the Middle East, some Caribbean islands, several South American countries including Brazil and in China, Laos, Cambodia, the Philippines and Indonesia. There are many reports of entire communities becoming infected due to large dams and associated irrigation projects. Heavily infected people become debilitated, with weakness and loss of energy, and are eventually unable to work at all. Production falls and lifespans are shortened. Attempts to prevent snail breeding in reservoirs and canals by engineering modifications or chemicals have met with limited success (Jobin, 1999). In fact, infestation of tropical irrigation systems in endemic zones is so common that it is more noteworthy if problems do not arise (Hunter *et al.*, 1993; Jobin, 2000).

Another important dam-induced infection is malaria, a disease spread even more widely than schistosomiasis. Other mosquito-borne infections associated with dams include the nematode worms that cause elephantiasis and several serious viral diseases, including Rift Valley fever, Japanese encephalitis, and dengue. In some areas of Africa and Latin America, black fly populations can breed on dam spillways and transmit the worm that causes river blindness.

Less acknowledged, but probably of greater importance, are diseases caused by poverty and poor sanitation, because they are all made worse by inadequate resettlement of people displaced and pauperised by dams. The potential list is long and includes maternal anaemia and mortality, malnutrition, and infections causing diarrhoea, pneumonia and tuberculosis. These diseases are usually present before a dam is built, often more so due to the poverty induced by the blight on private and public investment that descends on river valleys once a dam is considered, usually decades before it is built. Common diseases already present in affected populations are not usually attributed to large dams, even when they become worse after the dam is built (Sleigh and Jackson, 1998, 2001).

In addition to the infections above, the influx of construction workers and other migrants, such as fishermen or boatmen attracted by the reservoir, brings other microbial risks. Incoming migrants can introduce malaria or schistosome infection, if the vector mosquitoes or host snails are present. They also bring sexually transmitted infections, including syphilis and HIV. The influx of money and the large number of unpartnered males brings prostitution, making infection risks even higher. For a large project, the workforce may grow by 20,000 and the problems expand accordingly.

There are many other adverse health effects of large dams, but these will only be mentioned briefly as they do not involve infections. When harmless inorganic mercury in the soil of the reservoir bed is processed by bacteria feeding on decomposing vegetation, toxic methyl mercury may form; consequently, large fish at the top of the reservoir food chain accumulate dangerous levels of this neurotoxic chemical. Heavy metals and organic solvents may enter the water via run off from flooded factories. Algal blooms or cyanobacteria appear in eutrophic waters of tropical reservoirs soon after they fill, if flooded basins are not cleared of vegetation. Injury, often fatal, is a constant threat to construction workers. Drowning is also a risk after the reservoir forms, especially in tropical areas with no safety measures, and alcohol makes this risk higher. Less understood are the psychological problems induced by loss of land, home and work. Indigenous people are so deeply affected that they may not survive the displacement. Depression and suicide would be expected but are little studied. Violence and conflict have been reported among those adversely affected (World Commission of Dams, 2000; McCully, 2001). The conflict is thought to be a consequence of stress, poverty, communalism, and competition for resources, but is poorly documented because it is hard to trace those displaced, unless there are funds and the political will to do so.

There is also a possibility of catastrophic failure for all large dams. Reservoir-induced landslides are common and so is the seismic activity induced by the weight of the impounded water. Dam walls can collapse or be overtopped by floods or waves. One famous instance is the 1963 landslide into the reservoir behind Vaiont Dam in the Italian Alps north of Venice. A wave formed above the lake, ran rapidly in both directions, overtopped the dam, and killed 2,600 people located in several villages downstream (McCully, 2001).

Water and Development

Today, the world population is extracting 3,800 cubic kilometres (3,800 gigalitres) of fresh water every year from lakes, rivers and aquifers (World Commission on Dams, 2000). This accounts for over half the water available in rivers, and is six times the volume extracted 100 years ago, growing twice as fast as the population (UNDP, 2000). With world population set to increase another 50% over the next 50 years, bringing with it increased economic activity and wealth, we can expect the volume of extracted fresh water to increase much more. This means that more stress will be on hydrological resources and more people marginalised inside what UNDP calls "our fraying web of life".

Despite the large annual withdrawal of fresh water, nearly a quarter of the world population uses less than 50 litres per person per day, approximately the minimum amount needed to prevent infection. UNDP (2000) notes that irrigation uses 70% of water withdrawn from freshwater systems for human use. Today, 17% of agroecosystems depend on irrigation, with the irrigated area up by 72% from 1966 to 1996. Competition with other kinds of water use, especially for drinking water and industrial use, will be most intense in developing countries with fast growing populations and industries. Many of these countries are in Asia. Within Asia, several countries are already classified as water-stressed, withdrawing over 25% of annual water resources; water-stressed regions are also expanding rapidly within China and India. China, India, Pakistan and the USA account for > 50% of the world's total irrigated area. It is obvious that both agricultural water use and hydrological water stress will continue to grow within Asia, and we can expect that China and India will continue to build large dams to capture and manipulate water.

Dams and Politics

With 45,000 large dams already built, India and China continue to be the main players as they have been for decades. China reports that it is currently building 280 large dams, and India is estimated to be building somewhere between 695 and 960 (World Commission on Dams, 2000). Over the last 10 years, the most vigorous anti-dam protests have been directed at the Narmada river dams in India and the Three Gorges Dam in China. Both schemes continue to be built despite the massive negative publicity about their social and environmental impacts and considerable doubt about their economic utility (Morse and Berger, 1992; Pearce, 1992; Fearnside, 1994; Jackson and Sleigh, 2000, 2001; McCully, 2001). Over the last 20 years, the 'people affected by dams' (Declaration of Curitiba, 1997) and various environmental groups have joined together to fight many large dams. This battle is best described in McCully's comprehensive account. The World Bank withdrew from or avoided involvement in several major projects in the 1990s, including the Sardar Sarovar Dam in India and the Three Gorges Dam in China. The dam industry and governments feared the World Bank was withdrawing from large dams as a major development tool and this fear helped to bring the conflicting groups together for intensive dialogue and a search for evidence bearing on the debate.

In 1997, the World Conservation Union and the World Bank co-convened a productive meeting of industry and environmentalists in Switzerland (Dorcey *et al.*, 1997; Goodland, 1997) and this led on to an independent two-year World Commission on Dams that reported back in 2000. The report produced was excellent and constituted the greatest single advance of our knowledge base of the effects and performance of large dams, but it was not well accepted by the most active dam-building governments and the World Bank was accordingly cautious as well. The report confirmed that large dams vary widely in their benefits, and they usually have substantial cost overruns and construction delays, often failing to meet economic targets, especially in relation to irrigation. They also have more negative than positive environmental impacts, and have systematically failed to mitigate the many serious and inequitable adverse social effects. To help move dialogue on, the United Nations Environment Programme is convening a series of inclusive 'Dams and Development Forums', seeking consensus about instituting the 'rights, risks and negotiated outcomes' approach advocated by the Commission. This approach recognises that reconciling competing needs and entitlements is the single most important factor in understanding dam-related conflicts. There is a fundamental need to recognise rights and assess risks (especially rights at risk), and negotiate outcomes openly rather than impose decisions on legitimate stakeholders. Unfortunately, health effects did not feature prominently in the Commission's report but WHO did make a useful submission advocating Health Impact Assessment integrated into the design and construction of all large dams (World Health Organization, 1999).

Getting a Voice for the Health Sector

In the past, most large dams had no health appraisal in the design stage unless a well known risk was apparent. Thus, if schistosomiasis or malaria were present in the area, the dam builders were cautious, aware that these two diseases could severely embarrass them if they ignored the risk and epidemic infection broke out after the dam was built. For the Three Gorges Dam, the risks were assessed in a general sense by using a team of medical geographers who mapped rainfall and temperature, collected scanty information on infection in the reservoir area and made a crude evaluation of potential risks (Chen *et al.*, 1990). There was no direct study of the various affected populations and no involvement of the broader health sector already serving those populations. Central government and provincial health inputs were restricted to doing snail surveys in the area of the future reservoir to establish that the snail host was not present (Sleigh and Jackson, 1998). Thus, the 'health opportunity' approach advocated by Jobin (1999) and many others was missed, as usual. The same happened for Ertan Dam, upstream of Three Gorges, which was built near to an area previously endemic for schistosomiasis. Health assessment was restricted to managing the schistosomiasis risk (Gu *et al.*, 2001). The other health risks, including those arising from poverty induced or worsened by the planning blight, were not addressed. For both of these large dams, a narrow curative health service was developed during the construction phase, focused on incoming workers, not integrated with local health services, and not oriented to prevention or surveillance. Such health services are typical of those provided when building large dams.

Jobin points out that knowledge about dams and disease is fragmentary and often not available to the dam builders inside their organisation. Even outside the organisation, the (few) available experts often have a rather narrow field of view. Thus, entomologists will be aware of the infections related to their discipline (such as malaria) and malacologists will have a 'snail-view' of schistosomiasis or related parasites. Neither would know much about other infections such as diarrhoea, tuberculosis, syphilis and HIV, or other health problems unrelated to infection such as depression, suicide, violence, stress and injury.

As with the recommendations emerging from the World Commission on Dams (2000) on mitigating social impacts, integrated attention to health impacts will certainly require additional investment and make dams more expensive to design and construct. At present, it is not happening due to the unwillingness to invest such funds in advance as well as the lack of familiarity of dam managers, engineers and economists with the breadth of the health risks. Narrow single discipline (i.e. one expert) assessments will rarely be sufficient. Multidisciplinary health teams conducting comprehensive dam health impact and opportunity assessments are needed. In the near future, the emerging health impact assessment skill being developed by many national health departments may help create both the capacity and the will to make integrated assessments of health risks of large dams. It is sorely needed in Asia, especially given the population and hydrological dynamics and the certainty of many more large dams affecting millions of people.

References

Alvares C, Billorey R. (1988) *Damming the Narmada*. Third World Network/Appen, Penang, Malaysia.

Barber M, Ryder G (eds.). (1993) *Damming the Three Gorges. What Dam Builders Don't Want You to Know*. Earthscan, London.

Brody H. (2000) *Social Impacts of Large Dams Equity and Distributional Issues*. (Thematic Review, World Commission on Dams). Available at http://www.dams.org/docs/kbase/contrib/soc192.pdf, Accessed 24 September 2003.

Cernea MM. (1988) *Involuntary Resettlement in Development Projects: Policy Guidelines in World Bank-financed Projects. World Bank Technical Paper*: 80. World Bank, Washington, DC.

Cernea MM. (1999) *The Economics of Involuntary Resettlement: Questions and Challenges*. World Bank, Washington, DC.

Cernea MM, McDowell C (eds.). (2000) *Risks and Reconstruction: Experiences of Resettlers and Refugees*. World Bank, Washington, DC.

Chen Y, Shi M, Zhao M, Chen M, Huang X, Luo X, Lie B, Wu Y, Yang L, Yan J, Wang J, Zhong D, Yao S, Fan F, Wang D, Han A (eds.). (1990) *Atlas of the Ecology and Environment in the Three Gorges Area of the Changjiang River*. Science Press, Beijing.

Declaration of Curitiba. (1997) *Affirming the Right to Life and Livelihood of People Affected by Dams*. Approved at the First International Meeting of People Affected by Dams. Curitiba, Brazil, 14 March 1997. Available at http://www.irn.org/programs/curitiba.html, Accessed 24 September 2003.

Dorcey T, Steiner A, Acreman M, Orlando B (eds.). (1997) *Large Dams. Learning from the Past, Looking at the Future*. World Conservation Union (IUCN) and World Bank Workshop Proceedings, April 11,12, Gland, Switzerland.

Fearnside PM. (1994) The Canadian feasibility study of the three Gorges Dam proposed for China's Yangtze river: A grave embarrassment to the impact assessment profession. *Impact Assessment* 12: 21–53.

Goodland R. (1997) Environmental sustainability in the hydro industry, in T Dorcey, A Steiner, M Acreman & B Orlando (eds.), *Large Dams. Learning from the Past, Looking at the Future*, pp. 69–102, World Conservation Union (IUCN) and World Bank Workshop Proceedings, April 11, 12, Gland, Switzerland.

Gu YG, Xia LF, Li ZW, Zhao MF, Yang HY, Luo QY, Xia WH, Feng QY. (2001) Study on schistosomiasis control strategy in Ertan reservoir. *Chinese Journal of Parasitology and Parasitic Diseases. [Zhongguo Ji Sheng Chong Xue Yu Ji Sheng Chong Bing Za Zhi].(In Chinese, English Abstract)* **19**: 225–228. (In Chinese, English Abstract).

Hunter JM, Rey L, Chu KY, Adekolu-John EO, Mott KE. (1993) *Parasitic Diseases and Water Resource Development.* WHO: Geneva.

Jackson S, Sleigh A. (2000) Resettlement for China's three Gorges Dam: Socio-economic impact and institutional tensions. *Commun Post-Commun Studies* **33**: 223–241.

Jackson S, Sleigh AC. (2001) Political economy and socio-economic impact of China's three Gorges Dam. *Asian Studies Rev* **25**: 57–72.

Jobin W. (1999) Dams and disease. *Ecological Design and Health Impacts of Large Dams, Canals and Irrigation Systems.* E & FN Spoon, New York.

Landes D. (1998) *The Wealth and Poverty of Nations.* Little, Brown and Company, London.

Morse B, Berger T. (1992) *Sardar Sarovar. Report of the Independent Review.* Resource Futures International, Ottawa.

McCully P. (2001) *Silenced Rivers. The Ecology and Politics of Large Dams.* Zed Books, London (enlarged and updated edition).

Pearce F. (1992) *The Dammed. Rivers, Dams and the Coming World Water Crisis.* The Bodley Head, London.

Scudder T. (1997) Social impacts of large Dam projects, in T Dorcey, A Steiner, M Acreman & B Orlando (eds.), *Large Dams. Learning from the Past, Looking at the Future*, pp. 41–68, World Conservation Union (IUCN) and World Bank Workshop Proceedings, April 11, 12, Gland, Switzerland.

Sleigh AC, Jackson S. (2001) Dams, development and health: A missed opportunity. *Lancet* **357**: 570–571.

Sleigh A, Jackson S. (1998) Public health and public choice: Dammed off at China's three gorges? *The Lancet* **351**: 1449–1450.

Smith NAF. (1971) *A History of Dams.* Peter Davis, London.

UNDP. (2000) A Guide to World Resources 2000-2001. United Nations Development Program, World Bank, World Resources Institute, Washington, DC. Available at http://www.undp.org/dpa/publications/ExecSumWeb.pdf, Accessed 20 October 2004.

Wittfogel KA. (1957) *Oriental Despotism: A Comparative Study of Total Power.* Yale University Press, New Haven.

World Commission on Dams. (2000) *Dams and Development. A New Framework for Decision Making.* Earthscan Publication, London. Available at http://www.dams.org/, Accessed 3 May 2005.

World Health Organization. (1999) *Human Health and Dams.* WHO: Geneva (submission to the World Commission on Dams). Available at http://www.dams.org/docs/kbase/working/health.pdf, Accessed 3 May 2005.

5

The Impact of Imported Infection

Niels G Becker and Kathryn Glass

Introduction

There are two settings in which the importation of an infection is a major public health concern. The first arises when an infectious disease is managed by a routine vaccination schedule, and there is a constant threat of importation from neighbouring countries. For example, measles has been endemic in most nations and is currently managed by national immunisation schedules, with some nations achieving elimination and many others working towards it. In this setting, which we describe as *importation of a vaccine-preventable* disease, local success achieved by immunisation may be undermined by imported infection.

The second setting arises when a new infection emerges in one country and neighbouring countries want to prevent a local outbreak of the infection. The disruptions associated with the 2003 outbreaks of SARS illustrate the concerns from such an infection. In this setting, which we describe as *importation of an emerged infection,* an entirely susceptible population is placed at risk by imported infection.

Although the routes of importation of infection are the same, the control measures that may be applied to reduce the risks associated with importation vary considerably between the two settings. Vaccination coverage is a key factor in reducing risks from the importation of vaccine-preventable diseases. In the case of an emerged infection, there is no vaccine available and transmission must be reduced by traditional methods that aim to minimise infectious contacts. Due to the differences in control response, we consider the two settings separately. To keep the discussion specific, we will use measles as an illustrative example of a vaccine-preventable disease, and SARS as an example of an emerged infection. However, the discussion is relevant to all infectious diseases, for which person-to-person contact is the primary mode of transmission.

We use mathematical models to

(1) gain a better understanding of the factors, including control strategies, that affect the threat from imported infection and
(2) provide guidance on appropriate responses to these threats,

for both vaccine-preventable and emerged infections, and also to highlight the differences in the appropriate responses for these two settings.

Inportation of a Vaccine-Preventable Disease

Consider first the role of importation in the control of an endemic infection being controlled by mass vaccination. When elimination of a vaccine preventable disease has been achieved, or is close to being achieved by mass vaccination, there is concern that the importation of infection from neighbouring countries may lead to outbreaks of infection. We look at the relationship between vaccination coverage and the risks associated with the importation of infection, using measles as an example.

Regular importations of measles into a country, province or city are likely, while measles remains endemic in many parts of the world. The rates of importation into a location depend on the number and sources of its visitors. To see what a typical rate of importation of measles infection might be, we turn to countries or provinces where elimination has been achieved. We consider only outbreaks with at least two cases because importations that involve no secondary cases are likely to be underreported. In the United States, there were 41 such outbreaks in the period 1997–1999 (Gay *et al.*, 2004). Adjusting for the fact that we have excluded "outbreaks" without secondary infections, this corresponds to a rate of importation of ~27 per year, in a country with a population of 250 million. Victoria, a southern state of Australia, with a population of five million had 14 outbreaks with secondary transmission during 1998–2001, (Becker *et al.*, 2005a). Adjusting for exclusion of single-case "outbreaks", this estimates a rate of importation of 7 per year. On the basis of these observations, importation rates in the range of 0 to 10 per year seem most relevant for a population of one million, and importation rates greater than 100 per year seem irrelevant.

How much do these importations contribute to disease incidence? We look at this with the aid of appropriate mathematical transmission models when measles transmission is controlled by mass immunisation.

Transmission model

The transmission model is kept simple by including only those components that crucially affect the impact of importations. Briefly, as concerns measles, the model assumes that individuals fall into one of the following states:

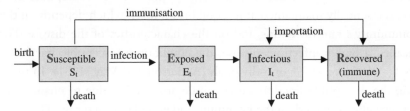

This is known as an SEIR model. We allow an element of chance in all possible transitions, because the chance component cannot be ignored when control is adequate to make the measles incidence small. Individuals are born susceptible, exposed individuals are infected but not yet infectious and individuals recovered from infection have life-long immunity. Current cases are taken to be those in the exposed and infectious stages, i.e. $E_t + I_t$.

Realisations of the stochastic model depend on the size of the community. The specific realisations depicted here are for a population, perhaps a city, of one million, unless otherwise indicated. The birth rate and death rate are equal and chosen to give a life expectancy of 60 years. We are guided by the Communicable Diseases Manual (Chin, 2000) in our choice of transmission parameter values. Specifically, the mean latent period is 10 days and the mean infectious period is 5 days, which are also used by Keeling and Grenfell (1997). The transmission rate is determined by setting the basic reproduction number R_0 to be 15, a value thought to be appropriate for measles (Anderson and May, 1991). Formulas for doing this are given by Hethcote (2000). Further details about the model are given in the Appendix.

A computer is used to simulate realisations of the model. Simulated realisations vary due to chance. Here, we summarise conclusions reached after many runs and present a few illustrative examples. In particular, probabilities and means for the stochastic transmission model are estimated from 5,000 realisations, i.e., from 5,000 chains of transmission generated by the chance mechanism of the model. A range of plausible parameter values is investigated to ensure that the conclusions are robust.

Sustained endemic transmission

A central quantity when considering the control of an infectious disease is the proportion of individuals circulating in the population who are susceptible (Anderson and May, 1991). We call this the *susceptible fraction*. Under sustained endemic transmission, in a large population, the susceptible fraction is essentially maintained at its equilibrium level, which depends on the community's rate of mixing and on the characteristics of the disease. For measles, a highly infectious disease, the equilibrium susceptible fraction is small, $\sim 100/R_0 = 7\%$ of individuals (Anderson and May, 1991). In practice, the susceptible fraction varies a little around 7%, due to chance and seasonal effects, including the beginning and end of school terms. The same susceptible fraction applies irrespective of the coverage achieved in regular immunisation, as long as the immunity coverage is below 93%. With an immunity coverage maintained above 93%, measles is eliminated and the susceptible fraction is one − (immunity coverage). Immune individuals are comprised of those who acquired their immunity from vaccination and those who acquired it by exposure to measles infection possibly before elimination was achieved.

Effect of importation while there is sustained endemic transmission

Our interest lies in the extent to which the number of individuals infected annually is affected by the rate of measles importation. This depends on the

Table 1. Annual number of measles cases as a function of percentage successfully immunised by routine immunisation and the rate of importation of measles infection (endemic transmission in a population of 1 million).

		Rate of measles importation (number per year)				
		0	10	20	50	100
	0%	15,576	15,587	15,597	15,630	15,684
	50%	7,232	7,243	7,255	7,290	7,347
Immunity coverage	80%	2,225	2,240	2,255	2,300	2,373
	90%	556	585	613	689	796
	93%	56	265	274	617	933
	96%	0	90	168	365	645

proportion of infants successfully immunised by the routine immunisation schedule. In Table 1, the annual number of measles cases as predicted by the model is given under the assumption that endemic transmission is in equilibrium. Results corresponding to 10 importations per year are thought to be the most relevant. It is seen that the effect of importation is minimal, while there is substantial endemic transmission in the population. In that situation, importation raises the annual number of cases by slightly more than the number of importations. Importation has a larger effect when the regular immunisation schedule is able to achieve a coverage near the critical immunity coverage. The annual incidences in Table 1 depend on population size, but they are stable when viewed as the number of cases per one million population, assuming the overall population size is ~1 million or more.

The explanation for the minimal effect lies in the central property of endemic transmission, namely that at endemic transmission, the susceptible fraction is essentially kept at a level such that infected individuals just replace themselves by each infecting, on average, one of the susceptible individuals. If an infected individual joins the current circulating infected individuals, it simply means that on average, they each infect *almost* one individual to keep the susceptible fraction at ~7%.

Interrupted transmission

Importations of measles infection are of greater concern when endemic transmission has been interrupted, because of the fear that endemic transmission may be re-established. We investigate whether this concern is warranted. Following interrupted transmission, the impact of an imported infection depends crucially on how many susceptible individuals are circulating at the time of the importation. This in turn depends on three factors:

(1) the number of susceptible individuals circulating when transmission is interrupted,
(2) the rate of replenishment of susceptible individuals, by un-immunised infants and immigration, and
(3) how long after interrupted transmission the importation occurs.

It is therefore necessary to look at the way interruption was achieved.

Achieving interrupted transmission

As mentioned, *sustained* interrupted transmission for a disease as infectious as measles requires the susceptible fraction to be maintained continuously below the small equilibrium value of ~7%. On the other hand, temporary interruption of transmission can be achieved more easily, by a sudden enhancement in immunisation. We briefly illustrate that

(1) any sudden enhancement in immunisation that takes the susceptible fraction temporarily below 7% stands a good chance of interrupting transmission, and
(2) when interruption occurs, the susceptible fraction is almost certainly below the equilibrium value of 7%.

The susceptible fraction is reduced rapidly by either (i) implementing a pulse immunisation campaign, or (ii) introducing an additional opportunity of immunisation to a routine schedule, or (iii) having a major measles epidemic.

Suppose that measles transmission is at endemic equilibrium and a pulse campaign of immunisation, implemented over a short time period, is able to immunise 30% of the susceptible individuals, i.e., the susceptible fraction of the population is reduced from 7% to 5%. This reduction in the susceptible fraction, which is modest in terms of what one hopes to achieve with a pulse campaign, has a very good chance of interrupting transmission. Without any routine immunisation of infants in place, the probability that this campaign interrupts transmission is ~0.8. When a program of immunisation is in place for infants, the probability is even greater because the rate of replenishment of susceptible individuals is then lower. Note that the probability depends on the population size.

Although enhanced immunisation by way of adding a routine dose to an existing immunisation schedule reduces the susceptible fraction more slowly than a pulse campaign, it can still interrupt measles transmission. For example, suppose that there has been no immunisation and a single dose of immunisation is introduced which renders 75% of the infants immune. This will tend to reduce the number of infectives and the probability that this number becomes zero before the susceptible fraction returns to 7% is ~0.7. Again, this probability depends on the population size.

An epidemic of measles, whatever the reason for its occurrence, can also lead to an interruption of transmission. This is because at the end of the epidemic, the susceptible fraction will be below its equilibrium value and the number of cases will be low. At this time, chance fluctuations can lead to interrupted transmission.

Whatever the reason for interrupted transmission, when it occurs it is almost certain that the susceptible fraction is below the equilibrium value, of about 7%.

Importation while the susceptible fraction is below its equilibrium value

It is helpful to discuss the typical effect of an importation with respect to a specific scenario.

Suppose that transmission has been interrupted and that the susceptible fraction is below the equilibrium level of 7%. The parameter values for birth rate, death rate, mean duration of latent period, mean duration of infectious period and population size are as specified above. Choose the time at which transmission is interrupted as time origin ($t = 0$). The number of cases when transmission is interrupted is zero. That is, $E_0 + I_0 = 0$. The remaining parameters are chosen as follows:

The susceptible fraction when transmission is interrupted

$$= 80\% \text{ of the equilibrium susceptible fraction}$$
$$= 0.8/15,$$

(which corresponds to 53,333 susceptible individuals in a population of 1 million)

Rate of measles importation = 10 per year;

Percentage of infants successfully immunised in a routine schedule = 50%.

Figure 1(a) shows two realisations of the probability model. In Realisation 2, transmission is interrupted after the first epidemic, whereas in Realisation 1, it is not. However, there is a second epidemic in both realisations. In Realisation 2, this occurred because of measles importation after

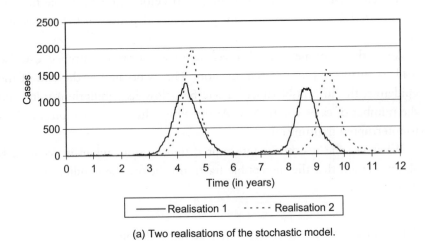

(a) Two realisations of the stochastic model.

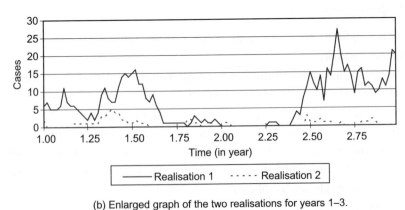

(b) Enlarged graph of the two realisations for years 1–3.

Fig. 1. Illustration of the typical transmission dynamics following interruption of transmission, in the presence of measles importation. (Cases = those currently in the Exposed or Infectious stages.)

the susceptible fraction returned to the equilibrium value. Figure 1(b) shows the graphs for the number of cases in the same two realisations from the end of year one to the end of year three, on a scale that makes it easier to see the minor outbreaks arising from importations of measles during the earlier period.

The following features of the realisation of cases shown in Fig. 1 are noteworthy, and will be elaborated upon in the following subsections.

(1) There is an initial period during which there are relatively few cases.
(2) After some time an epidemic breaks out.
(3) During the course of the first epidemic, the number of cases rises above the equilibrium number of cases.
(4) After the first epidemic, measles incidence returns to a low level. In one of the realisations shown in Fig. 1, transmission was interrupted at this point. This happens with a probability of 0.36 for the chosen parameter values.
(5) A second epidemic, somewhat smaller, then occurs.
(6) Over time, these epidemic waves dampen out, tending towards the equilibrium endemic transmission level (although in practice, periodic factors such as school terms may leave a seasonal component).

We now elaborate on these features under separate headings.

Effect of measles importation while the susceptible fraction is below its equilibrium value

The realisations in Fig. 1(a) illustrate that relatively few cases occur during periods when the susceptible fraction is below 7%. These cases stem from importations and subsequent secondary cases. Few secondary transmissions occur because on average, each infected individual replaces himself or herself, by less than one person as long as the susceptible fraction is below its equilibrium value.

The main message is that imported measles has a minor impact during periods when the susceptible fraction is below 7%. Let us quantify this impact more precisely. Suppose that the susceptible fraction is $100c\%$ of the equilibrium susceptible fraction, where c is less than 1. For example, $c = 0.5$ when the susceptible fraction in the population is 3.5%. It can be shown analytically that the mean size of an outbreak started by a single

Table 2. Mean outbreak size from a single importation and the 95% upper probability bound for outbreak size when the susceptible fraction is as shown.

Fraction susceptible in the population (%)	1.67	3.33	4.67	5.33	6.00	6.33	6.60
Susceptible fraction (as percentage of the equilibrium susceptible fraction), $100c$	25	50	70	80	90	95	99
Mean size of outbreak, $1/(1-c)$	1.3	2	3.3	5	10	20	100
k such that Prob(outbreak size $\leq k$) = 0.95	3	6	13	20	39	62	107

importation is approximately $1/(1-c)$. The mean outbreak size (including the imported case) is calculated from this formula for some values of c in Table 2. Table 2 also shows k, the smallest value such that we can be 95% sure that the outbreak size will be k, or less.

The model indicates a small outbreak size is assured if we can get the susceptible fraction below 5% (70% of the equilibrium susceptible fraction). These results on outbreak size apply to all large populations.

The delay until the first epidemic after interrupted transmission

The main part of the delay until substantial transmission is resumed in the community is due to the time needed to replenish the susceptible fraction up to 7% of the population. This time depends on two quantities, namely how far the susceptible fraction is below 7% when transmission is interrupted and the rate at which infants are successfully immunised by routine immunisation. This relationship is displayed in Table 3.

If the fraction of infants successfully immunised exceeds 93% indefinitely, then the susceptible fraction will never reach 7% and the pattern of the minor outbreaks arising from imported cases continues indefinitely, i.e. sustained measles elimination is then achieved. In the event that the susceptible fraction does reach 7%, it takes additional time for transmission to

Table 3. Time (in years) until the susceptible fraction returns to the equilibrium value of 7% as a function of the fraction of infants successfully immunised and the susceptible fraction when transmission is first interrupted.

Infants successfully immunised	Susceptible fraction when transmission is interrupted (as percentage of the equilibrium value)			
	80%	60%	40%	20%
0%	0.85	1.7	2.5	3.3
50%	1.8	3.6	5.3	7.0
80%	5.8	11.1	15.9	>20
85%	9.3	16.9	>20	>20

gather some momentum. The additional time can be 1 to 2 years, depending on chance and the coverage achieved by routine immunisation.

The first and later epidemics after interrupted transmission

When the immunisation schedule is not adequate to keep the susceptible fraction below its equilibrium level, there will inevitably be an epidemic some time after interrupted transmission is achieved.

Why does this epidemic occur?

The epidemic occurs because at the time when the susceptible fraction returns to its equilibrium value of 7%, the number of infectious individuals is too small to keep the susceptible fraction at that value. As a result, the susceptible fraction grows larger than the equilibrium value, allowing transmission to gather momentum. At the time when the number of cases reaches the equilibrium level corresponding to the immunisation schedule in place, the susceptible fraction is still above its equilibrium value. As a result, the number infected becomes even larger. The growth in transmission stops only when depletion in those susceptible takes the susceptible fraction back down to the equilibrium level. Then the number of cases starts to decline because they are less than replacing themselves.

Note that a single importation into a measles-free community at a time when the susceptible fraction is above the equilibrium value of 7% does not guarantee an epidemic. An importation in this situation tends to produce one of two possible outcomes. Either transmission fades out rapidly (we refer to this as a 'minor outbreak') or transmission gathers momentum and leads to a major epidemic. Outbreaks of intermediate size are very rare. Figure 2 shows the graph of the probability of an epidemic as a function of the susceptible fraction at the time of a single importation. The probability that an importation of measles into a large community results in a minor outbreak is approximately $1 -$ Prob(epidemic). The size of the first epidemic varies, with those slow to gather momentum tending to be of a larger size because the susceptible fraction has then grown larger. Figure 3 shows the mean size of the first epidemic as a function of the susceptible fraction at the time of importation. The epidemic is seen to affect a large fraction of the individuals susceptible at the time. While such an epidemic is not desirable, it should be noted that measles transmission before and after the epidemic is well below what is expected when transmission settles to its equilibrium endemic level. On balance, averaging transmission over the epidemic and non-epidemic period, one has the same number of measles cases per unit time as would result with transmission at equilibrium endemic level.

In Realisation 2 of Fig. 1, transmission was interrupted following the first epidemic. This tends to happen particularly when this epidemic is larger than average. The probability that transmission is interrupted immediately after

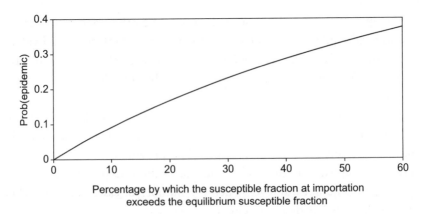

Fig. 2. Probability of an epidemic as a function of the percentage by which the susceptible fraction exceeds the equilibrium value of 7% at the time of an importation.

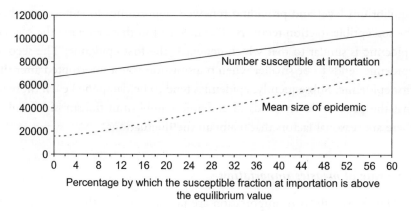

Fig. 3. Mean size of the first epidemic as a function of the percentage by which the susceptible fraction exceeds the equilibrium value of 7% at the time of importation.

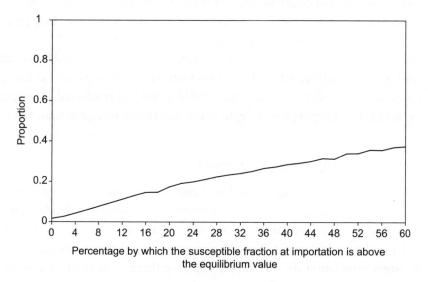

Fig. 4. Proportion of first epidemics immediately followed by interrupted transmission, as a function of the susceptible fraction at the time of an importation.

the first epidemic is shown in Fig. 4 as a function of the susceptible fraction at time $t = 0$, when transmission is first interrupted. Approximately, one in five of such epidemics are followed by interrupted transmission.

The second epidemic occurs because during the first epidemic, the susceptible fraction becomes low, driving the number of cases below the equilibrium level and providing renewed opportunity for infection when the susceptible fraction recovers. The mechanism that generates the second epidemic is similar to that which generates the first epidemic. The second epidemic tends to be smaller when transmission is not interrupted after the first epidemic. Subsequently, epidemics tend to be dampened even more so that the process slowly tends to endemic equilibrium transmission, unless there are seasonal factors that maintain the fluctuations.

Low rate of measles importation

The above effects of importation are not sensitive to the rate of importation in the range of plausible rates, estimated to be ∼ 5–15 per year with present global levels of control. As global control of measles improves, the rate of importation could drop to rather low levels. This creates the possibility that transmission is interrupted and no importation occurs for a long time. If immunisation levels are neglected over this time, there could be a very substantial growth in the susceptible fraction and then an importation could lead to a very substantial epidemic in which transmission gathers so much momentum that virtually every susceptible individual is infected. This can be avoided by keeping the susceptible fraction below its equilibrium value.

Comments on the simplifying asumptions

While some specific means and probabilities presented here might differ when there is spatial heterogeneity or heterogeneity among individuals, the impact of measles importation remains basically the same, as we now discuss.

Consider first the effect of population size. Most of the results carry over to larger population sizes by simply applying them to population proportions, rather than to population counts. For example, if measles is imported when the susceptible fraction is above its equilibrium value, then neither the probability that there will be an epidemic nor the proportion of cases in such an epidemic depends on the population size. One value that does depend on population size is the probability that transmission is interrupted by a pulse campaign of immunisation.

It is known that measles transmission is age-specific, so it is desirable to allow for different types of individual consisting of different age groups.

The epidemic threshold result still applies when there is plausible hetero-geneity among individuals. In other words, an importation of measles will result in a minor outbreak when the susceptible fraction is below its equi-librium value, although the different types of individual might contribute different numbers to the susceptible pool. The central conclusions reached from the above results continue to apply. The main effect of age-specific heterogeneity lies in the effectiveness of age-specific immunisation strate-gies. However, it is possible to construct a setting with an extreme form of heterogeneity where the results break down.

Spatial heterogeneity needs to be taken into account when the above results are applied to a large country. The best we can do to deal with spatial heterogeneity is to consider the country in terms of smaller population units such as cities or provinces, and to apply the above results separately to each of these. An important observation made by looking at a country in this manner is that a city, or province, with a routine immunisation schedule that succeeds in keeping the susceptible fraction below its equilibrium level enjoys all the benefits of measles elimination, irrespective of how well the rest of the country is managing its immunisation schedule. The main difference between two cities that have achieved measles elimination, where one is surrounded by cities and provinces with low measles incidence and the other has high incidence in its surrounding area, lies in the rate of measles importations. As we have seen, the effect of importation is not substantial when the susceptible fraction is maintained below the equilibrium value.

Importation of an Emerged Infection

We now turn to questions concerned with the effect of importation of a newly emerged infection. During an outbreak of such an infectious disease, there is considerable effort made to prevent the disease spreading to unin-fected regions. As vaccines are generally not available for such diseases, the control response in infected areas is directed towards reducing transmission by minimising contacts with infectious individuals by a number of means that include identification and isolation of new cases as quickly as possible. The SARS outbreak prompted such control measures to be implemented in infected countries and also prompted preparedness measures and border controls to be implemented in uninfected countries. We look at the effect of these responses in reducing the likelihood and size of an epidemic of a newly emerged infection, using SARS in Singapore as an example.

In Singapore, control measures rapidly reduced the time from onset of symptoms to the isolation of SARS cases from nine days in the last week of February 2003, to under two days at the end of April (Tan, 2003). During this period, six SARS cases arrived in Singapore, but only the first of these caused extensive secondary transmission (Wilder-Smith *et al.*, 2004). We use a mathematical transmission model to quantify the extent to which improvements in control measures can reduce the likelihood of secondary transmission of a newly emerged infection.

Transmission model

The transmission model is essentially equivalent to that of vaccine-preventable diseases, but we replace the "Recovered" class with a "Removed" class, which incorporates both recovered individuals and individuals who are removed from circulation by isolation.

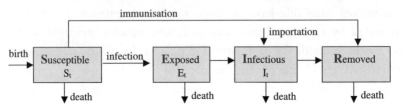

In the case of endemic infections, vaccination is used to reduce disease spread by ensuring that there are few individuals in the Susceptible class. When vaccination is not available, transmission is reduced, instead, by minimising exposure to infectious individuals, which includes making individuals pass from the Infectious to the Removed class as quickly as possible.

We again adopt a stochastic model of disease transmission that takes into account the effect of chance when the number of infected individuals is small. Results presented here will be broadly similar for any relatively large community (e.g. 50,000 or more individuals) because all realisations assume that control measures are successful in interrupting transmission, so that the vast majority of the population remains susceptible throughout the outbreak. For the same reason, births and deaths play very little role in the transmission dynamics, provided that the death rate of infectious individuals who have not yet been isolated does not greatly exceed that of the general population.

We assume a latent period for SARS of 6 days (Donnelly *et al.*, 2003). It is important to get an estimate of the basic reproduction number for SARS, which is the reproduction number in the early stages of an outbreak, before extensive control measures have been implemented. Using data for Singapore, the basic reproduction number has been estimated to be three (Lipsitch *et al.*, 2003). In this early stage of the outbreak, cases in Singapore were isolated about 9 days after onset (Tan, 2003), and we assume that nine days is the effective infectious period of the disease before control. The transmission rate is then calculated using these two estimates. As before, realisations of the model are simulated on a computer, and we present both example realisations and average statistics from many realisations of the model.

Probability of secondary transmission

As with importation of an endemic infection, not all arriving infected individuals will lead to secondary transmission. The probability of secondary transmission depends on the level of control in the region, and specifically on the time from onset of infection until isolation of a case. Figure 5 shows the probability that a single infected individual arriving in an uninfected region at the start of their infectious period will infect one other individual, and also the probability that there will be at least 10 local cases resulting from the single arrival, as a function of the time from onset to the isolation of cases in the arrival region. These results are based on 10,000 simulated realisations of the stochastic model for each value of the time from onset to isolation.

We see from the figure that even when individuals are isolated nine days after onset of symptoms, there is still a 25% chance that there will be no secondary case, although if there is a secondary case, there is a high probability that there will be at least 10 local cases. When control measures are stricter, the probability of a secondary case drops, and the probability of at least ten cases drops even further. If individuals can be isolated within ~ two days after the onset of symptoms, there is a high chance that there will not be many local cases, as is seen from the lower graph in Fig. 5.

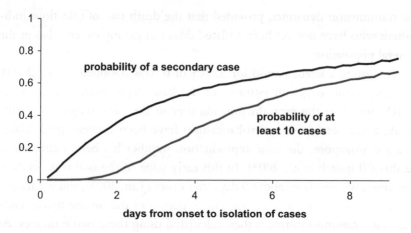

Fig. 5. Probability that a single infected individual arriving at the start of their infectious period will lead to secondary cases.

Epidemic size

We have seen that when a newly emerged infection is imported into a new region, the probability that local transmission will occur depends on the level of control in the region. The number of local cases will also depend on the level of control. If insufficient control measures are in place and they are not tightened on the discovery of cases, a large proportion of the population will be infected, and the outbreak will only cease when the numbers of susceptibles are sufficiently low. In the case of SARS, control measures in all affected regions became more effective over the course of the epidemic, and this enabled the disease to be controlled.

Importations into Singapore

Data from Singapore on the mean time from onset of symptoms until the isolation of cases show that control measures became increasingly effective over the period from the 25th of February until the 28th of April (Tan, 2003). We fit an exponential trend to these data [see Fig. 7(a)], and use it in our model to allow the effectiveness of control measures to improve over time. Infected individuals are assumed to incubate the disease for a period of 6 days, and then become infectious. Infectious individuals circulate in the community for a number of days determined by the Singapore data, and are then isolated. We assume that individuals do not infect anyone after being isolated. Using this model, we investigate the effect of the date of arrival of an infected individual on the likelihood of them infecting local cases, and on the size of the epidemic that they generate. As shown in Fig. 5, regardless of the date of arrival of the infected case, there is some chance that there will be no further transmission. In Fig. 6, we reproduce this graph as a function of the time of arrival of the initial infected individual.

In addition to knowing the probability that there will be at least one local case, we are interested in the mean epidemic size when this occurs. As there is a chance component in the model, the progression of the epidemic will be different every time we run the model, even when the date of arrival of the first infected case remains the same. Figures 7(b)–(d) gives examples of such epidemic outbreaks when the infected individual arrives on the 25th of February, the 4th of March, and the 11th of March. As we have seen from Fig. 6, both the probability of a secondary case, and the probability of at least 10 cases does not drop very much over this period; however, the example outbreaks involve markedly fewer cases as time progresses.

In order to look at the effect of increased control on the mean epidemic size, we generate 5000 realisations of the model and look at those in which there is secondary transmission. Figure 8 shows the mean epidemic size assuming at least one secondary case and assuming at least 10 cases occur.

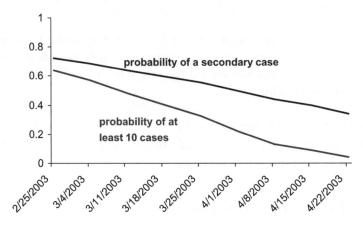

Fig. 6. Probability that a single infected individual arriving at the start of their infectious period on a given date will lead to secondary cases, or to at least 10 cases.

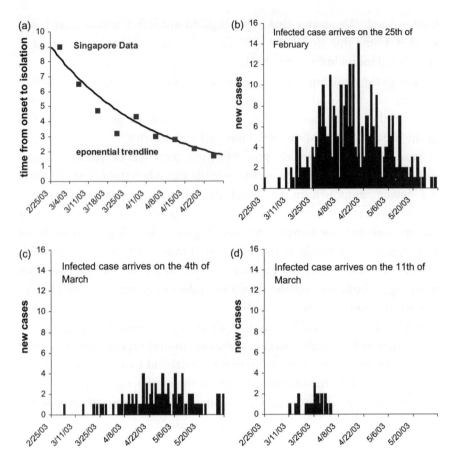

Fig. 7. The effect of control measures on the size of an epidemic: (a) shows data from Singapore on the time from onset to isolation of SARS patients; (b)–(d) gives illustrative realisations when an infected case arrived on the specified date and there was at least one secondary case.

We see that the mean size of the epidemic decreases very quickly over the first few weeks, so that by the middle of March, the mean size is ∼ one third that of the last week in February.

Effect of delays in control response

The response to SARS in Singapore was very prompt, so that the time from onset to isolation decreased rapidly. We investigate the effect of delays

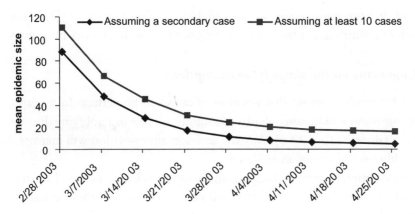

Fig. 8. Mean epidemic size resulting from one infected individual arriving into Singapore on the given date. The curves compare means for outbreaks in which there was at least one secondary case and outbreaks in which there were at least 10 local cases.

in the control response by assuming that the time from onset to isolation remained at nine days for one, two or three weeks before it declined as in Fig. 7(a). In other words, the introduction of effective intervention was delayed by one, two or three weeks. Figure 9 shows the mean epidemic size of outbreaks in which there is a secondary case and outbreaks in which there are at least 10 cases. For each additional week's delay in response, we

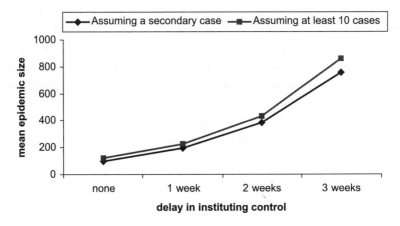

Fig. 9. Mean epidemic sizes assuming a delay before control was instituted.

find that the mean epidemic size doubles, so that a delay of three weeks before instituting control leads to ∼ eight times as many cases on average.

Comments on the simplifying asumptions

Our model assumes that isolation of cases can be perfect. In Singapore, transmission within hospitals played a significant role in amplifying the spread of the disease (Tan, 2003). Any transmission after isolation will increase the likelihood and size of an epidemic.

In addition to prompt diagnosis and isolation of cases, increased awareness of the disease in the community will play some part in reducing transmission of the infection. Individuals will take steps to avoid infection in the community by wearing masks, reducing the rate of making close contacts with individuals, reducing hand-to-mouth contacts and increase the washing of hands more regularly. Previous work has identified that these measures can interrupt transmission if the rate of making close contacts is reduced to between 40% and 50% of its natural value (Becker et al., 2005b).

Discussion

We have used mathematical transmission models to quantify the impact of imported infection in two settings: that of a vaccine-preventable disease such as measles, and that of a newly-emerged infection such as SARS. The results indicate that the most appropriate public health response to imported infection is quite different in these settings.

When controlling an infection by a routine vaccination schedule, there is generally no need for a response to an imported infection, if the immunity coverage achieved is below the threshold required for sustained elimination. The number of extra cases resulting from importation is generally so small that more cases are prevented by focusing effort on improving the immunity coverage. There is also no need to respond to imported infections when the immunity coverage achieved comfortably exceeds the threshold required for elimination, uniformly over the community. This is because outbreaks cannot gather momentum and are nearly always very small. However, there is a risk that a major epidemic will result from an imported infection in periods after achieving elimination, if the coverage achieved by the immunisation schedule is not adequate to maintain the susceptible fraction below the threshold. This risk requires careful management because temporary elimination can arise relatively easily and evidence that routine immunisation is adequate to maintain sustained elimination is often lacking. As a consequence, it is essential to monitor the susceptible fraction during periods of elimination. Some methods for doing this are discussed by Farrington *et al.* (2004) and Becker *et al.* (2005b).

In contrast, to prevent a major outbreak from an emerged infection, the public health response should focus primarily on preparedness. One should be ready to initiate traditional interventions such as early diagnosis, both promptly and effectively. The model results demonstrate that in the early days of an outbreak, while the number of cases is low, early isolation of these cases can avert an epidemic.

Acknowledgement

The study of the impact of measles importation was supported by the Western Pacific Region Office of WHO.

References

Anderson RM, May RM. (1991) *Infectious Diseases in Humans: Dynamics and Control.* Oxford University Press, Oxford.

Becker NG, Li Z, Hsu E, Andrews R, Lambert SB. (2005a) Monitoring measles elimination in Victoria. *ANZJ Public Health* **29**: 58–63.

Becker NG, Glass K, Li Z, Aldis GK. (2005b) Controlling emerging infectious diseases like SARS. *Math Biosci* **193**: 205–221.

Chin J (Editor). (2000) *Control of Communicable Diseases Manual.* 17th edition. APHA, New York.

Donnelly CA, Ghani AC, Leung GM, Hedley AJ, Fraser C, Riley S, Abu-Raddad LJ, Ho L-M, Thach T-Q, Chau P, Chan K-P, LamT-H, Tse LY, Tsang T, Liu S-H, Kong JHB, Lau EMC, Ferguson NM, Anderson RM. (2003) Epidemiological determinants of spread of causal agent of Severe Acute Respiratory Syndrome in Hong Kong. *Lancet* **361**: 1761–1766.

Gay NJ, De Serres G, Farrington CP, Redd SB, Papania MJ. (2004) Assessment of the status of measles elimination from reported outbreaks: United States, 1997-1999. *J Infec Dis* **189**: Suppl 1: S36–S42.

Hethcote H. (2000) The mathematics of infectious diseases. *SIAM Rev* **42**: 599–653.

Keeling M, Grenfell B. (1997) Disease extinction and community size: Modeling the persistence of measles. *Science* **275**: 65–67.

Lipsitch M, Cohen T, Cooper B, Robins JM, Ma S, James L, Gopalakrishna G, Chew SK, Tan CC, Samore MH, Fisman D, Murray M. (2003) Transmission dynamics and control of Severe Acute Respiratory Syndrome. *Science* **300**: 1966–1970.

Tan CC. *National Response to SARS: Singapore.* WHO Presentation, available at http://www.who.int/csr/sars/conference / june_2003/materials/presentations/en/sarssingapore170603.pdf.

Wilder-Smith A, Goh KT, Paton NI. (2004) Experience of Severe Acute Respiratory Syndrome in Singapore: Importation of cases, and defense strategies at the airport. *J Travel Med* **10**: 259–262.

Appendix (Transmission Model)

Let N_t denote the number of individuals in the community at time t. Consider an SEIR model (Hethcote, 2000) in which an individual passes from the susceptible state to the exposed state upon infection. After some time in the exposed state, the individual becomes infectious and subsequently recovers, having acquired permanent immunity.

The number of individuals who are susceptible, exposed and infectious at time t are S_t, E_t and I_t, respectively. At any time, there can be a birth, a death, an infection, a transition from exposed to infectious, a recovery or an importation of an infectious individual. A birth gives an increase in the number of susceptible individuals. The probability for each of these events in the time increment from time t to time $t + h$, is approximately as follows:

Event / Transition	Probability
Birth	$\lambda N_t h$
Infection	$\beta I_t (S_t/N_t) h$
Becoming infectious	$\sigma E_t h$
Recovery	$\gamma I_t h$
Importation of an infective	$\delta N_t h$
Death (susceptible)	$\lambda S_t h$
Death (exposed)	$\lambda E_t h$
Death (infective)	$\lambda I_t h$

Note that the birth rate is equal to the death rate, so that the mean growth of the population size is zero.

## 6

Demographic and Epidemiological Transitions in Asia: Comparative Health Policies for Emerging Infectious Diseases

Phua Kai Hong and Vernon JM Lee

Introduction

In the decades preceding the 1990s, the economies of East Asia underwent such dramatic growth and rapid development that the phenomenon was commonly termed "the East Asian Miracle." Particularly, Japan and the "Four Tigers", i.e. Hong Kong, the Republic of Korea, Singapore and Taiwan, formed the initial wave of countries to exhibit remarkably high and sustained GNP growth rates. Today, they enjoy standards of living comparable to those of industrialised, high-income nations. Other newly industrialising economies (NIEs), those of Malaysia, Thailand and Indonesia, have been quick to follow in their stead. In the past 30 years, per capita incomes in East Asia have nearly quadrupled, while absolute poverty has fallen by about two thirds (World Bank, 1993). However, despite areas of "miraculous" growth, Asia encompasses considerable economic diversity, including low-income developing economies and former socialist economies that recently opened up to market forces.

Significant demographic and epidemiological shifts have paralleled the economic transitions throughout Asia. Larger numbers of people continue to migrate from rural to urban areas and it is predicted that by 2020, 55%

of Asians will live in urban centers (Peabody *et al.*, 1999). Since 1960, life expectancy has increased and child mortality has fallen in all Asian countries. Nevertheless, population growth has already slowed due to declining fertility rates. These concurrent changes in mortality and especially fertility rates have the effect of population aging. By 2030, the proportion of Asia's population over 60 years old will have more than doubled since 1990, reaching 16% (Phillips, 2000). Furthermore, the demographic shift in age structure is accentuated in some NIEs, which face the prospect of even higher percentages of elderly. By 2030, Hong Kong's proportion of pensioners is expected to reach 34%, Singapore's 29%, and Taiwan's 26% (Phillips, 2000). As a whole, East Asia is the world's most rapidly ageing region.

Population aging is driving an epidemiological shift towards a disease burden dominated by chronic non-communicable diseases. However, in lower-income countries and rural areas, communicable diseases remain a prevalent threat, and some governments are saddled with the "double burden" of addressing these epidemics, even as non-communicable illnesses are on the rise. Similar to the concept of "dual economy" used to explain uneven economic development, for instance, between rural and urban areas, "epidemiological polarisation" has resulted within these countries because of growing inequities between geographical regions and social classes. Moreover, such disparities of access are not limited to the urban–rural divide; for example, the protracted epidemiological transition is also manifested in the disease burden of poorer city slum-dwellers, compared with their far more affluent urban counterparts. Many countries still have large segments of poor people who bear the brunt of illnesses, including communicable diseases and malnutrition (Phua and Chew, 2002).

Additionally, potent new health threats have developed in the form of resurgent strains of communicable diseases that are resistant to common antibiotics. New behavioural diseases with high infection rates such as HIV/AIDS and STDs, have already seriously affected Asian countries such as Thailand and Cambodia, and threatened to spread rapidly in others. The spread of these communicable diseases is compounded by rural-urban as well as transnational migration patterns. Thus, in contrast to the classical epidemiological transition that took place in Western Europe, in which communicable diseases lost significance and were replaced by a rising burden of non-communicable diseases, lower-income countries of Asia faced an overlapping transition weighed by both burdens. Even the reversal of health gains remains a possibility, given the re-emergence of certain communicable diseases.

Along similar lines, trends in population ageing vary unevenly. Country to country, proportions of population over age 65 currently range from 3% to above 10%, and will grow at a variety of rates over the coming decades. Japan, the Four Tigers, Thailand and China are projected to have the largest proportions of elderly throughout the next 25 years; in contrast, Cambodia and Laos are still experiencing an increase in the numbers of youths and will have a smaller percentage of elderly in 2010 compared with 1990 (Phillips, 2000). Old-age mortality in low-mortality countries has plummeted to levels lower than ever previously recorded, and today's population ageing estimates that do not account for mortality may prove too conservative (Phillips, 2000). Those countries with rapid ageing can expect related challenges in healthcare financing and provision. However, even where families with more offspring are still the norm, such as in the Philippines or rural China, rural-urban migrations may elicit younger generations who, working far from their parental homes, are unable to care for their own elders directly (Kinsella, 2000).

The pressures placed on national healthcare systems by these recent demographic and epidemiological transitions are amplified by the growing demands of a more educated and affluent population for high quality healthcare and the supply of the latest medical technology. An expanding middle class in many higher-income NIEs has pushed their demand for higher quality care into a booming private sector. According to World Bank estimates, the East Asia-Pacific region has an estimated 1.4 elasticity of demand for healthcare prior to the regional financial crisis (Prescott, 1993).

The relative burden of non-communicable versus communicable diseases across Asia illustrates the world-wide trend of rapid epidemiological transition. Mortality declines in combination with fertility declines are bringing about a demographic transition that is the driving force behind the steep projected increase in the burden of non-communicable disease among the rapidly ageing populations. Yet, a significant component of the burden of disease in Asian countries, however, still remains attributable to communicable disease. This is especially so for many countries in the region, where such

diseases still constitute approximately half or more of all diseases. (Bobadilla
et al., 1993).

There have been several recent emerging and re-emerging infectious diseases in Asia, and these have had significant epidemiological and demographic impact on the local population. The effects of these diseases are made
more significant because of the social, economic, and political impact within
the region and throughout the world. Globalisation has brought about
increases in travel and economic cooperation, but has also increased the
likelihood of transmission of infectious diseases and the economic impact on
neighbouring and even global economies. What are the significant emerging
infectious diseases in the region and the potential impact they have on the
region and global front? How can healthcare systems and policies respond
to the new challenges posed by these emerging infectious diseases?

Effects of Emerging Diseases

Since 1990, there have been several infectious disease outbreaks and the
few that will be showcased in this chapter are chosen for their epidemiologic,
economic, and political significance. These include the purported outbreak
of plague in India in 1994, the Nipah virus outbreak in 1999, the severe
acute respiratory syndrome (SARS) outbreak in 2003, and the ongoing avian
influenza outbreak.

The outbreak of plague in India in 1994 was one instance where the
re-emergence of a disease resulted in greater indirect effects than warranted. The events started in a hospital in Surat, India, where seven patients
were admitted and two died from a pneumonia-like disease (Cash and
Narasimhan, 2000). Although no confirmatory diagnosis of the plague was
available, this event, coupled with reports of similar incidences across the
state prompted the government to declare an outbreak. The national and
international reaction resulted in significant economic damage, with estimates of the total direct and indirect economic costs approaching US$2 bil-
lion (Ramalingaswami, 2001). Local reaction constituted primarily of large
numbers of people fleeing the affected areas, while international reaction
included increased surveillance of travellers from India, restriction of travel
and airline cancellations, as well as restriction of trade (Cash and Narasimhan,

2000; Campbell and Hughes, 1995). Much of the international reaction was fuelled by media publicity, as admitted by foreign authors (Mansotte, 1997; Slimani, 1997). The effect of the decision in this case to report an outbreak resulted in widespread economic and social damage that was out of proportion to the actual threat from the outbreak, with many actions taken outside of the World Health Organization's (WHO) recommendations (Cash and Narasimhan, 2000). Some experts have even noted that the outbreak did not meet the epidemiological or clinical standards to be declared as an actual outbreak of plague (Deodhar, Yemul and Benerjee, 1994; Mudur, 1995). Sporadic outbreaks of the plague have been reported occasionally with less significant outcomes (Levy and Gage, 1999), and the effect of the 1994 outbreak in India is a reflection of the economic damage that can result, if adequate information and rational decision making are not emphasised.

The Nipah virus outbreak in 1998–1999 had similar widespread effects on regional economies. The outbreak was attributed to a new strain of virus for which the transmission to humans was through direct contact with infected pigs, the carriers of the virus (Harcourt *et al.*, 2000). The virus was responsible for 257 cases of encephalitis and recorded more than 100 deaths in Malaysia (MMWR, 1999; FAO and APHCA, 2002), and one death in Singapore (Paton *et al.*, 1999) during that outbreak. Although there was no human to human transmission, the high fatality rate of the disease, coupled with fear of further transmission, prompted the Malaysian government to cull more than one million pigs across the country. The costs to the economy due to the destruction of pigs and the closure of farms, the loss of trade in pigs between Malaysia and the neighbouring countries, and the decrease in consumption of pork due to public sentiment during this period, was estimated to be in the region of US$350 million (FAO and APHCA, 2002). The additional cost to the government of Malaysia was estimated to be ∼ US$275 million of subsidies, revenue loss and costs in controlling the outbreak (FAO and APHCA, 2002; Nor and Ong, 2000b). Additional intangible costs to the local economy and trade may be equally sizeable. While further spread of the outbreak was averted by timely action, and the direct epidemiological effect of the disease was limited, the resultant cost to the economy further emphasises the impact that infectious diseases can have on the local economy. Even Australia, which was relatively unaffected by the outbreak at that time, calculated the possible economic effects of an epidemic of Nipah and other similar virus in the country. It concluded that the direct costs from a limited epidemic would amount to AUD$10 to 30 million, with greater indirect and intangible costs on the economic and society in general (Garner *et al.*, 2001).

An economic model to assess the full costs due to infectious disease epidemics should not only address the direct but also the indirect effects on the rest of the economy and society (Fig. 1). Most of the apparent costs affecting the health sector in an epidemic would be the direct costs of medical care and public health services. There are also indirect costs attributable to the loss of productivity resulting from mortality, morbidity and disability, besides the costs of related medical and public health interventions. The total impact on the economy could be imputed from the aggregated loss of industrial productivity in all other sectors, in addition to the direct and indirect costs to the health sector.

Economic Impact of Infectious Disease Epidemics

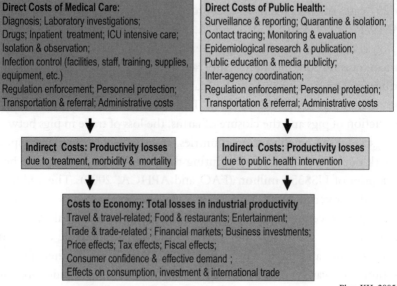

Phua KH, 2005

Fig. 1. A model to cost the economic impact of infectious disease epidemics. Modified from "Socio-economic effects of SARS", Source: KH Phua and J Killingsworth (May, 2003).

The SARS epidemic from late 2002 to mid 2003 is another situation where the direct epidemiological impact of the disease is limited due to a combination of factors, including concerted international efforts at preventing the spread of the disease. However, the economic impact is far greater due to the severity and impact of the disease, resulting in a change in the socio-economic landscape during that period. The direct and indirect costs of controlling the outbreak in one hospital alone in Canada amounted to more than CAN$12 million, with opportunity cost accounting for the bulk (Worrall, 2003). The outbreak resulted in more than 8,000 cases of probable SARS and 774 deaths worldwide (World Health Organization, 2003), which is relatively small compared with many common infectious diseases that affect millions globally. However, the high case fatality rate and the lack of a cure created larger ripples affecting trade, travel and societal interactions. The overall economic cost of the SARS epidemic worldwide has been estimated at US$30 billion or greater (Achonu, Laporte, Gardam, 2005; Wall Street Journal, 2003), but the actual cost remains unknown. The East Asian economies were hit particularly hard by the outbreak and the longer-term impact on the people and future policies will be felt in the years to come. In addition to the economic costs, the social effects are shown in a study in Taiwan, where healthcare demands during the SARS epidemic fell by 17% to 35%, reflecting fear by the public of utilising healthcare facilities, which affected their access to healthcare (Chang *et al.*, 2004).

Even smaller and less severe outbreaks such as the hand, foot, and mouth outbreak in Singapore in 2000 resulted in significant socio-economic effects. From September to October 2000, there were 3,790 cases of hand, foot, and mouth disease caused by enterovirus 71 with four fatalities. Although the epidemic was limited, the closure of preschool centres for more than two weeks in October would have resulted in indirect and intangible costs, especially arising from the need to care for the children, and from the panic that arose from the situation.

Finally, the ongoing avian influenza outbreak has the potential to cause severe socio-economic damage within the Asian region. Control of an unrelated smaller scale avian influenza outbreak in the United States resulted in the destruction of US$65 million worth of livestock. The current Asian outbreak has had case fatalities above 50% in certain regions (Trampuz *et al.*, 2004) and the overall costs of the epidemic could be more than US$100 billion by the end of 2005 (Centre for Infectious Disease Research and Policy, 2004). In Vietnam, there have been 41 cases of avian influenza and 16 deaths up to April 2005 (World Health Organization, 2005). The costs could increase significantly in the coming years with no end to the outbreak in sight. In addition, the effect on certain segments of society, especially on the agricultural industry could have severe socio-economic outcomes, changing the fabric of Asian society. And the potential for the avian influenza strain to mutate, resulting in high human-to-human transmission rates and a global pandemic, continues to create fear of the potential outcome.

Potential effects of infectious diseases

The potential of infectious diseases to spread across geographical and national boundaries are a growing concern, especially with global travel aiding transmission. The impact of diseases is also made more significant with the inter-connectivity of economies, where the effect within one region could send ripples which affect other regions. While the social and economic impact of infectious diseases is important, the clinical effects of infectious diseases are also equally significant and cannot be ignored by regional policy makers. An influenza pandemic similar to the 1918 pandemic is estimated to cause more than 25,000 deaths in Singapore at a cost to the economy of more than S$45 billion, excluding intangible costs such as loss of trade and travel. The effects on critical services such as healthcare are also important because a pandemic can be expected to result in an enormous number of hospitalisations which will overwhelm current healthcare capacity. Policy makers worldwide have thus embarked on various preparedness plans for emerging and re-emerging infectious diseases, including plans for influenza pandemics and bioterrorism.

Recent developments have seen several countries building stockpiles of anti-viral drugs for use in prophylaxis and treatment for influenza (van Genugten, Heijnen and Jager, 2003). Neuraminidase-inhibitors are often chosen because of their proven effectiveness in the treatment of influenza and their good safety profiles (Turner *et al.*, 2003; Kaiser *et al.*, 2003). While these agents are effective during a pandemic, the costs of stockpiling are extremely high and the benefits are not immediately apparent, especially when the probability of a future pandemic is unknown. The important policy decision in such an instance is the amount of insurance a nation should purchase to build its resistance against future infectious disease epidemics. This does not only include stockpiling on therapeutic agents, but also on building surveillance networks, barriers to entry, infection control and other measures. These are all costly endeavours for which the costs are immediate but the accrued benefits are unknown and will not be apparent until the event is over. The amount of investment in such strategies is a factor of the importance national policy makers place on the perceived severity of the outcome of infectious disease epidemics and the risks they are willing to take. The investment will be similar to purchasing insurance policies, the greater the perceived probability of an outcome and the more severe each outcome is, the larger is the investment.

In the regional context, the above argument is not as straightforward as it may seem to be. In addition to the perceived risks and benefits of investments against such threats, each nation has its limitations of the amount of resources it can pour into such an endeavour. This is especially true in Asia where there is a significant disparity in the resources available to different nations. As such, the perceptions of risk may only guide the investment in preventive measures, but in any particular nation, the decision will be affected by the availability of resources, and the presence of other more urgent concerns that may require immediate attention. However, as previously mentioned, due to the intertwined economies and societies in this region, the effect that an infectious disease epidemic has on a nation can easily spread to its neighbouring nations. This may be enough cause for wealthier nations to invest in the surveillance and disease control programs in less privileged nations because the spill-over effects can be felt by all. This complicates the decision-making process that policy makers must undergo in deciding on their investment.

There remains the question of whether such investments to guard against the effects of infectious diseases should be regarded as a public or private good. Certain measures such as national surveillance are seen as a necessity for the public good and are items that governments invest in by utilising public resources. Other measures are less clear, such as the treatment and prevention against influenza. In the yearly epidemics, most countries regard influenza treatment and vaccination as a private good, where the individual pays for vaccination against influenza and treatment in the event of illness. The exception to this would be certain segments of the population such as healthcare workers, where the nature of their work would place them at higher risk of exposure to the disease and transmission of the disease if they are infected. However, in an influenza pandemic where the hospitalisations may overwhelm the healthcare system and when the overall costs are much higher than the costs of personal prevention and treatment, then it may be argued that providing prevention and treatment in such an instance is a public good and should be spearheaded by the relevant national bodies. However, in influenza pandemic planning, where stockpiles have to be built before the actual pandemic, it is unclear where the line between public and private good should be drawn. It is the degree of severity of a perceived pandemic that makes prevention and treatment a public good rather than a private good.

The above trade-offs will require further studies within the region on the threshold for public intervention where the public's interests are at stake, and also the amount of investments that nations should make within their own boundaries and also across boundaries to build a regional preparedness network against infectious diseases. Thus, the public health control of communicable diseases could even be regarded as an international public good and a basic responsibility of all governments. National health systems would normally be expected to cover the functions of provision, financing and regulation involved in the prevention and treatment of infectious diseases for their own populations. When provided by governments and financed from taxation, such public health services would represent a form of income distribution from higher to lower income groups across the population, or as foreign aid from richer to poorer countries.

Policy Issues and Implications

Rapid economic development in Asia is requiring tremendous social, behavioral and policy adjustments, and certain demographic, epidemiological, and socioeconomic shifts are particularly accelerated for many newly industrialising economies. The provisionary, financing and regulatory functions of the public sector must adapt accordingly to the aforementioned transformations. The need to restructure health care delivery and financing systems also becomes critical for balancing new demand and supply equilibriums against the changing disease burden. Current trends towards greater privatisation and private health care would have to be re-examined against the expected challenges posed by infectious diseases. Previous arguments in favour of individual responsibility for health and health care are now eroded by the externalities of sharing the social costs (or benefits) for infectious disease control on a collective basis.

The World Health Organization has attempted to assess national health systems performance according to the criteria of health attainment, responsiveness and fairness in financing (World Health Organization, 2000). Responsiveness is not just about how a health system meets the health needs of the population it serves, but it is also about non-health aspects of the system, meeting the population's expectations of how it should be treated in terms of basic amenities, social support, respect, confidentiality, autonomy, choice and communications. Based on the concept of fairness in financing to achieve vertical equity, a progressive system is one in which lower income groups pay a lower proportion of their income than higher income groups, depending on local value systems, i.e. to what extent the less well-off should be subsidised by the better-off. This principle could not be more relevant in the case of infectious disease control.

Almost all countries have traditionally depended on taxation as the main source of financing public health services, especially for infectious disease programmes. However, the rising costs of providing health care to rapidly ageing populations with chronic degenerative conditions, due to harmful lifestyles and individual behavioural risks, have led governments to introduce more cost-sharing and other alternative methods of financing. Many health systems in Asia have also undergone reforms including increasing private provision, corporatising hospitals and contracting services out to the private sector. With increasing privatisation and cost-containment, questions of affordability, equity, social solidarity and the role of government have been raised. The regional fiscal crisis and the rapid emergence of new infectious diseases such as SARS and Avian flu have thrown the vulnerabilities of Asian healthcare systems into sharp relief.

What are the costs of the burden arising from these newly emerging diseases for national health systems? How should national health systems respond to these new challenges through the implementation of disease control policies? What could be the alternative forms of providing, financing and regulating health services for the control of newly emerging diseases in Asia? A comparative analysis of national health policies and systems in selected countries is strongly needed to identify the different approaches taken and their respective outcomes. A more rigorous analysis of the regional experiences in response to newly emerging diseases should provide useful lessons for public policy and future development of health systems in Asia.

References

Achonu C, Laporte A, Gardam MA. (2005) The financial impact of controlling a respiratory virus outbreak in a teaching hospital: Lessons learned from SARS. *Can J Public Health* **96**(1): 52–54.

Bobadilla JL, Frenk J, Lozano R, Frejka T, Stern C. (1993) The epidemiological transition and health priorities, in Jamison DT, Mosley WH, Measham AR, Bobadilla JL (eds.), *Disease Control Priorities in Developing Countries*. World Bank, New York.

Campbell GL, Hughes JM. (1995) Plague in India: A new warning from an old nemesis. *Ann Intern Med* **122**(2): 151–153.

Cash RA, Narasimhan V. (2000) Impediments to global surveillance of infectious diseases: Consequences of open reporting in a global economy. *Bull World Health Org* **78**(11): 1358–1367.

Center for Infectious Disease Research and Policy. (2004) University of Minnesota. News- Avian Flu Could Cost Asia $130 Billion. Accessed in April 2005 at http://www.cidrap.umn.edu/cidrap/content/influenza/avianflu/news/dec0304avian-flu1.html

Chang HJ, Huang N, Lee CH, Hsu YJ, Hsieh CJ, Chou YJ. (2004) The impact of the SARS epidemic on the utilization of medical services: SARS and the fear of SARS. *Am J Public Health* **94**(4): 562–564.

Deodhar NS, Yemul VL, Banerjee K. (1998) Plague that never was: A review of the alleged plague outbreaks in India in 1994. *J Public Health Policy* **19**(2): 184–199.

FAO and APHCA. (2002) The emergence of nipah virus, in *Manual on the Diagnosis of Nipah Virus Infection in Animals*, Food and Agriculture Organization of the United Nations Regional Office for Asia and the Pacific Animal Production and Health Commission for Asia and the Pacific (APHCA).

Garner MG, Whan IF, Gard GP, Phillips D. (2001) The expected economic impact of selected exotic diseases on the pig industry of Australia. *Rev Sci Tech* **20**(3): 671–685.

Harcourt BH, Tamin A, Ksiazek TG, Rollin PE, Anderson LJ, Bellini WJ, Rota PA. (2000) Molecular characterization of nipah virus, a newly emergent paramyxovirus. *Virology* **271**(2): 334–349.

Kaiser L, Wat C, Mills T, Mahoney P, Ward P, Hayden F. (2003) Impact of oseltamivir treatment on influenza-related lower respiratory tract complications and hospitalizations. *Arch Intern Med* **163**(14): 1667–1672.

Kinsella K. (2000) Demographic dimensions of ageing in east and southeast asia, in Phillips DR (ed.), *Ageing in the Asia-Pacific Region: Issues, Policies and Future Trends*, Routledge, London.

Levy C, Gage K. (1999) Plague in the United States, 1995–1997. *Infect Med* 54–63.

Mansotte F. (1997) Plague epidemic in India from september to october 1994: What lessons can be learned from a study of press coverage? *Sante Publique* **9**(2): 135–144.

MMWR. (1999) Update: Outbreak of nipah virus: Malaysia and Singapore. *MMWR Morb Mortal Wkly Rep* **48**(16): 335–337.

Mudur G. India's pneumonic plague outbreak continues to baffle. *BMJ* **311**(7007): 706.

Nor M, Ong B. (2000b) The nipah virus outbreak and the effect on the pig industry in Malaysia, in *Proceedings of the 16th International Pig Veterinary Congress*, pp. 548–550, International Pig Veterinary Congress, Ocean Grove, USA

Paton NI, Leo YS, Zaki SR, Auchus AP, Lee KE, Ling AE, Chew SK, Ang B, Rollin PE, Umapathi T, Sng I, Lee CC, Lim E, Ksiazek TG. (1999) Outbreak of nipah-virus infection among abattoir Workers in Singapore. *Lancet* **354**(9186): 1253–1256.

Peabody JW, Rahman MO, Gertler PJ *et al.* (1999) *Policy and Health: Implications for Development in Asia*. Cambridge University Press, Cambridge.

Phillips DR (ed.). (2000) *Ageing in the Asia-Pacific Region: Issues, Policies and Future Trends*. Routledge, London.

Phua KH, Chew, AH. (2002) Towards a comparative analysis of health systems in the Asia-Pacific region. *Asia Pac J Public Health* **14**(1): 9–16.

Prescott N. (1997) A Script — How to Manage Rising Healthcare Costs in East Asia, in *HealthCare Asia*, 4th Quarter 1997, Economist Intelligence Unit, London.

Ramalingaswami V. (2001) Psychosocial effects of the 1994 plague outbreak in Surat, India. *Mil Med* **166**: 29–30.

Slimani D. Plague in India in 1994: Is there a world threat from this focus? *Sante Publique* **9**(2): 123–134.

The Wall Street Journal. (2003) Across the globe, A race to prepare for SARS Round 2. *Wall Street* **CCXLII**(113): 1

Trampuz A, Prabhu RM, Smith TF, Baddour LM. (2004) Avian influenza: A new pandemic threat? *Mayo Clin Proc* **79**(4): 523–530.

Turner D, Wailoo A, Nicholson K, Cooper N, Sutton A, Abrams K. (2003) Systematic review and economic decision modeling for the prevention and treatment of influenza A and B. *Health Technol Assess* **7**(35): 1–182.

van Genugten MLL, Heijnen MA, Jager JC. (2003) Pandemic influenza and healthcare demand in the Netherlands: Scenario analysis. *Emerg Infect Dis* **9**(5): 531–538.

World Bank. (1993) *The East Asian Miracle: Economic Growth and Public Policy, World Bank Policy Research Reports*, Washington, D.C., Oxford University Press, New York.

World Health Organization. (2000) Health *Systems: Improving Performance. The World Health Report 2000*. World Health Organization, Geneva.

World Health Organization. (2003) Summary of probable SARS Cases with Onset of Illness from 1 November 2002 to 31 July 2003. Accessed in April 2005 at http://www.who.int/csr/sars/country/table2003_09_23/en/

World Health Organization. (2005) Avian Influenza- Situation in Vietnam-Update 16. Accessed on 14 April 2005 at http://www.who.int/csr/don/2005_04_14/en/

Worrall M. (2003) The Economics of SARS in East Asia. Accessed in April 2005 at http://www.edc.ca/ProdServ/Economics/regions/sars/SARS-2003-05-05_e.htm

DEVELOPMENT AND INFECTIOUS DISEASES IN ASIA

7

Control of Infectious Diseases and Rising Life Expectancy in Shanghai: 1950–2003

Zhongwei Zhao, Feng Zhou, Guixiang Song,
Shengnian Zhang and Tingkui Zhou

Introduction

Shanghai is located on the east coast of China and occupies an area of more than 6,000 square kilometres. Its population has increased from five million in 1950 to 17 million (including temporary migrants) in 2003. Since the late 1970s, Shanghai has experienced rapid social changes and economic development and has once again become a major economic centre in East Asia. Shanghai also made extraordinary progress in controlling infectious diseases and improving mortality in recent history, which led to a dramatic increase in life expectancy from 44 years in 1951 to 80 years in 2003. This latest figure is only one year lower than that for Japan, where the highest life expectancy in the World has been recorded.

In order to gain a better understanding of these great changes, this chapter analyses data collected by Shanghai Municipal Centre for Disease Control and Prevention (Shanghai CDC) over the last half century and examines the following issues: the impact of infectious diseases in the past and control of infectious diseases since 1950; the reduction in death rates of major infectious diseases over time and its impact on the improvement in life expectancy; recent changes in the patterns of infectious diseases and major challenges. Since Shanghai has led China's socio-economic development, epidemiological transition and demographic changes in many respects, the study also sheds light on the current and the future happening in the Chinese population as a whole.

Changing Patterns of Infectious Diseases in Shanghai

Before 1950, health and medical services available to the general population were rather limited, the coverage of diseases surveillance was poor, and effective death registration systems did not exist. For these reasons, records made during this period often suffered from severe under-registration and had poor quality. In spite of this, however, a number of observations about infectious diseases could be made through the examination of available data.

Due to the lack of effective control and prevention, many infectious diseases were endemic and widespread, breaking out on a regular basis. For example, cholera epidemics appeared 12 times (with six of them very severe) in Shanghai between 1912 and 1949. One outbreak was recorded in 1949, when 11,365 cholera cases and 2,246 cholera-related deaths were reported. Smallpox was also a problematic infectious disease, and its severe outbreaks were recorded in 1927, 1933 and 1940. The situation was so devastating in 1933 that Shanghai was declared as a serious smallpox transmission area in the world. Paratyphoid, another major infectious disease, also broke out frequently, once in every two to three years. According to available but incomplete records, more than 15,000 people were infected and nearly 10,000 people died because of paratyphoid during the period between 1931 and 1943 (Editorial Committee of Shanghai Local Historical Health Archives, 1998).

Both incidence and death rates of infectious diseases were high during the 1930s and 1940s. In 1938, for example, the recorded incidence rate was 2,122 per 100,000 and the infectious disease death rate was 565 per 100,000 (Editorial Committee of Shanghai Local Historical Health Archives, 1998). While these rates were already high, they considerably under represented the magnitude of infectious diseases at the time. The actual incidence and death rates would be much higher. This suggestion is supported by other evidence.

Some studies reported that, *Pu Shan Shan Zhuang*, a non-government charity organisation, for instance, collected 127,000 corpses from the streets in Shanghai during the period between 1946 and 1949, or an average of 42,000 bodies per year. The annual death rate of this particular type of deaths alone reached 7 per thousand (Hu *et al.*, 1987). Many of these deaths might have been caused by infectious diseases, but have never been characterised. The situation similar to that described above did not change until 1950. According to a recent study, in the late 1940s, "the crude death rate was above 20 per thousand. Deaths due to infectious diseases accounted for more than 40% of the deceased." "Average life expectancy was only 35 years" (Shanghai Municipal Bureau of Health and Population Research Institute of Fudan University, 2003).

After 1950, death registration has been gradually introduced in Shanghai. Diseases surveillance, especially the surveillance of infectious diseases, has made remarkable progress. Health and mortality statistics have in general become more reliable than those produced in the first half of the 20th century. According to available statistics, infectious diseases remained a major health threat to the population in the early 1950s. Even in urban areas, the death rate of infectious diseases was as high as 696 per 100,000 in 1951. Infectious diseases were still the most common cause of deaths and accounted for nearly 40% of the total. During this period, infectious diseases (excluding TB) that resulted in a large number of deaths included paratyphoid, meningitis, diarrhoea, diphtheria, measles, rabies and epidemic encephalitis B (Shanghai Municipal Bureau of Health and Population Research Institute of Fudan University 2003, Peng *et al.*, 2003).

Figure 1 shows recorded incidence rates of infectious diseases in Shanghai over the last half century. Data used in this and other figures are derived from the health statistics collected by Shanghai CDC, and their sources will be specified otherwise. It is important to note that because there have been changes over time in both the type of reported infectious diseases and the size of geographic area from which these statistics were obtained, some results are not strictly comparable. However, they are reliable and effective in indicating major changes and clear trends of the epidemiological transition in Shanghai.

According to this figure, changes in the incidence rate of reported infectious diseases can be broadly divided into three stages. From the early 1950s

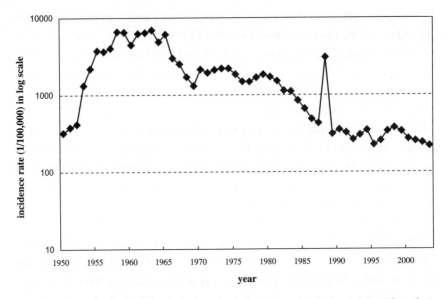

Fig. 1. Changes in incidence rates of reported infectious diseases in Shanghai, 1950–2003.

to the mid 1960s, the incidence rate of infectious diseases remained high. During the first few years of observation, the recorded incidence rate was relatively low, but this was a result of under-reporting rather than a low rate of infectious diseases. From 1955 to 1965, the incidence rates were all above 3,500 per 100,000. The highest was recorded in 1963 at 6,955 per 100,000. The progress in reducing incidence rates of infectious diseases seemed to have been slow or moderate.

A considerable fall in the incidence rate of infectious diseases was observed over the period between the mid 1960s and the early 1990s, from about 3,000 per 100,000 to 300 per 100,000. However, there was a noticeable exception in 1988 when the incidence rate bounced back to 3,078 per 100,000 due to an enormous outbreak of Hepatitis A, which was caused by contaminated shellfish. The outbreak started in January and was under control by March in the same year. At its peak, the number of new cases of Hepatitis A reached more than 10,000 per day. The total number of recorded new Hepatitis A cases was 352,048 in 1988. The incidence rate was 2,803 per 100,000 or 7 times of that in previous year. The death rate of Hepatitis A, however, was close to that observed in 1987 and slightly more than 1 per 100,000. Since the early 1990s, the incidence rates of infectious diseases have fluctuated at a relatively low level between 200 and 400 per 100,000.

These changes are closely related to the control and elimination of some infectious diseases and the changing composition of major infectious diseases. This is indicated by Fig. 2, which shows the percentage distribution of the reported number of major acute infectious diseases.

During the 1950s and first half of the 1960s, the spread of measles, diarrhoea, malaria, and pertussis was a major health threat. Altogether they accounted for more than 90% of new cases of acute infectious diseases. This pattern changed considerably in the next two decades. From the mid 1960s to the mid 1980s, the incidence rate of measles decreased from more

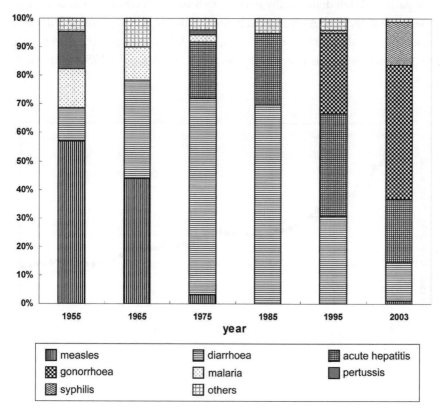

Fig. 2. Percentage distribution of major acute infectious diseases in Shanghai, 1955–2003.

than 1,000 per 100,000 to less than 1 per 100,000. Malaria fell from 717 per 100,000 in 1965 to 2 per 100,000 in 1985. However, it is worth noting that there has been an increase in the incidence rate of measles in recent years.

In the 1970s, 1980s, and perhaps the early 1990s, diarrhoea had the highest incidence rate among all infectious diseases and acute hepatitis ranked the second. Since the mid 1990s, further changes have taken place. The incidence rate of diarrhoea continued to decline from 70 per 100,000 to 30 per 100,000 by the end of the century. However, this period witnessed a noticeable increase in the spread of sexually transmitted diseases such as gonorrhoea and syphilis, which became the most prevalent infectious diseases, while acute hepatitis remained in the second place.

Changes in the death rate of reported infectious diseases showed a different pattern. It fell dramatically in the 1950s and then continued to decline in the last few decades. As illustrated by Fig. 3, the death rate of recorded infectious diseases dropped by nearly 90%, from 696 deaths per 100,000 people in 1951 to 86 deaths per 100,000 in 1960. In the early 1950s, infectious

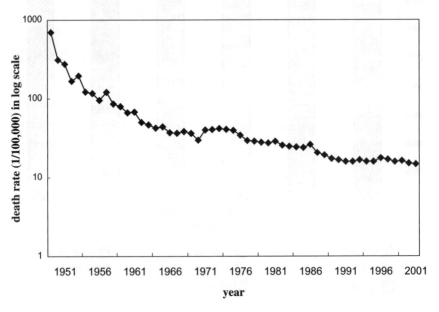

Fig. 3. Changes in death rates of reported infectious diseases in Shanghai, 1951–2003.

diseases with relatively high fatality rates included meningitis, paratyphoid, rabies, diarrhoea and epidemic encephalitis B. By the end of the decade, deaths caused by most of these diseases decreased to a moderate or low level. Infectious diseases, which were the major killer in the first half of the twentieth century, became the second major cause of death at the beginning of the 1960s and their leading position was replaced by circulatory diseases. In the 1960s, the death rate of infectious diseases fell further from nearly 100 to less than 50 per 100,000. In the 1970s, it declined from approximately 50 to 30 per 100,000. Since then, it decreased steadily from close to 30 to 15 per 100,000.

Epidemiological Transition and Rising Life Expectancy

According to the statistics published by Shanghai CDC, the five major causes of death were infectious diseases, circulatory system diseases, digestive diseases, respiratory diseases and injury in 1952. Infectious diseases alone accounted for 37% of deaths. By the early 1960s, the proportion of deaths caused by infectious diseases fell to less than 15%. Their proportion further decreased to less than 6% in the next decade, and now stays at about 2%. Due to the remarkable reduction in the death rate of infectious diseases and other achievements made in improving survival, mortality has fallen considerably during the last half century. This is clearly indicated by changes in life expectancy at birth in Shanghai over the period between 1951 and 2003, which is shown in Fig. 4.

A number of observations can be made from the figure. Life expectancy in Shanghai has risen considerably from 44 years in 1951 to 80 years in 2003. Since the mid 1950s, changes in life expectancy in Shanghai have been similar to those observed in Hong Kong and Taiwan, with Hong Kong's life expectancy slightly higher and Taiwan's life expectancy slightly lower than that of Shanghai. As was mentioned earlier, at present life expectancy in Shanghai is only about one year lower than that for Japan, which is the highest in the World. As in many areas, Shanghai's female life expectancy has been longer than that of males. This gap was relatively small before 1960, and has been relatively stable around 4 years in the last four decades.

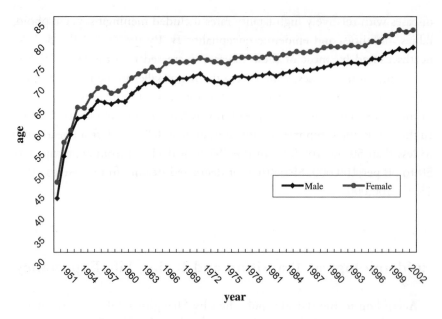

Fig. 4. Changes in life expectancy at birth in Shanghai, 1951–2003.

Rapid mortality decline took place largely in the 1950s and 1960s. In the first decade, the life expectancy increased for more than 22 years from 44 to 67, and for another five years in the second decade. Although these results were likely to have suffered from under-registration, the trend and magnitude of the mortality change were generally credible. According to reported figures, the improvement in mortality was relatively slow between the early 1970s and mid 1990s, but it has accelerated after 1996. The life expectancy at birth has increased nearly four years during the last seven years. This is an impressive improvement given that the mortality has already reached a very low level.

As indicated by these results, the age structure of deaths has changed considerably during this period. In the early 1950s, around one third of people died before reaching age 30, nearly half of them died before 50, and more than three quarters before 70. In 2001, the number of those who died before age 30 accounted for only 2%. Those who died before 50 consisted of 10% and those before 70 about 30%.

Major causes of death have changed considerably during this process, which has been regarded as both a main reason and an important characteristic of the mortality transition. This change has been largely brought about by the successful control of diseases, of which the control and prevention of infectious diseases played an extremely important role in the early period.

The impact of controlling infectious diseases on mortality decline and the changing age structure of death can be illustrated by the following examples. In the early 1950s, reported infant mortality was as high as 80 per thousand and the actual figure was most likely to have been higher. Half of these deaths were due to infectious diseases. This situation changed rapidly in the 1950s and 1960s. For instance, the number of deaths caused by measles was rather high and stayed at 491 per 100,000 among infants in 1953. However, it fell to 106 per 100,000 in 1963 and further dropped to 6 per 100,000 in 1973. Similarly, meningitis death rate was 31 per 100,000 among infants in 1953, but it declined to 7 per 100,000 in 1963 and 1 per 100,000 in 1973, displayed in Fig. 5.

Similar changes have been recorded among children and teenagers. As shown in Fig. 6, the measles death rate was 191 per 100,000 for those aged 1 to 19 in 1953. It fell to less than 10 per 100,000 in 1963 and below 0.5 per 100,000 in 1973. During the same period, the diarrhoea death rate declined from 10 per 100,000 to 1 per 100,000. These and some other similar changes greatly improved the survivorship of young people. It is due

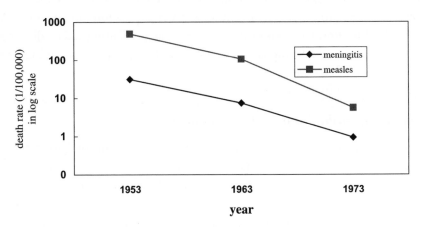

Fig. 5. Infant death rate of measles and meningitis in Shanghai, 1953–1973.

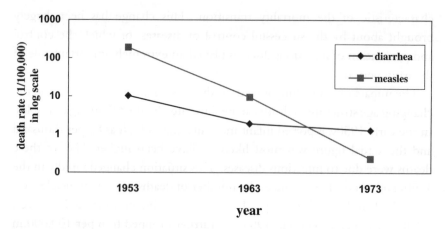

Fig. 6. Children and teenage (1–19 years) death rates of measles and diarrhoea in Shanghai, 1953–1973.

to these improvements that life expectancy at birth could have increased dramatically in Shanghai during the 1950s and 1960s.

Control of Infectious Diseases in the Last Half Century

Both incidence and death rates of infectious diseases fell considerably in the past 50 years. How did this happen, and could Shanghai's experience offer any lesson to other areas in China or other populations in the world? A considerable effort has been made in controlling, preventing and eradicating infectious diseases in Shanghai since 1950, which can be broadly summarised as follows.

Improving medical infrastructure for disease control

Strengthening the capacity of disease control is crucial in combating infectious diseases. One of the major steps taken by the Shanghai municipal government is to establish and consolidate a three-tier (street community, district and municipal levels) medical and health service network. The network consists of hospitals, clinics, health service stations, specialised institutes for diseases prevention and control, and health facilities of other types. There were 358 such institutions which employed 12,983 medical professionals in 1949. By 1966, the number of the institutions rose to 2,270 and that of medical professionals rose to 48,298. In the year 2003, although the number of medical and health institutions largely remained unchanged at 2,319, the number of medical professionals further increased to 133,000 (Shanghai Municipal Bureau of Health and Population Research Institute of Fudan University, 2003; The Information Centre of Shanghai Municipal Bureau of Health, 2004).

Another major step of building up the capacity for disease control and prevention, especially for infectious diseases, is to establish an effective disease surveillance network and a death registration system. The disease surveillance network, including the infectious disease notification system, was set up in the early 1950s and it has been responsible for monitoring changes in disease patterns, especially the outbreak of infectious diseases. The number of reported infectious diseases increased from 12 types in 1950 to 35 types in 2003 (Editorial Committee of Shanghai Local Historical Health Archives, 1998). In addition, Shanghai municipal government began registering births and deaths in urban areas in 1953. Since then, death registration became routine in urban districts and it further extended to all rural areas in 1973.

The establishment of the medical and health service network and the diseases surveillance system played an important role in controlling infectious diseases. This was particularly the case in the 1950s and early 1960s when timely and effective treatments became widely available to those affected by infectious diseases. Because of the considerable improvement in the accessibility to medical and health facilities, there was a great reduction in the mortality of infectious diseases. By the mid 1960s, infant mortality had already fallen from more than 80 per thousand (as recorded in the early 1950s) to 15 per thousand.

Promoting vaccination

This has been a major strategy in preventing infectious diseases since 1950. Shanghai Municipal Bureau of Health issued the first document to promote vaccination so as to control smallpox in 1951, and more related instructions and documents were issued thereafter. Vaccination of DPT (Diphtheria, Pertussis and Tetanus) started in the 1950s. In 1958, a network

responsible for managing vaccination was established and it has been organising the annual vaccination throughout Shanghai and kept detailed vaccination records for every child since. The OPV (Oral Poliomyelitis Vaccine)
has been used from 1962 and the MV (Measles Vaccine) from 1966 (Editorial
Committee of Shanghai Local Historical Health Archives, 1998).

During the 1970s and 1980s, major efforts were concentrated on improving the immunisation program and increasing its coverage. The Expanded
Program of Immunisation (EPI) was widely implemented and specialised
vaccination clinics were set up in many areas. The success of this program
was partly due to the wide-establishment of medicare systems, which played
an important role in improving public health at the time. From late 1980s,
further actions have been taken to prevent and eliminate infectious diseases.
A standard and scientific model was introduced to strengthen the program
management and to increase the rate of vaccination.

As a result of these efforts, the vaccination rate for DPT, OPV and MV
reached more than 90% in 1986. The coverage further increased to 99% in
1989 (Editorial Committee of Shanghai Local Historical Health Archives,
1998) and has since remained at this high level. The success and the effectiveness of the immunisation program are indicated by the remarkable decline in
the incidence rate of some infectious diseases. For example, incidence rates
for measles and pertussis were 3,510, and 1,150 per 100,000 respectively in
1958; however they both fell to less than 20 per 100,000 in 1978. Incidence
rates of diphtheria and poliomyelitis were high in the early 1950s, but they
all decreased to a very low level, 0.1 and 0.2 per 100,000 by 1973. Death
rates of these diseases fell to an even lower level.

Containing environmental and other risk factors

In addition to the wide use of modern medical technology, controlling
risk factors is also crucial in preventing the spread of infectious diseases.
The first groups of such factors are largely environmental, such as poor and
crowded living conditions, contaminated water and food, and the capacity
and effectiveness of confining infectious diseases or their agents.

Notable achievement has been made in improving living and working
environment in Shanghai in recent history. One such example is the progress
made in water supply in suburban areas and the countryside. While tap–water

was already widely accessible in urban areas in the early 1950s, drinking water for the overwhelming majority of the rural and suburb population came from wells or rivers. Improving the water supply and preventing water-borne infectious diseases were given a priority even at that time. In the early 1960s, coordinated by Shanghai Municipal Bureau of Public Utilities, several government departments, which were responsible for disease control and prevention, city planning and construction, jointly set up the plan of constructing water supply plants in the suburban areas and countryside. Although progress was made in the next decade, the project was considerably affected by the political turmoil caused by the Cultural Revolution. The proportion of those having access to tap-water was still low in the early 1980s, as shown in Fig. 7. Since then, there has been a rapid increase in village-level water supply factories. By 1995, Shanghai became the first out of China's 32 centrally controlled metropolitans, provinces and autonomous

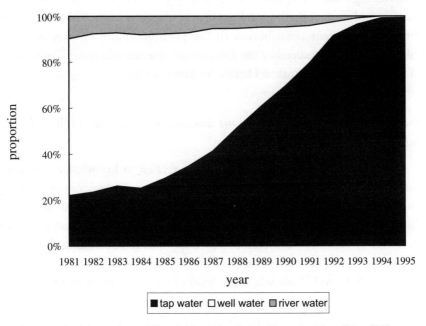

Source: Editorial committee of Shanghai local historical archives of public utilities, 2000.

Fig. 7. Percentage distribution of suburb and rural population by types of drinking water in Shanghai, 1981–1995.

regions, where tap-water supply was available for the entire population in urban and rural areas (Editorial Committee of Shanghai Local Historical Health Archives, 1998; Editorial Committee of Shanghai Local Historical Archives of Public Utilities, 2000). This change has been very important in controlling water-borne infectious diseases, which is clearly indicated by the marked reduction of diarrhoea.

Another example is the establishment of the inspection network for monitoring and controlling food production and distribution. This network was initially formed in the 1950s and consisted of a wide range of government departments at both municipal and district or county levels. It also included some specialised institutes responsible for food hygiene, production, and distribution and the system has issued a series of regulations and practice guidelines since then. To implement these regulations and guidelines, they also provide supervision to and audit the practice of the food production and distribution. In addition, the system is responsible for issuing the license, undertaking routine physical examinations for people involved in food production and inspecting the food quality on a regular basis. This system has made an important contribution to the prevention and control of acute infectious diseases, especially the food-borne diseases (Editorial Committee of Shanghai Local Historical Health Archives, 1998).

Increasing awareness of infectious diseases and reducing high-risk behaviour

Another group of risk factors is largely related to knowledge, attitude, and behaviour of the population with respect to disease control such as knowledge of disease prevention and behaviour vulnerable to infectious diseases. Improving people's awareness of infectious diseases and reducing their risk behaviours are therefore also important in controlling the spread of diseases and in lowering mortality.

In the 1950s and 1960s when the level of medical service and healthcare was still low, Shanghai municipal government organised numerous educational programs to improve people's knowledge of infectious diseases and their awareness of health risks. They also launched many patriotic health campaigns to promote public hygiene and to improve the working and living environment through reducing or eradicating various health hazards and sources of infection. These efforts helped people develop healthy behaviour such as drinking boiled water and washing hands before meals or before food preparation, which played a noticeable role in preventing and controlling infectious diseases.

Besides promoting healthy behaviour, controlling and eradicating certain risk behaviour also contributed to the rapid reduction of some infectious diseases. One such example is government campaigns of eradicating drug use and prostitution. Drug use and prostitution were very common in Shanghai in the first half of the 20th century. The prevalence of prostitution directly contributed to the spread of sexually transmitted diseases (STDs). During the period between the early 1950s and the early 1980s, both drug use and prostitution were strictly prohibited and severely punished. Their threat to public health fell to an extremely low level and many STDs disappeared in the population. However, these problems have returned since the 1980s and STDs have been on the rise in recent years. They will be further addressed in the next section where recent patterns of infectious diseases and their challenges are discussed.

Recent Patterns of Infectious Diseases and Challenges

Shanghai has achieved a great success in controlling and preventing infectious diseases. The incidence rate of all reported infectious diseases fell to 220 per 100,000 in 2003 and their death rate was 15 per 100,000. These levels are very similar to or even lower than those recorded in many advanced countries. Despite these achievements, however, Shanghai is facing some new challenges in combating infectious diseases, which are summarised below.

Incidence rates of a number of infectious diseases are still relatively high, although they have been under control for decades. In the second half of the 1990s, the incidence rate of tuberculosis (TB) showed a slight increase, from 12.8 per 100,000 in 1995 to 15 per 100,000 in 2000 (Peng *et al.*, 2003). The recorded incidence rate of hepatitis was 41 per 100,000 in 2003, which was considerably higher than that recorded in some other populations, for example, Hong Kong and Singapore. Moreover, the incidence rates of certain sexually transmitted diseases have risen rapidly and become the leading infectious diseases in recent years. For example, the incidence rates of syphilis and gonorrhoea rose substantially from 1.5 per 100,000 and 73.1 per 100,000 in 1994, to 27 per 100,000 and 230 per 100,000 in 1998 (Peng *et al.*, 2003). While the incidence rate of gonorrhoea has decreased in recent years, it is still 100 per 100,000. Syphilis has further increased to more than 30 per 100,000 (Shanghai Municipal Bureau of Health, 2005). These rates are rather high in comparison with those recorded in other areas. This makes Shanghai different from China as a whole where the incidence rate of sexually transmitted diseases is markedly lower. In addition to the threat of these old (in some cases) resurfaced infectious diseases, certain new infectious diseases have increased noticeably. One such example is HIV/AIDS. There were only nine cases in Shanghai in 1990, but the number increased to 42 in 1995 and 106 in 2001 (Peng *et al.*, 2003).

China's national population is facing similar and perhaps more serious challenges. In recent years, China has been one of the areas with the highest risk of TB infection in the world. The incidence rate was 52 per 100,000 in 2003. TB kills many more people each year than most other infectious diseases. China also has a high incidence rate of hepatitis, which is ranked at the top of all reported infectious diseases. The hepatitis incidence rate was 69 per 100,000 in 2003, and the number of people whose hepatitis B antigen is positive was about 120 million (National Bureau of Statistics of China, 2004; Qiu and Ying, 2004). Like Shanghai, the new cases of sexually transmitted diseases have also increased recently in China. Its incidence rate rose considerably during the 1990s. Sexually transmitted diseases have now become one of the leading infectious diseases after having largely disappeared in many areas for more than a quarter of a century. As for new infectious diseases, HIV/AIDS has spread quickly in China. According to the figure published by the Ministry of Health, more than 800,000 people have been infected by the virus since it was first identified in China. The figure estimated by the WHO is much higher. Despite such differences, most researchers believe that if no action is taken in the next few years, the number of people being infected could rise to 10 million by 2010 (Lü, 2004). It is particularly noteworthy that the threat of infectious diseases on public health has increased in recent years. For example, according to the Ministry of Health, the incidence rate of 26 types of reported infectious diseases increased from 186 to 192 per 100,000 and the death rate rose from 0.26

to 0.45 per 100,000 during the period between 2000 and 2003. While this may be partly due to improvements in data collection, the increase in certain infectious diseases is real.

Recent increase in the incidence rates of a number of infectious diseases are clearly related to some major population changes which have taken place in recent years. The first change is the increase of migration. During the last decade, migration and the number of floating population have greatly increased. Many peasants have left their home villages and worked in cities or coastal areas. According to recent estimates, the number of migrants has reached 4 to 5 million in Shanghai. For China as a whole, it has reached 150 million or more than 10% of the national population. The volume of such population movements is still growing. It has been found that the incidence rate of TB has been on the rise among migrants in recent years. This is largely due to the fact that they often live and work in crowded and poor conditions. As migrants move around frequently, it is often difficult to provide proper treatment to those who are infected by the disease. For the same reason, they can easily carry the bacterium to other areas such as their home villages or new workplaces, thereby causing further infection (Sleigh *et al.*, 2004). Data recently published by Shanghai Bureau of Health have provided further evidence. They show that incidence rates of a number of infectious diseases (e.g. meningitis, measles, TB, hepatitis, and diarrhoea) for people without Shanghai *Houkou* (permanent residence permit) are much higher than those for the population with such status (Shanghai Municipal Bureau of Health, 2005).

Another demographic change or change in demographic behaviour has been observed in people's attitudes and practices toward marriage and sex. Since the 1980s, a 'sex revolution' has been taking place in Shanghai and other parts of China, where people adopt a more liberal attitude towards marriage and sex. Although marriage remains an important social institution and the proportion of people marrying is still very high, pre-marital sex is no longer a taboo. Divorce is far easier and more common than before. Having more than one sexual partner or an extra-marital affair has increasingly become acceptable. This is particularly the case in the floating population where the percentage of people having extra-marital affairs is much higher than in non-migrant population. In addition, the number of prostitutes and people engaged in the sex trade has grown rapidly (Nan, 2003). Drug use has also been on the rise in recent years. All of these are closely related to the rapid increase of sexually transmitted diseases, and to some extent, the increase of HIV/AIDS.

The third major change is rapid population ageing. According to the 2000 census, the proportion of people aged 65 and above had already reached 12% among Shanghai's 13 million permanent residents. The number of 65 and above will increase from 1.5 million in 2000 to 3.5 million in 20 years time. If the number of migrants and floating population were added, the total number of old people would be greater. A similar trend has been and will continue to be observed in China, although its development will be somewhat slower than that in Shanghai. There is evidence showing that the TB incidence rate has been higher among people aged 65 and above in Shanghai. As their TB is likely to have been complicated by diabetes or other diseases, it is more difficult to be effectively treated (Lin *et al.*, 1998). The elderly population is also vulnerable to other infectious diseases such as influenza and pneumonia, and often suffers more when these diseases strike. This will become more observable given that the growth of the elderly population will accelerate in the near future.

Acknowledgement

This research is partly supported by research grants from the Wellcome Trust and University of Cambridge. The authors also like to thank Li Li for her assistance in preparing this paper.

References

Editorial Committee of Shanghai Local Historical Health Archives. (1998) *Shanghai Local Historical Health Archives*. Shanghai Social Science Institute Press, Shanghai.
Editorial Committee of Shanghai Local Historical Archives of Public Utilities. (2000) *Shanghai Local Historical Archives of Public Utilities*. Shanghai: Shanghai Social Science Institute Press.
Hu H, Zhang K, Pan J. (1987) *China's Population: Shanghai Volume*. China Finance and Economics Publishing House, Beijing.
Lin S, Shen M, Sun Y. (1998) Epidemiological characteristics of tuberculosis patients complicated diabetes in Shanghai. *Zhonghua Jiehe Huiyi Zazhi* **21**(8): 504–506.

Lü Y. (2004) *AIDS in China: Threat, Challenge, and Opportunity*. Available at http://www.usembassy-china.org.cn/shenyang/pas/c/dvc/Aids%20in%20China.html, Accessed October 2004.

Nan X. (2003) *A Survey of Sexuality in China*. Available at http://www.sexstudy.org/article.php?id=88, Accessed October 2004.

National Bureau of Statistics of China. (2004) *2004 China Statistics Yearbook*. China Statistics Press, Beijing.

Peng J, Zhang S, Lu W, Chen ATL. (2003) Public health in China: The Shanghai CDC perspective. *Am J Pub Health* **93**(12): 1991–1993.

Qiu L, Ying Q. (2004) *Viral Hepatitis is Still the Leading Infectious in China*. Available at http://news.163.com/2004w04/12536/2004w04_1083120603348. html, Accessed October 2004.

Shanghai Municipal Statistical Bureau. (2004) *Shanghai Statistical Yearbook 2004*. China Statistics Press, Shanghai.

Shanghai Municipal Statistical Bureau. (2005) *Types A and B Infectious Diseases in Shanghai 2004*. Available at http://wsj.sh.gov.cn/node2/xxgk/gkml/ywl/jbyf/userobject7ai743.html, Accessed April 2005.

Shanghai Municipal Bureau of Health and Population Research Institute of Fudan University. (2003) *Preliminary Health Care in Growing Urban Population and Ageing Society*. Unpublished research report.

Sleigh A, Jackson S, Wang G, Liu X. (2004) *Risk of Pulmonary Tuberculosis and Out-migration Work Among Rural Workers of China's Hunan Province*. Paper presented to International Workshop on Population Dynamics and Infectious Diseases in Asia, Singapore.

The Information Centre of Shanghai Municipal Bureau of Health. (2004) *Major Health Statistics, Shanghai 2003*. Shanghai Municipal Bureau of Health, Shanghai.

8

Social Change and Infectious Diseases in Northern Mountain Vietnam

Tran Lam Nguyen

Introduction

Over the last two decades, Vietnam's Northern Mountain Region (NMR) has undergone important changes such as the allocation of land to individual households and economic liberalisation, including opening to external markets. Although the Renovation since 1986 has some positive effects on this region, the disparity in economic growth benefits between the delta zone and NMR is likely to grow during the next decade (Castella and Quang, 2002). Lower school enrolment rates and poorer access to health services by minority households reflect the widening gap in living standards between the ethnic minorities and the majority population (Baulch *et al.*, 2002). Some authors have attributed the predicted rise in poverty in the Northern Mountain Region to the vicious circle of increasing population, environmental degradation, increasing poverty, and the marginalisation of ethnic minority groups (Dorovan *et al.*, 1997; Cuc and Rambo, 2001). These changes negatively affect the living conditions of particular poor communities of ethnic minorities in the Northern Mountain Region (Castella and Quang, 2002). By creating risk environments, these processes may also contribute to the spread of infectious diseases (Barnett and Whiteside, 2002).

The interconnections among agrarian change, risk environment, livelihood, and infectious disease are complex and poorly understood (McGranahan *et al.*, 1999; Waltner-Toews and Lang, 2000; Koren and Brown, 2004). Little attention has been paid to the implications of infectious disease (ID) on rural livelihoods and the resultant social responses. For various reasons, the methodologies for measuring infectious disease and their socio-economic vulnerability have developed independently. However, it is imperative to consider a move to a more integrated approach, which will incorporate biomedical and social sciences, taking account of the ecological, cultural and socio-economic contexts in which infectious disease are taking place. This chapter presents results of a case study conducted in Vietnam's Northern Mountain Region to illustrate how infectious diseases spread and affect people under specific socio-political conditions. The contention is that changing socio-political and ecological conditions in NMR affect the lives and livelihoods of particular minority people in ways that significantly influence the spread of infectious disease and condition the shape of infectious disease epidemics. In turn, the infectious disease morbidity and mortality affect people's livelihoods and lead to social and cultural reactions to mitigate these negative effects.

Chronic Poverty, Livelihood, and Infectious Disease

Although research shows that there are strong relationships between chronic poverty and disease (Streefland, 2004; Stillwaggon, 2000; Farmer, 1996), little is known about the complex interplay between chronic poverty, livelihood, and ID. The livelihood approach is useful in this regard, as it permits the tracking of household assets in relation to its vulnerability context over time (Ellis, 2000; Hulme, 2003; Chambers, 1989). Livelihood is often conceptualised as the capabilities, assets (natural, physical, human, financial, and social capitals) and activities required for a means of living (Chambers and Conway, 1992; Scoones, 1998; Ellis, 2000). Livelihood is considered sustainable when the outcome of the processing of different types of capital is meaningful in terms of human well-being and viable in terms of securing people against shocks and stresses (Ellis, 2000; De Haan and Van Ufford,

2001). Poor people infected with infectious diseases are most vulnerable since they have limited access to assets and limited abilities to respond to risk and uncertainty; this may have severe consequences on one or more of the vital capitals, thus increasing the probability of experiencing a life-threatening loss in the future (Chambers, 1989). To understand the nature of such adversities, in particular, the impacts of infectious diseases, it is important to look at the forms and contents of different kinds of narratives about the epidemics and their contexts, focusing on the metaphors and images used (Scott, 1985; Streefland, 1998; Nichter, 1992; Briggs and Briggs, 2003) and to examine how these interpretations change overtime (Farmer, 1990; Streefland, 1998).

Method

The research context

Mountainous areas represent 75% of Vietnam and contain about 20% of the nation's population. The Northern Mountain Region is home to more than 30 different ethnic groups and is characterised by very high levels of ecological and social diversity, as well as a rapid but unevenly distributed process of change (Jamieson *et al.*, 1998). Most mountainous people subsist on agriculture, suffer poor living conditions and have limited access to social services. The poverty rate in this region is expected to rise from 28.1% in 1998 to 34.4% by 2010 (World Bank *et al.*, 2001). Pneumonia, viral encephalitis, acute bronchitis, diarrhoea, and respiratory TB are the leading causes of mortality in Northern Mountain Region (MOH, 1998).

Previous studies show that mountain people are less likely to use public health services except for severe conditions (Population Council, 1999; Toan *et al.*, 2002). The lack of trust in modern medicine is due to the lack of medicines, equipment and skilled medical staff. Mountain people prefer private traditional medicine because they are able to pay in-kind instead of cash or they may defer payment (MOH, 1998). Often, the use of herbs is combined with magic beliefs and rituals (Hanh, 2000; WHO, 2003). The influence of religious principles on health actions among some Christian and Protestant minorities is substantial (UNFPA, 1999).

The study site

The study was carried out in four communities of Lao Cai province of the Northern Mountain Region from January 2002 to March 2004. The province lies on the border with China in the extreme northwest of the country, consisting of 10 districts and 165 rural communes, with a total land area exceeding 8,000 square kilometre (Que *et al.*, 1996). Mountainous communes are scattered among numerous ridges and secluded valleys. Areas with steep slopes exceeding 25° occupy 84% of the land area and the elevation ranges from 80 m to 3,143 m above sea level. The province belongs to the monsoon tropical climate region. The winter season (November to March) is cold and mostly dry while the rainy season (April to October) is hot. The average annual rainfall is 1,750 mm.

Lao Cai is home to 33 ethnic groups, with complex patterns of land use systems and socio-cultural particularities. While Hmong, Dao, and some other ethnic groups tend to live at the higher elevations, Kinh and Tay predominate in the midland areas. In 1999, the province had 594,345 inhabitants with rural population densities, varying from 30 persons per square kilometre in some upland communes to 200 persons per square kilometre in the midlands. With nearly 70% of the population belonging to ethnic minorities, Lao Cai has one of the highest rates of illiteracy in Vietnam. The Lao Cai economy is primarily agricultural and subsistence based on nearly 90% of the labour force in self-employed farming. While upland peasants are more reliant on rain-fed agriculture, midland farmers often practise mixed farming systems, (including wetland rice and rain-fed hill crops), and intensive home garden and forest-garden production systems, combining livestock, horticulture, and gathering. The province's proximity to China and the potential for tourism development have attracted people and stimulated a variety of activities connected to development and growth. For instance, this is reflected in the rapid increase in the rate of sexually transmitted diseases during the last three years.

The household survey

This study is based on an earlier phase comprising an ethno-epidemiology household survey and a later phase of ethnographic fieldwork. The purpose of the survey was to assess the magnitude of IDs in the Lao Cai region. Four villages (V1 = Supai; V2 = Tava; V3 = Taho; V4 = Tavon) were selected, based on two criteria: accessibility and reported prevalence/incidence of major IDs. A convenience sample of 40 households (ten in each village) was selected for pre-test interviews (open-ended and following no rigid format). Other methods were used to study local knowledge related to infectious diseases such as free listing of infectious disease categories, pile sort exercises, vignettes, interviews about the signs/symptoms of specific infectious diseases, recent infectious disease events common to their village, and the severity of major infectious diseases. Open-ended interviews were also conducted with health personnel and healthcare providers to assess their perceptions of the prevalence/transmission of infectious diseases. Based on this pre-test phase, a structured questionnaire was administered to 210 households out of 365 households in the four villages (Table 1).

A team of six local research assistants were recruited to help with the questionnaire distribution. An additional questionnaire was also sent to the representatives and health workers at both district and village levels. The questionnaire covered topics such as the presence of diseases with obvious manifestations such as malaria, pneumonia, diarrhoea, flu, tuberculosis (TB), and acute respiratory infections. Where present, an estimated number of people affected were asked. Each household was given a calendar containing pictures of common symptoms which are usually treated at home. Each family received a small incentive for noting down on a daily basis all the illnesses in the family during a four-month period. Each illness episode was later probed for symptoms, severity (number, type, and duration of symptoms) and causes, the drugs used, the sources and cost of drugs, and health workers' attitude during consultations. In total, data were obtained for 1,970 illness episodes. Table 1 provides details on the survey.

As the patterns of morbidity observed in primary care may represent a good proxy for knowledge of morbidity in the general population, we decided to gather additional data for all outpatients' visits from the two general clinics and two district hospitals during 2002. For each visit, basic information of the patient was recorded and in-depth interviews were conducted if informed consent was obtained. Questions asked were similar to those of the previous survey. The research was conducted in collaboration with six health workers (two doctors specialised in infectious diseases and

Table 1. Details of the villages and the household sample.

	V1	V2	V3	V4
Village				
Population	543	567	468	529
Major ethnic groups	Hmong Dao	Hmong Dao	Hmong	Hmong
Population density (persons/km2)	123	146	159	57
Topography	Mountain-valley realm	Mountain-valley realm	High rocky mountain	High rocky mountain
Education (% of people aged 6 or older who have attended school)	Low (31%)	Low (39%)	Very low (11%)	Very low (10%)
Major occupation	Farming	Farming	Farming	Farming
# of village health centre	1	1	1	1
Distance from VHC to nearest district hospital (km)	34	26	19	23
Distance from VHC to the remotest household	10.2	7.8	8.4	11.4
Average distance from hhs to VHC	3.2	2.7	3.7	2.8
Poor hhs (%)	33	21	41	56
# of hhs	108	97	76	84
# of children 1–5 yrs	87	93	109	121
# of doctors	0	1	0	0
# of elementary nurses	2	3	1	2
# of hamlet health workers	4	2	3	3
# of private practitioners	2	1	0	0
Sample				
Households sampled	53	41	67	49
Average of pre-school children per hhs	1.3	1.1	1.5	1.6
Average family size	4.6	4.1	5.3	5.5
Mean age	37.4	41.3	31.1	33.7

V = Village; VHC = Village health centre; # = number; hhs = households; yrs = years.

four nurses), who helped in interpreting health records and questionnaires. The clinical examination by health professionals was valuable for objectively assessing the occurrence of infection. In addition, two local people were recruited to serve as guides and as interpreters for translating local dialect into Vietnamese.

The ethnography

After the situation analysis phase, ethnographic fieldwork was conducted during two years 2003 and 2004, aiming to understand the nature of infectious disease context and impact, structured around sanitation and environment hygiene, food, housing, migration, seasonality, and health services. In each village, 25 households were recruited for interviews using a convenience sampling method. Study participants included men, women, young and old, sick persons, in-patients, outpatients, and children. Nobody refused to participate. All interviews were conducted in the local language (90% of the conversation time) and then simultaneously translated into Vietnamese by the local research assistants. Informed consents were obtained with all respondents and all names were changed for confidentiality. Interviews generally lasted 60–90 minutes and were recorded by tapes and note taking. All households visited were offered money or gifts as a token of thanks according to Vietnamese etiquette. Different methods were used to assess infectious disease frequency (e.g. illness calendar, agricultural calendar, cause tree, body mapping, and disease problem ranking, social network analysis). Key informants include: district and village health workers and personnel, village leaders and folk healers. Participatory mapping was conducted concurrently during all focus group discussions, of which 11 sessions were with health workers and villagers and four sessions were with mothers of children under five. In-depth interviews were also used in these group discussions. Extensive observations were conducted at the beginning of the fieldwork, covering various themes such as daily routine, housing conditions, water use, storage practices, defaecation, sewerage disposal, food preparation, animal contacts, self care, patient records, and health workers-patients interactions. As there was no electricity, daily hand analysis was used instead of computer.

Findings

From the data collected on 1,970 illness episodes in the four villages (VI, V2, V3, and V4), it was noted that there was a marked difference in the number of episodes between V1 and other villages. This might be explained by the fact that the local research assistants in V1 were not familiar with primary care research and the population there were also less willing to collaborate with the research team. Another difficulty was the translation of some symptoms into western medical terms, as the local people often defined diseases in their own terms, covering a wide range of symptoms. Although these factors may limit the interpretation of the survey, the data are still useful for the purpose of this study.

Frequency of major infectious diseases

The most common infectious diseases reported by respondents in the four villages are diarrhoea, pneumonia, acute bronchitis and influenza. On average, these four infectious diseases represent 67.3% of all reported illnesses. Other infectious diseases which are much less prevalent (6.8% of all cases), include malaria, dengue fever, dysentery, hepatitis, reproductive tract infections (RTIs), respiratory tuberculosis, and acute encephalitis (mainly Japanese encephalitis). The remainder ('Others' in Table 2) consists of minor infectious diseases and non-infectious diseases, accounting for 25.9% of all reported illnesses (Table 2).

Table 3 lists the leading 10 diagnoses for outpatient visits made by residents of the four villages during 2002, representing over half of all visits. Among these 10 infectious diseases, the "top four" i.e. influenza, diarrhoea, acute bronchitis and pneumonia are much more prevalent in comparison with the rest such as dysentery, hepatitis, RTI, dengue fever, TB, and malaria. These are the four commonest reasons for seeking healthcare. From Table 3, it is noticeable that the proportion of the "top four" is somewhat similar in all four villages. However, there are few notable differences among the villages in the frequency of each type of illness, namely, dengue fever, TB and encephalitis. In-depth interviews with the local health workers also showed that these are the three "emerging phenomena" in the region.

Table 2. Percentage distribution of ten reported infectious diseases.

Illness	V1 (n = 296)	V2 (n = 435)	V3 (n = 678)	V4 (n = 561)
Diarrhoea	21.3	15.7	24.1	27.2
Pneumonia/Acute bronchitis	18.6	34.7	22.2	21.8
Influenza	19.8	15.6	12.8	17.7
Dysentery	9.8	7.5	7.3	5.2
Dengue fever	0.7	0.4	1.3	0.6
Malaria	0.4	0.2	1.2	1.4
Hepatitis	0.4	0.2	0.9	0.7
RTI	1.2	0.9	0.4	0.5
TB	0.8	0.3	1.1	0.5
Acute encephalitis	0.0	0.2	0.5	0.3
Others	27.0	24.3	28.2	24.1

V = Village; TB = Respiratory tuberculosis; RTIs = Reproductive tract infections.

Table 3. Leading ten IDs diagnoses for outpatient visits, Lao Cai, 2003. (% of total visits).

	V1 (n = 296)[a]	V2 (n = 435)[b]	V3 (n = 678)[c]	V4 (n = 561)[d]
Influenza	39.7	39.2	33.1	39.1
Diarrhoea	20.6	19.3	24.6	19.8
Acute bronchitis	16.1	16.7	15.6	14.4
Pneumonia	13.5	13.5	15.3	17.5
Dysentery	4.2	3.6	3.6	2.3
Hepatitis	2.4	1.9	1.8	1.5
RTI	1.3	1.9	1.3	1.1
Dengue fever	0.9	1.7	1.5	1.8
TB	0.7	1.5	1.8	1.1
Malaria	0.6	0.7	1.4	1.4
All causes	100.0	100.0	100.0	100.0

[a]Represents 62.5 % of all visits.
[b]Represents 60.1 % of all visits.
[c]Represents 77.8 % of all visits.
[d]Represents 68.3 % of all visits.

Diarrhoea

Diarrhoea is prevalent not only among children but also adults. Table 3 shows the proportion of the total visits for this disease in the four villages, which is 20.6%, 19.3%, 24.6% and 19.8% respectively. The data shows that the prevalence of diarrhoea is high during the winter months from November to February. A greater concern is the high frequency of diarrhoea among children below 5, especially in V1 (29.4%), V3 (23.2%), and V4 (31.6%) (Table 4). On the average, these figures are ten times higher than those reported among children living in urban and semi-urban areas, where the incidence of reported diarrhoea has sharply declined over the last 20 years (World Bank *et al.*, 2001). These differentials in the rates of disease might be explained by socio-economic variables such as preparation of weaning foods, boiling of drinking water, or personal hygiene. It is interesting to note that more than 90% of mothers believed that diarrhoea occurs naturally and is associated with stages of the child's growth and development. Parent's inability to effectively monitor their children's eating habits due to their busy schedules is a factor frequently mentioned. Observations also show that both diarrhoea and dysentery are the most commonly cited problems resulting from people using dirty water from streams and water tanks, and especially from children eating unclean food. In the villages that suffer annual water shortages and which lack wells, diarrhoea is a frequent occurrence (McGranahan *et al.*, 1999).

Table 4. Percentage distribution of infectious diseases among children below five years of age.

Illness	V1 ($n = 87$)	V2 ($n = 93$)	V3 ($n = 109$)	V4 ($n = 121$)
Diarrhoea	29.4	8.7	23.2	31.6
ARI	12.1	52.8	10.9	23.5
Pneumonia	18.7	11.5	19.5	9.8
Bronchitis	14.3	5.1	24.4	12.7
Dysentery	7.3	5.6	7.8	6.2
Others	18.2	16.3	14.2	16.2

V = Village; ARI = Acute respiratory infections.

Acute respiratory infections (ARIs)

Table 4 shows the distribution of acute respiratory infections including pneumonia and acute bronchitis among 410 children (under five years old) in the four villages. There are some marked differences between villages for each infection, especially in V2 where 52.8% of children suffered from acute respiratory infections. However, these figures are only part of the real situation as most of the mothers are unable to distinguish symptoms and causes of these three infections. For example, although most of them know that rapid breathing is abnormal, based on their own judgement, they do not always recognise it as a sign of pneumonia, tending to relate it with fever instead. Acute respiratory illnesses are universally thought to be caused by "coldness" and therefore treated with home remedies, largely antibiotics, thereby increasing the chance for drug resistance. The increase in drug resistance and the result of irrational antibiotic use have compromised the successful treatment of ARIs and contributed to the rise in ARI-related mortality (World Bank *et al.*, 2001).

Influenza

There is a high occurrence rate of influenza in all four villages. Table 2 shows the frequency of influenza based on the number of cases reported by the respondents in four villages (19.8%, 15.6%, 12.8%, and 17.7%). In Table 3, influenza ranks top (nearly 40%) among the leading ten infectious diseases diagnosed for outpatients. While these figures reflect the severity of the disease, it is considered by the local people as a "natural illness" or "minor illness" and is often confused with a common cold. The neglect of influenza is also expressed by healthcare workers who considered it of little significance in relation to the severe burden of other infectious diseases such as acute respiratory infections and diarrhoea. At the national level, influenza is not a priority issue of public health and is rarely reported. However, my observations show that the situation is becoming worse. The fact that large populations of poultry (chickens, ducks, pigs) are in close contact with the farmers' residence could serve as avian influenza reservoirs for the virus. This poses a constant threat. Experience from China has shown that human agricultural practices, in particular combined pig and duck farming, further increase the opportunity for the recombination between avian and human strains (Schrag and Wiener, 1995).

Malaria

Figures in Table 2 and Table 3 show that malaria is not as worrisome, compared with the "top four" mentioned above. In general, the occurrence rate of malaria in the Northern Mountain Region is lower than that in the Central Highlands where the prevalence of falciparum malaria could reach as high as 67% (GFATM, 2003). Falciparum malaria is the most virulent strain, transmitted mostly by two species of *Anopheles* mosquitoes, *An. dirus* and *An. minimus*; the first is an efficient and highly adaptable vector which bites at night and rests out of doors and is thus not exposed to indoor surfaces of houses sprayed with residual insecticide, which has been a usual means of reducing vector numbers (Prothero, 2002). In Vietnam, the disease has been controlled in the lowlands but remains intractable in these forested highlands. With high population movements and deforestation, vector breeding is continuous with resultant intense malaria transmission. For example, in recent years, malaria epidemics have occurred in some northern and central provinces, owing to the migration of the Hmong people (World Bank *et al.*, 2001). Even in areas where malaria has decreased, the immunity to the disease has also declined after three to five years; thus epidemic outbreaks and resurgence of malaria are possible if preventive measures are not sustained. In two of the four study villages, impregnated bed nets were provided for the local people through a European Union project, but many were torn after two or three years and people did not have enough money to buy replacements. Another problem is that drug resistant falciparum malaria is now widespread in Vietnam. Chloroquine resistance *in vivo* currently ranges from 30–85 per cent, while sulphadoxine/pyrimethamine resistance is encountered in 30–80 per cent of patients depending on location (GFATM, 2003).

Hepatitis

The frequency of hepatitis in the four villages is still low, so is the number of outpatients with hepatitis diagnosed by the district health workers (Table 2 and Table 3). The highest occurrence rate is found in V3 (0.9%, Table 2) where I also conducted interviews with six cases diagnosed with liver cancer. As blood samples have not been collected, these figures may underestimate the real situation. However, in–depth interviews with healthcare workers and local people reveal that many people in this region have liver diseases and some of them suffered from liver cancer, which is one of the predictors of hepatitis prevalence. This is expected as hepatitis B and hepatitis C have been reported as endemic in Southeast Asia where liver diseases are the major health problems (Ishida *et al.*, 2002). In future, hepatitis C may become epidemic in Vietnam, given the fact that the prevalence rate already ranges from 2.6% to 2.9%.

Reproductive tract infections

Reproductive tract infections are a major problem for ethnic minorities. The frequency of reproductive tract infections was found to be 1.2%, 0.9%, 0.4%, and 0.5% in the four villages respectively (Table 2). While RTIs are not as prevalent as the "top four" (Table 3), ethnographic work reveals that a great number of local people, both men and women, complain of reproductive tract infection-related problems. The gynaecological rate is especially high. Nurses in V2 and V4 reported that about 90% of women claimed to have gynaecological problems, whose severity can be explained by poor sanitary conditions, infrequent and poor bathing habits due to women's heavy work schedules, and a lack of access to clean water sources. The figures in Table 2 and Table 3 might be underreported, as women are too embarrassed to talk about sex and seek medical treatment. Most of the local women have no knowledge of menstruation sanitation or reproductive health, including prenatal, delivery and post-partum care, and safe sex.

It is also important to take into account socio-cultural factors that shape sexual practices. Hmong youth can have sex at a very young age, as this ethnic group has the custom of getting married young. Although virginity is important, pre-marital sex is not strongly forbidden in the Hmong community. Many people accept the fact that their spouse might have sex with others before marriage and that premarital sex is natural and permissible in Hmong custom. Given their low education, poor access to information, the need for cash and the lack of communication between parents and children regarding sex matters, most Hmong youth are oblivious to the prevention of HIV/AIDS. Although the district hospital records give a very modest number of HIV cases (only two cases in 2002), my findings indicate a much more serious situation.

Tuberculosis (TB)

The frequency in percentage of TB cases in four villages is 0.8, 0.3, 1.1, and 0.5 (Table 2), while the rate based on number of total visits for outpatients is 0.7, 1.5, 1.8, and 1.1 respectively (Table 3). These figures seem to conflict with the government report, which gives a very modest incidence rate in some Northern Mountain Regions (ranging from 29 to 36 new TB cases per 100,000 population per year). In fact, the rate of detected TB has increased during the later part of the 1990s (Johansson and Winkvist, 2002). There are a number of factors contributing to the current rise in TB incidence, including the aging of the population, rising levels of air pollution, overcrowding in urban areas and high levels of cigarette smoking (World Bank *et al.*, 2001). Moreover, the rate of TB patients and undetected cases in remote areas is much higher than in urban areas. The resurgence of TB is complicated by the high rate of drug resistance, thus making TB control more difficult. District hospital doctors in Lao Cai report that about 60% of the patients resisted anti-tuberculosis medicine. The supervision and monitoring of treatment is also very flexible in the district hospital. DOT (directly observed therapy) is not used; patients often receive medicines once a month even though this interval may change at random. Doctors rely on x-ray for the diagnosis of TB rather than sputum smear, and they often prescribe inappropriate treatment regimens.

Encephalitis

Among four villages, only V1 did not report any cases of encephalitis. However, four cases (0.5%) are found in V3. In V2 and V4, the frequency is lower with 0.2% and 0.3% respectively (Table 2). Although these figures are low, the local people reported that this "local disease" was new to them and that they knew many others, including small children, who also contracted the same disease. These cases may reflect a broader picture of encephalitis, which has been reported to occur mainly in the northern and central high-lands, during the wet season (World Bank *et al.*, 2001). Japanese encephalitis (JEV) was first detected in Vietnam in 1952 and occurred mainly in children below five. Most infections with JEV have no symptoms. Less than 0.1% develops into severe encephalitis, with clinical signs of spinal-cord involvement (Solomon *et al.*, 1998). As a result, the number of JEV in Lao Cai might be seriously underreported.

Dengue fever

The frequencies (in percentage) of reported dengue fever in the four villages are 0.7, 0.4, 1.3, and 0.6 respectively (Table 2); while the frequencies for outpatient visits are 0.9, 1.7, 1.5, and 1.8 respectively (Table 3). Like encephalitis, these figures might be underreported because respondents are unaware of the disease symptoms, which are often confused with fever or common malaria. According to the local health workers, large outbreaks of the virus tend to occur periodically. This comment is congruent with some studies which report that dengue first appeared in Vietnam in the 1960s and that there are major epidemics every three to four years (Solomon *et al.*, 2000). The disease continues to be among the top ten causes of mortality in Vietnam, with the incidence rate per 100,000 population increased considerably from 65.8 (1994) to 105 (1996) and 312.3 (1998) (World Bank *et al.*, 2001). In Southeast Asia, this is a disease predominantly of children and characterised by increased vascular permeability, plasma leakage, haemorrhagic manifestations and thrombocytopenia (Solomon *et al.*, 2000).

Primary drivers of infectious diseases

Sanitation and environmental hygiene

Water is a very important concern for the minorities in Lao Cai (Table 5). In these villages, domestic drinking water is the main difficulty. In V1 and V3, for example, during the dry season, people were spending considerable amount of time searching for water. Water tanks and wells have been constructed in all 4 villages, but the supply may not be sufficient to last throughout the year. Low land cover, a harsh, cold and dry climate, and the fact that limestone cannot retain water, are factors that directly affect the

Table 5. Major types of environment risks in the four villages. (% of respondents mentioning risk as occurring in their village).

	V1	V2	V3	V4
Water	87.2	78.6	69.7	74.1
(water pollution, scarcity of clean drinking water)				
Forest	89.6	79.8	84.5	88.1
(forest destruction, scarcity of fuel wood, shortage of timber, scarcity of wild plants, scarcity of wild animals)				
Natural disasters	43.6	65.4	57.2	55.8
(landslides, drought, flood, storm)				
Agricultural problems	59.9	61.2	76.2	45.9
(decline of soil fertility, increase in number of weeds, scarcity of land to make swiddens, diseases of livestock)				

Adapted from Cuc and Rambo (2001).

supply of water (Cuc and Rambo, 2001). In addition to the limited access to clean water, the contamination of water is worrisome as well. Water shortage requires people to collect water from far away sources which are often unclean.

Lifestyle is also a factor conducive to ill being. People in these areas have a habit of drinking unboiled water. Observations show that different types of water are stored in different wooden tanks, but are left open and are thus exposed to mosquitoes, flies and other disease-bearing insects. In these villages, local people keep their livestock such as buffaloes, cows, pigs, chickens and ducks along with their manure within or close to the house. They do not build pens and sties. Pigs, chickens, ducks and cattle are free ranging. In the evening, animals are kept in the house to prevent theft. Nearly 90% of households in this study do not have fixed latrines or toilets. People defecate freely, often near the water sources, which might also be additionally contaminated by cattle dung and other types of waste. Thus, it is evident that the poor sanitary environment has created favourable conditions in which animal and human diseases may quickly spread.

Deprivation

The depth of poverty among these ethnic groups is hard to define. More than 95% of the households in the study suffered food shortage in all of the last ten years. Approximately 90% of the households had food shortages for three to six months in 2002. In general, chronically hungry households are those that have a severely limited resource base in terms of cultivable land, livestock (buffalo, cow, pig, duck etc.) and family labour capacity (number of people that need to be fed). The following story is an illustration of deprivation:

Cases 1 — There are 14 members in Mr Sung's family. They do not have any paddy land or a vegetable garden. Neither do they have a cow, a buffalo, nor a pig. The only land they have is some maize fields located some 17 km away from their home village. Each year they plant around 15 kg of seed. They also plant cassava and cana (*dong rieng*) there. This gives enough food for about three months. To make up the shortfall, they borrow maize from their uncle in exchange for ploughing and splitting wood. Mr Sung also sent his eight-year-old daughter to work for a cousin. Sometimes they go to the forest to seek brown tubers (*con giong*) and yam (*con pua*) to eat. During times of shortage (from May to July), the food runs out and the crop has yet to be harvested, they seek honey, roots and medicinal plants (*thao qua*) to sell in the markets in order to buy oil and salt etc.

In the well-being ranking exercise, housing was given a heavy weighting by the respondents. In these poor villages, having a permanent solid house that is close to the field and equipped with basic furniture is considered of utmost importance. Many people live in a dark and unclean house made of earth with no windows and wooden poles to hold up the roof. The kitchen is often arranged near the fire and the bed. Minorities in this region have very limited property, with a typical household having a cooking pot, a pan, a knife, a narrow bed, a ladder and a stone mortar to grind maize. They do not own a stove, table or chairs. Many households cannot afford to buy basic supplies such as mosquito nets or warm clothes for infants. It is difficult to assess the total genuine assets, but a 1999 survey of four ethnic minorities communities in the Northern Mountain Region found that the average total value of all household assets (land, house, and material possessions) range from US $200 to US $700 (Luong, 2003).

Seasonality

Data shows that seasonal deprivation is not only an indication of hunger but also an important determinant of illness. The existence of a hungry period is used by respondents as a criterion in defining poverty. According to the well-being ranking, those who are "well off" are those with enough food for the whole year and some savings; "the poor" are those who have nearly enough food for the whole year (9–10 months); and "the hungry" are those who have enough food for only 6 or 7 months. In general, food shortages are mostly prevalent during the lean months (from June to September) when the food stock from the previous harvest is almost exhausted, while scanty savings are destined for investment in the coming crop. Humans and livestock are both half-starved. It is also a time of the wet season when insect vectors and micro-organisms prosper. My observations and data showed that the peak of some illnesses is closely related to seasonality factors. For example, diarrhoea often occurs during rainy season in the summer (April–October), pneumonia is a frequent endemic during winter months (November–March) when the weather is cold and mostly dry, and influenza often strikes during the spring and autumn months.

Migration

One of the major sources of household vulnerability in the Northern Mountain Region stems from the fact that for the last 20 years, so many households have moved locations, both within and between provinces. The reasons for these movements vary. Many thousands of people were relocated during the military conflict with China in 1979. There has also been a massive migration of landless households from lowland areas to new economic zones in the north, and the movement of people within the mountain region primarily as a result of pressure on land resources. Recently, thousands of people in Lao Cai have migrated to the South due to the conflicts over land ownership and religion among fellow villagers, contributing to the increased "spontaneous migration" throughout the country. The construction of the Hoa Binh reservoir in the 1980s forced 56,000 villagers off their land (Cohen, 2004). The proposed 2,400 megawatts hydroelectric dam in Son La province will force more than 100,000 minority people to move to much less desirable areas (Luong, 2003; Cohen, 2004). Consequently, these movements may have unpredictable effects on the demography of the region and exert profound impacts on the environment and on health. In the two villages of this study, nine farmers reported that they got malaria after returning from Daklak, a province in the central highlands with high prevalence of malaria. In certain provinces of the north, over 90% of the confirmed cases of malaria occurred in visiting travellers or settlers returning from the central highlands (World Bank *et al.*, 2001).

Health services

The geographical distribution of health services is a major problem for the ethnic minorities in Lao Cai. Although access to health facilities in the province has improved during the last decade, real geographical access to health facilities is still quite limited for ethnic minorities due to a variety of reasons such as mountainous areas, long distances, bumpy roads, lack of transportation means, difficult walking tracks, etc. The coverage of village health centres has increased substantially over the last ten years, with village health centres established in more than 90% of all communes in Vietnam, in tandem with the development of the hamlet health worker network. Despite these efforts, many farmers in Lao Cai need several hours or even a day to reach a village health centres. Thus, even if health services are available and the community members know their location, there may still be barriers to overcome in order to receive the timely care they need. Consequently, opening hours are important since distances and travelling time can be substantial.

Drug resistance

Data from this study (as analysed above for TB, acute respiratory infections and malaria) show that drug resistance is very frequent. This finding is partly a reflection of strong traditions of self-medication in the Vietnamese culture as a whole. In the four villages, 76% of the children with respiratory infections are treated with antibiotics. In 67% of the cases, the antibiotics are given by the patient's family. Antibiotics were administered for all kinds of symptoms such as cough, bronchitis, headache, malaria, influenza, and so forth. Cotrimoxazole, erythromycin, ampicillin, gentamycin and tetracycline are the most commonly used medicines, as these are considered as 'panacea' for various illnesses. One of the consequences of the overuse of these antibiotics is the termination of treatment by the farmers themselves, regardless of illness stage and severity. Another serious consequence is self-medication, particularly the overuse of antibiotics, since this leads to spread bacterial resistance to antibiotics. My observations also show that the abuse and overuse of antibiotics are practised not only by patients, but also by doctors themselves. When the main symptom is diarrhoea, 47% of the cases are given antibiotics only and none of them are given oral dehydration solution. Irrational prescribing practices by health care providers are not only due to their insufficient knowledge and profit motives, but to bureaucracy as well. Doctors in the hospitals tend to prescribe expensive antibiotics without caution so as to enhance their "capacity". In many cases, the mother's strong belief in antibiotics also reinforces this tendency.

The impact of crises

A serious illness or death in the family is one of the main reasons for a household suddenly becoming much poorer. Illness is a double-edged sword for poor people, affecting labour capacity, and thus threatening daily subsistence. Treatment costs can also be a great burden on the already meagre resources. As a result, many households cannot afford adequate medical treatment, and are not patient enough to follow treatment periods. This early termination again puts them at a greater risk for medical complications and recurring illness. A number of households in this study spoke about chronic illness as preventing them from working their way out of poverty, as shown by the following story:

Case 2 — Mrs Vang has five children, four daughters and one son. Her family used to be a rich family in the village but now they are one of the poorest. Her husband has got liver cancer for five years. He cannot work. Mrs Vang faced a lot of difficulties after he fell ill. Two years ago, she had to take him to the provincial hospital for an operation. She had to sell one buffalo and two pigs for the surgery. The doctor said he should stay in the hospital for three months. She did not know what to do. The children were still young; their house was damaged due to a storm. She had only four chickens left and could not buy good food and medicines for her husband. Her husband had to leave the hospital and is now very weak.

The family goes hungry through the year. In times of food shortage, she has to work for other families for 2 kg of maize to eat. She has also sent two children to work for a richer family in return for a small buffalo.

Households that have the greatest difficulties are those for whom several shocks and crises piled up in addition to a generally limited resource base. These households may become involved in a series of events that may plunge them into spiralling debt of one kind or another, loss of assets and lack of independence. The following story may be extreme but it is not unique in the region:

Case 3 — Mrs Phu is a widow with seven children; the eldest daughter being 29 years old and the youngest son being three years. Her husband died three years ago due to tuberculosis. At that time, she was about to give birth. Mrs Phu said that before her husband died, her family situation was much better. Then they had one cow, two pigs, eight ducks, five chickens and enough food to eat all the year round. When he died, she had to face a lot of difficulties for many years. She had to sell the cow for the funeral and withdraw her two daughters from the primary school. After that, her son got married and went to the south with his wife, bringing two pigs with them. Later, she bought four small pigs but all of them died in one day due to a local epidemic. She said she is not sure now how to survive through the winter months. She needs some cash to buy pigs and poultry to raise and to get manure but she is frightened of epidemics and not being able to pay off the debt. She feels weak now and has to rely on support from her relatives and neighbours. She intends to borrow a buffalo from an aunt to do the ploughing but the aunt is also in great trouble given her child's recent death due to diarrhoea. Mrs Phu has to send her 11-year-old daughter to work on other people's land, 12 km away.

Of the most common shocks and crises, illness, the death of a main labourer, and livestock disease appear to be particularly prevalent and destabilising. As above examples show, poor households have to work out a variety of tactics to deal with crises. The first source of assistance would be family, then relatives, and then the community. Within the family, selling assets is often the first action. Buffaloes and cows, although considered the greatest asset for the households, would be sold. The second action might be to withdraw children from school, which in turn has longer-term consequences for the household's opportunities for upward mobility. Selling labour by sending the children to work afield is also a possibility. As for relatives or neighbours, borrowing money, food, livestock, and even manure are common responses, but borrowing is not simple since it requires paying back. Many poor farmers expressed strong fears of borrowing money because of the risks they present amidst already miserable situations. Community, which is the last resource, may give a hand, but in these poor areas where most are poor, the level of assistance available is often limited and unsustainable. At this point, the household has to re-look at its own resources.

Conclusion

The changing infectious disease in the NMR, evidenced by the resurgence of some infectious diseases, forces us to re-consider the nexus of both natural and anthropogenic factors underlying infectious disease contexts. The study contributes to our understanding of how infectious diseases in different forms spread and affect people under specific conditions.

Upland systems in northern Vietnam are undergoing major changes, many of which are negative. Population is increasingly rapidly, forcing pressure on an already degraded environment. Biodiversity has plummeted. The length of swidden fallow periods is substantially shortened, undermining the sustainability of existing agricultural systems. Soil erosion has reduced fertility on millions of hectares of land (Luong, 2003). The high incidence of food shortage poses a constant threat to the health of the poor people, not only plunging them deeper into poverty, but also making them more susceptible to myriad infections. In Lao Cai, there are a number of contributing factors responsible for the spread of endemics and epidemics of infectious disease, including declining accessibility to fertile land, poor accessibility to and contaminated water, poor sanitation and hygiene awareness, under-nutrition and hunger, material and seasonal deprivation, poor housing conditions, seasonal migration, migration due to dam constructions and religious issues, drug resistance owing to antibiotic overuse antimicrobial resistance, due to early termination of prescribed courses of antibiotics by the patients themselves, and the uneven distribution of health services.

Data show that there are many similarities in terms of the contextual determinants of infectious diseases among the four villages, irrespective of different levels of social and cultural changes. There are also a few notable issues with respect to the types of illness episodes. In particular, the resurgence of TB, Japanese encephalitis and dengue fever deserves special attention. Although there are some limitations regarding symptom interpretations and technical issues, the study is an initial step towards a deeper epidemiology-anthropology analysis on the emerging infectious diseases in the Northern Mountain Region.

Of great concern is the impact of infectious diseases in combination with other multiple crises. The presence of an illness can lead to the depletion of household assets and social support systems, thus reducing temporarily or permanently the household's ability to devise strategies, allowing it to respond to future changes; yet the effects of crises and illness do not stop at individual and household levels. Where infectious disease epidemics spread in a large scale, they also affect farming system and the environment through their effects on the human population (Barnet and Whiteside, 2002). Thus, the results of this study are but the tip of an iceberg; they reach deep into the rural livelihood systems of the NMR.

References

Barnett T, Whiteside A. (2002) *AIDS in the Twenty-First Century: Disease and Globalisation*. Palgrave Macmillan.

Baulch B, Chuyen TTK, Haughton D, Haughton J. (2002) *Ethnic Minority Development in Vietnam: A Socio-economic Perspective*, Research Working Paper Series, The World Bank, No. 2836.

Briggs CL, Mantini-Briggs C. (2003) *Stories in the Time of Cholera: Racial Profiling during a Medical Nightmare*. University of California Press.

Castella JC, Quang DD. (2002) *Doimoi in the Mountains: Land Use Changes and Farmers' Livelihood Strategies in Bac Kan Province, Vietnam*. The Agricultural Publishing House, Hanoi.

Chambers R. (1989) Vulnerability, coping and policies. *IDS Bull*, Institute for Development Studies, Brighton, **20**(1): 1–7.

Chambers R, Conway G. (1992) *Sustainable Rural Livelihoods: Practical Concepts for the Twenty First Century*, Discussion Paper No. 296, IDS, Brighton.

Cohen M. (2004) Vietnam: Development poker. *Far Eastern Econ Rev*. 8 January.

Cuc LT, Rambo AT. (2001) *Bright Peaks, Dark Valleys: A Comparative Analysis of Environmental and Social Conditions and Development Trends in Five Communities in Vietnam's Northern Mountain Region.* National Political Publishing House, Hanoi.

De Haan L, Van Ufford PQ. (2001) The Role of Livelihood, Social Capital and Market Organisation in. Shaping Rural-urban Interactions, in Baud I, Post J, De Haan L and Dietz T (eds.), *Re-aligning Government, Civil Society and the Market. New Challenges in Urban and Regional Development,* pp. 283–308, AGIDS, Amsterdam.

Dorovan D, Rambo T, Fox J, Cuc LT, Vien TD. (1997) *Development Trends in Vietnam's Northern Mountain Region, Vol. 1,* National Political Publishing House, Hanoi.

Ellis F. (2000) *Rural Livelihood Diversity in Developing Countries: Analysis, Policy, Methods.* Oxford University Press, Oxford.

Farmer P. (1996) Social inequalities and emerging infectious diseases. *Emerg Infect Dis* **2**: 259–70.

Farmer P. (1990) Sending sickness: Sorcery, politics, and changing concepts of AIDS in rural haiti. *Med Anthropol Q* **4**: 6–27.

GFATM Global Fund to Fight AIDS, Tuberculosis and Malaria. (2003) Malaria Proposal Vietnam Submitted to the GFATM, March 2003.

Hanh TH. (2000) The Prevention and Cure of Disease Among the Dao Quan Chet. *Vietnam Social Sciences,* National Center for Social Sciences and Humanities, **6**(80), pp. 52–74.

Hulme D. (2003) Conceptualising chronic poverty. *World Dev* **31**: 403–423.

Ishida T, Takao S, Settheetham-Ishida W, Tiwawech D. (2002) Prevalence of Hepatitis B and C virus infection in rural ethnic populations of northern Thailand. *J Clin Virol* **24**: 31–35.

Jamieson NL, Cuc LT, Rambo T. (1998) The Development Crisis in Vietnam's Mountains. East-West Centre Special Report No. 6, East-West Centre, Honolulu, HI.

Johansson E, Winkvist A. (2002) Trust and transparency in human encounters in tuberculosis control: Lessons learned from Vietnam. *Qual Health Res* **12**: 473–491.

Koren HS, Brown DC. (2004) A framework for the integration of ecosystem and human health in public policy: Two case studies with infectious agents. *Environ Res* **95**: 92–105.

Luong HV. (2003) *Postwar Vietnam: Dynamics of a Transforming Society.* Rowman and Littlefield Publishers, Institute of Southeast Asian Studies, Singapore.

McGranahan G, Lewin S, Fransen T, Hunt C, Kjellen M, Pretty J, Stephens C, Virgin I. (1999) *Environmental Change and Human Health in Countries of Africa, the Caribbean and the Pacific.* Stockholm Environment Institute, Stockholm, pp. 214.

Ministry of Health (MOH). (1998) *Health Statistics Yearbook 1997.* Health Statistics and Informatics Division, Planning Department, MOH, Hanoi.

Nichter M. (1992) Of ticks, kings, spirits and the promise of vaccines, in Leslie Ch. and A. Young (eds.), *Paths to Asian Medical Knowledge*, pp. 224–257, University of California Press, Berkeley.

Population Council. (1999) Factors Behind Low Use of Public Health Care Services Among Ethnic Minority Groups in Kontum Province, Unpublished Report, Population Council Hanoi.

Prothero RM. (2002) Population movements and tropical health. *Global Change Hum Health* **3**: 20–32.

Que TT, Phan NTH, Tuan TD. (1996) *Population Data of Sparsely Populated Areas in Vietnam*. Statistical Publishing House, Hanoi.

Schrag S, Wiener P. (1995) Emerging infectious disease: What are the relative roles of ecology and evolution? *Tree* **10**: 319–324.

Scoones I. (1998) Sustainable Rural Livelihoods: A Framework for Analysis, Working Papers No. 72, IDS, Brighton.

Scott JC. (1985) *Weapons of the Weak: Everyday Forms of Peasant Resistance.* Yale University Press, New Haven and London.

Solomon T, Kneen R, Dung NM *et al.* (1998) Poliomyelitis–like illness due to Japanese encephalitis virus. *The Lancet* **351**: 1094–1097.

Solomon T, Dung NM, Vaughn DW, Kneen R, Thao LT, Raengsakulrach B *et al.* (2000). Neurological manifestations of dengue infection. *The Lancet* **355**: 1053–1059.

Stillwaggon E. (2000) HIV Transmission in latin America: Comparison with Africa and policy implications. *South African J Econ* **68**: 985–1011.

Streefland P. (1998) Epidemics and social change, in Streefland P. (ed.), *Problems and Potential in International Health: Transdisciplinary Perspectives*, pp. 33–39, Het Spinhuis, Amsterdam.

Streefland, P. (2004) *Chronicity, Poverty and Care in Zambia: A Health Social Science Study in Mongu.* Study Report, University of Amsterdam & Royal Tropical Institute, Amsterdam.

Toan NV, Tong LN, Hojer B, Persson LA. (2002) Public health services use in a mountainous area, Vietnam: Implications for health policy. *Scandinavian J Pub Health* **30**: 86–93.

UNFPA (1999) The Situation and Role of Mother-children Protection/Family Planning Teams, Hamlet Health, Population Collaborators in the Reproductive Health Work in Yen Bai, VIE 97/P03 Project Report, UNFPA, Hanoi, (in Vietnamese).

Waltner-Toews D, Lang T. (2000) A new conceptual base for food and agricultural policy: The emerging model of links between agriculture, food, health, environment and society. *Global Change Hum Health* **1**: 44–58.

World Bank, SIDA, AUSAID, and Royal Netherlands Embassy. (2001) *Growing Healthy: A Review of Vietnam's Health Sector*, VDIC, Hanoi.

World Health Organization (WHO). (2003) *Health and Ethnic Minorities in Vietnam.* VDIC, Hanoi.

9

Ngos and the Re-Organisation of "Community Development" in Northern Thailand: Mediating the Flows of People Living with HIV and AIDS

Vincent J Del Casino Jr

Introduction

It is October in Chiang Mai Province, Thailand. The rainy season is coming to an end. Porn, a woman in her late 20s, is sitting on the second floor of her house with her parents and son. She has recently met someone, a new *faen* (boyfriend), who works in a distant province. She contemplates the future. A local non-governmental organisation (NGO), with the help of a larger international NGO, has recently set up a small development project for the local women's organisation in her *tambon* (sub-district). She discusses this project with her family as well as her own lack of participation. She feels ambivalent about her involvement. She is frustrated because the organisation operates at the behest of the local *kamnan* (sub-district headmen) and is being overseen by his wife. Like other NGO projects that have come to her *tambon*, this is mediated by politics and economics. While Porn has found opportunities working for the local NGO, she has also been frustrated by the limitations inherent in the local systems of power and authority.

As she examines her situation and discusses her options with her family, it becomes clear that employment opportunities in her village are limited. She feels she has little option but to migrate, despite the efforts of the NGOs.

She thinks about her son and his future. Like many others in her circle of friends, she wants her son to have the opportunities that she does not have. She wants him to study beyond the 9th grade and to enjoy more chances. She wants a "modern," urban life for him, or at least for him to have more choices, so she ultimately decides to migrate from her village to find work with her new *faen*. She leaves her son with her parents and begins a cycle that she has engaged in before seeking wage employment in the growing urbanity of northern Thailand and beyond.

There is another part to Porn's story. She is HIV positive. Her mobility is limited by the disease's impact on her ability to work. Her health and healthcare options are also inextricably linked to her locale because it is only near her village that she is eligible to receive the less costly services provided by the public sector. Migration thus poses a risk not only in terms of Porn's physical health, but also in terms of her economic health and well-being. If she falls ill during her migration experience, it is much more likely that she will have to attend a private clinic, which would be significantly more costly than public care. In the context of Porn's health concerns and economic instability, an NGO outreach effort which focuses on local development appears to make sense. If people living with HIV and AIDS (PLWHA) can remain local, they have the benefits of public healthcare, extended family support and the potential for consistent follow-up by medical and social service agencies. The "local" is situated as the logical place in which to invest resources for people like Porn: healthy, HIV positive, single parents with a strong aspiration to work. The Thai government in fact endorsed such a plan in the mid 1990s, funnelling money directly to NGOs to support home-based care initiatives (Del Casino, 2001b). Since then, the government has continued to provide small grants to women with children interested in developing local economic initiatives.

The dynamic relationship between mobility and locality raises the question of how the embodied experiences of living with HIV/AIDS in and through a myriad of identity and subject positions, healthy and ill, mobile and immobile, global and local, simultaneously complicates a set of discursive practices that privilege one side of these binaries (e.g., NGO's outreach for HIV focuses on the local, ill and the immobile). Following on the important cultural critique on the gendering of HIV outreach offered by Chris

Lyttleton (2004), my contention is that NGOs spatially fix HIV outreach in ways consistent with their discourses of locality and human development. This fixing of HIV identities and spaces in the local and the home ignores the mobile nature of this disease and marginalises the people who choose to continue operating within the complicated globalised economy of circular migration that is part and parcel of everyday life in many rural northern villages. These issues are the focus here because the contested nature of PLWHA subjectivities and identities impact not only those who have contracted HIV, but also those affected by HIV/AIDS such as children and grandparents, who are positioned within the wake of the epidemic's impact on working-age people. NGOs have 'stepped in' to provide both care programmes and community development support as a way of enhancing local development. Their goal is to 'keep people local' by focusing on community development. They provide outreach in PLWHA support groups, skills training and small grants for business initiatives, which are intimately tied to a particular discourse of local, human development. However, it is perhaps best, in the current *milieu* of Thai politics, economics and cultural change to think of outreach in ways that are more consistent with the nomadic, mobile subjectivities of many of those people who are at most risk of contracting HIV and for those already living with AIDS.

Background and Methodology

"It is now well over ten years since the Thai government began its wholehearted response to the dire prescription that HIV and AIDS forecast both for this country and the region as a whole. Since then AIDS has become an ever-present nightmare facing people throughout Southeast Asia. And yet, after years of programming, it is clearer than ever that alleviating the *impact of HIV/AIDS still remains a highly politicised project* full of contradictions and complex issues of identity and responsibility" (Lyttleton and Amarapibal, 2002, my emphasis).

As Lyttleton and Amarapibal aver, and the literature supports (e.g. Tanabe, 1998, 1999; Del Casino, 2001a, 2001b, 2004; Knodel, Saengtienchai and

Im-Em, 2001), those living with HIV and AIDS in Thailand have to negotiate a number of complex socio-spatial relations, while addressing their
own health and healthcare. Issues of identity and subjectivity are central
to those relations, in both prevention and healthcare outreach programmes
(Whippen, 1987; Treichler, 1992; Gatter, 1995; Craddock, 2000). Access to
resources and information is complicated by gendered identities, language
differences, economic conditions and socio-cultural locations. Issues such
as who is targeted for prevention and for what purposes are contingently
related to the historical constructions of models of transmission, which are
themselves embedded in western notions of risk and risk groups (Patton,
1990, 1994). Following Craddock (2000),

> "it is possible to argue that diseases...are cultural products, given a
> specific moral lexicon depending upon symptomology and the ide-
> ological needs of a society at a given moment. HIV/AIDS, which
> has been widely interpreted to be a sexually transmitted disease, thus
> tends to be framed through the trope of sexual deviance, bring pur-
> ported 'risk groups' such as prostitutes into the punitive spotlight."

Thailand has been subject to the deployment of similar tropes of health and
illness (Lyttleton, 2000; Whittaker, 2000; Del Casino, 2004).

The use of medicalised and moralised epidemiological models extends
beyond HIV prevention programmes and into the organisation and deployment of healthcare programmes (Takahashi, 1998). Healthcare programmes,
complicated by local and global flows of health and healthcare discourses and
practices (Farmer 1992, 1999; Farmer *et al*, 1996), mediate who is given control and access to healthcare, psychosocial and social welfare resources. As
such, these programmes are contingently organised around and through a
myriad of processes, many of which are tied into sedimented constructions of
gendered, sexed and classed identities (Treichler, 1992; 1999; Patton, 1994).
Determinations as to who "deserves" healthcare and support may depend on
who remains "innocent" in the cultural constructions of particular diseases,
as well as who remains immobile and situated in particular "reachable" contexts. In the case of HIV/AIDS, HIV positive children or "AIDS orphans"
are obvious choices of the "ultimate victim," since their serostatus and family status are considered to be "beyond their control" (Patton, 1994). Such

discourses and practices extend to the development of programmes by non-governmental and governmental organisations, such as support groups for PLWHA in Thailand, and thereby mediate who does and who does not participate (Tanabe, 1998, 1999; Del Casino, 2001a; Lyttleton, 2004).

Organisations are thus important sites through which epidemiological discourses flow, are practised, reconstructed, and sometimes sedimented (e.g. Chiotti and Joseph, 1995; Brown, 1997; Del Casino *et al.*, 2000; Takahashi, 2001),

> "Organisations do not simply produce geographies; they are, rather, infused with them, and these spatial ontologies are mapped onto their rules, procedures, and practices" (Del Casino *et al*, 2000).

Public healthcare organisations, non-governmental organisations (NGOs), and community-based organisations (CBOs) all play a role in the *development* and *location* of PLWHA activities, focusing and channelling particular agendas into various places of outreach (Altman, 1994). In Thailand, NGOs have been central to the government's and international donors' attempts to mediate the political-economic and socio-cultural effects of the HIV epidemic (Pokapanichwong *et al*, 1991; Pothisiri *et al*, 1998; Pramualratana, 1998; Rojanapithayakorn *et al*, 1998; Del Casino *et al*, 2000). In the Upper North of Thailand where the impact of HIV/AIDS epidemic was felt earliest and hardest, the organisational efforts of government agencies, NGOs and CBOs resulted in the proliferation of support groups for PLWHA — currently more than 250 such groups exist across the region (Tanabe, 1999). These groups are important sites for the reorganisation of local healthcare and social welfare politics, as PLWHA struggle to gain control over healthcare regimens and the resources needed to maintain them. Women have been at the forefront of this movement, participating in disproportionate numbers in PLWHA support groups at all levels (Lyttleton, 2000, 2004; Del Casino, 2001b).

At the nexus of the epidemiological and organisational geographies, PLWHA support groups are therefore situated as one of the key sites for the distribution of healthcare services and psychosocial support in the upper north of Thailand. As Brown (1995) and others (Wilton, 1996; Cochrane, 2000; Takahashi, 2001), argued, geographic studies historically focused on the diffusion of the epidemic fail to capture the nuances of HIV/AIDS epidemiology that construct particular peoples and spaces as "diseased" or as "targets of intervention." Moreover, such studies fail to investigate the organisational and cultural politics that converge around providing and developing care programmes for PLWHA (e.g., Gould, 1993,). This chapter interrogates the ways in which organisational and epidemiological intersections construct particular places and peoples as *the* sites for the promotion of healthy bodies among PLWHA in the upper north of Thailand. PLWHA support groups are not dominated by women simply because men die earlier and more quickly as Lyttleton (2004) has stated in his socio-cultural analysis. Rather, the cultural practices associated with PLWHA support groups are gendered (sexualised and classed) through the convergence of a particular epidemiological narrative about health and illness in Thailand with a historically contingent organisational formation, i.e. the local Thai NGO in the upper north of the country.

Data for this chapter were collected as part of a larger ethnographic study of one non-governmental organisation, AIDS Organisation (a pseudonym) in Chiang Mai Province, Thailand between 1997 and 1999. Two subsequent trips were undertaken to Thailand in 2001 and 2004. The longer ethnographic project was structured around two distinct phases. In the first phase, I collected data at AIDS Organisation itself, attended meetings, followed staff to the field, participated in the social functions at the organisation, and worked with staff in the translation of documents for grants and other outreach activities. In the second phase, I lived in one of AIDS Organisation's outreach areas, focusing on and what happened locally when the NGO was not present. I compared AIDS programmes and policies in three *tambon* in two bordering districts in Chiang Mai Province (Del Casino 2000, 2001b). In addition to participant observation data collected in both phases of the project, extensive interviews were conducted with AIDS Organisation employees, people living with HIV and AIDS, community health workers, *mor muang* (local village healers), and other key AIDS-related personnel in both the NGO and government sectors in the region. This work was conducted in Central and Northern Thai (*kham muang*). Interviews conducted with PLWHA in Northern Thai were translated by a research assistant present at the interviews, who then transcribed all Northern Thai-based interviews into Central Thai, highlighting words in Northern Thai in those transcripts if they were difficult to translate directly. I then used my

own knowledge of Northern Thai to find appropriate Thai or English equiv-
alents. These interviews provide the basis of examining the importance of
how NGOs operate in relation to the shifting nature of the AIDS epidemic
in Thailand and the tensions that emerge around local development, health
and mobility. My goal, however, is not to recount the experiences of this
particular NGO, or interrogate its operational practices in depth. Rather,
I seek to analyse how particular tensions emerge around the mobility of
PLWHA in relation to this particular organisation and the larger context in
which it is operating.

Spacing HIV/AIDS

The epidemiology of HIV/AIDS has always been about its spatialities, as
some of the first geographers noted at the end of the 1980s and in the early
1990s in their diffusion studies of the epidemic (Shannon, Pyle and Bashur,
1991; Ulack and Skinner, 1991; Smallman-Raynor, Cliff and Haggett, 1992;
Gould, 1993; Killewo, Dahlgren and Sandström, 1994; Lam and Lui, 1994;
Pyle and Gross, 1997). Where HIV originated has been a central concern
of much scientific explication of the disease and such inquisitions maintain
powerful markers of what Farmer (1992) has called "geographies of blame."
While the origins were critical in constituting particular nations and continents as key sites of disease, the early identification of HIV among gay men
made important and lasting epidemiological links between a rigidly defined
gay identity and an apparently deadly disease. The global power of the image
of HIV/AIDS as a "gay plague" maintained its hegemony throughout the
Western world, despite the fact that other modes of transmission were identified very early on among self-identified heterosexuals in the United States,
Africa, and shortly thereafter, in parts of Asia.

In Thailand, the twin model of HIV/AIDS as a "Western" and "gay"
plague was incredibly powerful, not only because the Thai government
(and the general populace) were able to place HIV/AIDS in particular western cities among gay men, but also because Thais could maintain a distinct
socio-spatial barrier between themselves and the disease. "Gay" and "Western lifestyles" remained outside *khwampenthai* (or Thai-ness) and therefore
HIV/AIDS remained at the margins of Thailand's nationalised geographical

imagination (Thongchai, 1994). The powerful constructs of HIV/AIDS was made even more secured when the first person living with HIV and AIDS was identified in 1984 as being a gay man who had lived abroad (for some, being "gay" itself was a western import and not an identity, or practice, that Thais themselves had historically engaged).

Relying on early epidemiological models of HIV/AIDS that emerged from the United States, the Thai government, in concert with the United States' Centers for Disease Control, began to test for HIV antibodies among male commercial sex workers in the mid 1980s. Those tests revealed a one in 101 seropositive rate, much lower than that which had been found among gay men tested in San Francisco, Los Angeles, and New York. In this early period (1985–1987), continued testing among epidemiologically constructed risk groups such as commercial sex workers, intravenous drug users and haemophiliacs, and in particular places such as large cities known for male and female commercial sex work, illustrated a limited spread of HIV. It is important to note that testing in Thailand began, and was maintained until 1990, almost exclusively in the country's major urban contexts and among very selected populations. Lyttleton (2000) argued that such early linkages between HIV and the city meant that many Thais, who considered themselves living in rural areas, did not believe that HIV was a personal concern. Not only was it something that could only be found among the country's "deviant" populations, but it was also an illness of some distance from their everyday lives.

Of course, while Thailand actively pursued a course of rapid economic development over the past 20 years, many Thais began living dual lives as both urban and rural dwellers. Moreover, a particular image of urban living, as modern and autonomous, permeated many rural places, and as Mary Beth Mills (1999) explained, some began to see urban life as a way of leaving behind a more conservative rural experience. This, coupled with rampant land speculation, construction of new suburban subdivisions from farm land and the experience and aspirations of those living in rural areas, has changed rural places dramatically in the last 20 years (see also Rigg and Ritchie, 2002).

Increased migration patterns, particularly circular migration in and between regions, enhanced the possibilities for viruses such as HIV to spread. However, HIV remained largely ignored by regional and national health officials, despite the fact that by 1988, a rapid and dramatic increase in HIV rates among intravenous drug users (IDUs) tested in Bangkok illustrated that the epidemic had entered a "new phase." In this model, most intravenous drug use was presumed to be an independent risk which only took place in Bangkok among the urban poor. Some misconceptions elided complex issues into a linear, simple narrative. In particular, Northern Thailand is the place through which heroin has been trafficked in large amounts since the 1970s and it is also a site of significant intravenous drug use. People incarcerated for drug use in the north intermingled with those incarcerated in Bangkok, creating an ideal place for the transmission of HIV. Lyttleton (2000) noted a correlation between incarceration and HIV seropositivity, with a high level of IDU in those who were tested positive for HIV and spent time in prison where needle sharing is also common.

While HIV/AIDS was constructed as an "urban phenomena" among gays, intravenous drug users, and westerners in the early days of the epidemic, the complex interrelationships between urban and rural life meant that HIV transmission was almost immediately both an urban and rural phenomenon. The statistics also bore this out (Nelson *et al.*, 1994). The upper north of Thailand, centred on the city of Chiang Mai, would quickly become the epicentre of the country's HIV epidemic. National testing revealed a dramatic shift in the epidemiology of HIV with high rates of HIV seropositivity reported among a sample of female commercial sex workers (CSWs) in Chiang Mai City (44 out of one hundred testing positive for HIV) (Beyrer, 1998). The sex workers tested worked predominantly in inexpensive brothels that served local clientele. Many reported low rates of condom usage and low levels of other preventative measures such as post-coitus genital cleansing against HIV or other sexually transmitted diseases (STDs) and high levels of genital ulcer diseases. By 1991, the HIV seropositivity rate was as high as 70% in some of the brothels in the Upper North where testing was conducted.

The "explosion" of a Northern Thai epidemic with the constructed "epicentre" centred on commercial sex work, questioned the presumptive model of a Bangkok-based urban gay and drug-using epidemic. It did little, however, to challenge the larger risk group model that permeated the imaginations of Thai bureaucrats, health officials and the larger general population. In addition, because most people, particularly the rural poor, did not have access to appropriate information, HIV transmission remained an enigma, spreading due to a lack of knowledge. As HIV continued to spread and was found to be transmitted through the practices of men and women who engaged in commercial sex work (as clients and workers), the Thai government organised the "100% condom" campaign in Thailand's brothels as a way to increase safer sex practices in the industry. These government education campaigns effectively linked HIV transmission to promiscuity and promiscuity directly to paying for sex. As such, commercial sex workers were labelled as the"pool" of HIV infection in Thailand, particularly female commercial sex workers (CSWs). Safer sexual practices were thus linked more or less exclusively to sex in formalised commercial settings. The connections made between HIV transmission, commercial sex work and the use of condoms in sexual relationships between individuals in commercial settings, made condom campaigns in "non-commercial" settings more complicated. What remains outside the socially imagined boundaries of HIV transmission, therefore, is the "general population", i.e. that group of all others who did not fit neatly into the categories of deviance (i.e. gay men, IVDU, commercial sex workers). Watney (1989) explained:

> "In this manner a 'knowledge' of AIDS has been uniformly constituted across the boundaries of formal and informal information, accurately duplicating the contours of other, previous 'knowledges' that speak confidently on behalf of the 'general public,' viewed as a homogeneous entity organised into discrete family units over and above all the fissures and conflicts of both the social and the psychic. This 'truth' of AIDS resolutely insists that the point of emergence of the virus should be identified as its cause. Epidemiology is thus replaced by a moral etiology of disease."

In the Thai moral etiology, those individuals who practised sex with non-commercial partners or who were monogamous (even serially monogamous), considered themselves less at risk and part of a general (and "risk free") population.

As HIV was detected in larger numbers among pregnant women, the epidemiology again shifted, and now women who had no other risk except having married a man, were now considered at risk. With this epidemiological shift, so did the geography of blame. Married men, who were thought to be the link between the HIV positive population of high-risk commercial sex work and drug use, now became the source of infection. At the same time, HIV was now considered to be entering the general population (i.e. married women who could be identified as "innocent"). As more people started to die, it was clear that a critical mass of PLWHA had to emerge to challenge the government's lack of support for those living with the disease; a shift had to occur that placed some emphasis on those who were already infected. The same moral etiology that constructed HIV as an "other" also constituted married rural women and their children as victims, bodies to be pitied and protected, places for the organisation of a new form of healthcare outreach. What emerges from this discourse is that HIV was moving rapidly from urban to rural spaces, from the nondescript city, where HIV transmission was occurring, along routes of relatively anonymous sex between heterosexual men and women working as commercial sex workers, to the homes of rural Thailand. Thailand's rural-ness and thus its own feminised national identity was under attack, and the marker of that national identity, the heterosexual mother, was the key target of that attack.

The epidemiological trail thus ends in the "home," in the "community," and in the "rural," which was now being devastated by a disease not of its making. If rural Thailand were to collapse, so too would one of the key nodes of the country's national identity. To "stop the bleeding," something had to be done in those rural villages. The Thai government offices in the upper north of Thailand where the epidemic appeared most severe, worked in conjunction with PLWHA and NGOs to devise a home-based health care programme and a support group network. The goal of these efforts was to facilitate dialogue, providing a means for HIV positive people and AIDS patients to actively engage each other. A quotation from an AIDS Organisation funding proposal avers:

"AIDS is affecting every aspect of life in rural communities; from earning a living to interaction between community members. *Rural communities, already struggling with problems of land tenancy, over dependence on market forces beyond their control and migration of family members to urban areas in search of employment, find that their hard-earned*

*progress and long-standing traditions are being overwhelmed by the pres-
ence of AIDS.* Current estimates place the number of HIV infected
people in Thailand anywhere between 400,000 and 600,000 people,
and about 500 new HIV infections occur each day. Experts estimate
that by the year 2000, in the absence of any significant behavioural
change, two to four million people in Thailand will be HIV positive... The six provinces of upper northern Thailand represent 50%
of all HIV positive or AIDS cases in the country" (AIDS Organisation Source Document, Project Proposal 1995–1997, original in
English, emphasis mine).

As the representatives of this organisation argued in another proposal,
as an NGO, they are best situated to act because of their relative location
to community culture and politics. It is thus important to consider how
NGOs construct themselves and their outreach programmes. To do this, I
will focus on the NGO movement in the upper north of Thailand and then
specifically discuss AIDS Organisation.

NGOS as a Bridge

NGOs are organisations that do not have the same approach as the
government. They have independence in their work, which means
they can speak about justice, the rights of the people, and other
issues. NGOs are also a choice for people who want to make a living.
Finally, NGOs are a bridge of society (*saphaan chuam sangkhom*)
(response to a survey question, "What is an NGO?" provided by
an employee of AIDS Organisation).

If you asked an NGO worker what made their organisation "non-
governmental", the answer they would give might be similar to the one
offered here. Firstly, NGOs are organisations that do not work directly for
the government. They therefore have "independence" from the centralised
bureaucracy of the Thai State. Independence means that NGO workers
are not bound by the same sets of strict policy guidelines that government
workers negotiate on a day-to-day basis. Their work has the potential to
be more adaptable, since they are not bound by the government-designed

development guidelines (often termed "cookbooks").[1] NGO workers see themselves and their work as more loosely structured than that of workers in the government sector and more adaptable to local circumstances. NGO "independence" does not suggest, however, that these organisations do not work in conjunction with the state apparatus. Rather, as Wolch (1990) argued in her discussion of voluntary sector, what this suggests is that NGOs may "provide new constituencies with opportunities to participate in service provision and social action, and to decentralise political power and decision-making."

In constructing those new constituencies, NGOs have focused on a number of key strategies and approaches in a Thai context. Somchai, an NGO worker who has been at the forefront of the NGO effort in the upper north for almost 20 years, explains,

> "We [have] worked on issues of *planning*. In the past we worked on ideas that had to do with *community culture and economy*. Economic politics was an issue for Marxism and of the communists, but they [the communists] didn't believe in *community economics* at all" (my emphasis).

Focusing on "community culture and economy" and "planning" has resulted in an intensely focused activism limited to rural development activities (such as co-operative farming groups and community banks) in specific villages and on building the capacity of local villages to participate in the mechanisms of government, infusing local knowledge into national agendas. Networking between projects occurs, but only to the extent to which community members exchange experiences in their rural development projects. Networking (and the localisation of outreach activities) has not been seen as a means to create a challenge to the Thai State at the regional or national levels. In so doing, NGOs potentially reinforce the authority of local officials to control project resources. Perhaps more importantly, they do little to challenge the hegemony of local leaders and officials, most of whom are men. Resources thus remain in the hands of the few and are focused around

---

[1] The term "cookbook" is a term that was used by NGO workers in northern Thailand when they described governmental work. It is similar to what we might call a "handbook," providing guidelines, for example, for holistic medical or community organisation practices.

issues of importance to men's economies, such as infrastructure development, political organisation and other sites of local power.

Despite the growing interconnections between the governmental and non-governmental sectors in Thailand, NGOs in the country still define themselves as autonomous of the government sector. More importantly, NGOs also define themselves in distinction from charity organisations, community-groups and business associations. Thus, in the Thai context, NGOs are limited by organisational politics. According to a pamphlet titled, "NGOs: Society's Bridge," printed by the Upper Northern Branch of NGO-CORD (Coordinating Committee on Rural Development) in 1997:

> "NGOs are organisations that are not of the state or of for-profit industries, but organisations that build and carry out activities for groups that have the intention to address the problems of society. Specifically, we address the problems of quality of life of the poor and those people who suffer from inappropriate development visions. NGOs try to search for knowledge and a number of choices for developing the nation with the intention of promoting for the population the ability for self-development in order to establish a sustainable environment and society for everyone. This approach to development is different from the current national approach to development that is focused more on [economic] development goals than on the quality of life and the progress of humanity."

The definition offered here limits the boundaries of the NGO not only to those organisations that are non-state and non-profit, but also to organisations that are ideologically associated with an alternative development strategy that places "human development" above "economic development." NGOs work for the protection of "local culture" and autonomy, and they are one of the voices representing an oppressed rural working class in Thailand.

The demarcation of a boundary around an organised NGO movement also excludes other NGOs, particularly CBOs. Whether PLWHA support groups, a farming cooperative, or a local sub-district administrative organisation, the target group is a necessary component (and often an organising principle) of NGO practice. NGO activities need organisation and CBOs provide an easy organisational base from which NGOs can offer their expertise and assistance. In the context of AIDS, support groups for PLWHA are that key CBO. The difference between NGOs and CBOs is thus representative of a dualistic notion of service providers (NGOs) and target populations (CBOs). In the process of identifying and demarcating the boundaries of NGOs, they construct an objective (and rational) intervention into the development landscape is constructed. As self-defined "facilitators and mediators", NGOs are constructed as a necessary, but not an essential part of the development process, as NGOs want development to be the product of local people (perhaps problematically, however, CBOs are targets of NGO experience and training).

The position of NGOs as facilitators also allows them to construct *chaaw baan* (villagers) as both the "backbone" of Thai society and targets of their development efforts. It is through the organisation of *chaaw baan* in and through CBOs that NGOs may facilitate the revitalisation of a traditional Thai society, i.e. a society that is co-operative, self-sustaining and cognisant of local knowledge. This approach is intentionally anti-urban and anti-industrial. Industry should be local and meet the specific needs of those in particular locales.

With the AIDS crisis firmly defined, the governmental and non-governmental sectors have developed more projects that are closer together in terms of target populations and broad policy agendas. For the first time, non-governmental organisations are being funded in large amounts by the Thai government. Cooperation has followed in both planning and implementation of AIDS awareness and care programmes. AIDS-related NGOs have developed as a service sector of some government programmes for caring for PLWHA. This has produced a unique opportunity for the state to further intervene in the workings of NGOs. At the same time, co-operation has opened up the spaces of the state, which have historically been closed off to those outside the military, bureaucratic and business elite, to a politically active and often alternative set of voices.

The extent to which NGOs can achieve these goals is dependent on a number of factors including their ability to negotiate the mechanisms of the state apparatus (e.g. public healthcare and social welfare systems) and the local power relations that mediate outreach in particular locales. Yet, these same organisations are mediated by their relationship to the mechanisms of the state, or what Foucault (1997) understood as the "regimes of practices of government" or governmentality. In similar ways to the Andean case context that Bebbington (1997; see also Bebbington and Thiele, 1993) has analysed, NGOs in Thailand are facing an "identity crisis" as they struggle to determine what role they should take and whom they "represent." In a more cynical world view, we can ask, following Commins (1999), the question "have NGOs become a global soup kitchen?" Or, as Bryant (2002) has argued in the context of the Philippines, we can examine now NGOs are reproducing governmentality effects through their adoption of the language of citizenship. NGOs in Thailand utilise similar tropes in their work, which have the potential to reproduce and reinforce particular gendered constructs within local politics and at home. I will now examine some of these processes by focusing on one NGO in particular.

AIDS Organisation: Situating Outreach in the Local

The emphasis of AIDS Organisation, like other involved NGOs, is to create networked structures of social support and strengthen the position of *chaaw baan* in relation to the structures of local governance. The development of groups is a central component of AIDS Organisation's work and is the site through which most of its outreach has historically been organised. In creating groups and networks, the aim of AIDS Organisation is to organise *chaaw baan* to discuss their needs and structure themselves in relation to the services that might meet those needs. This might include developing organisational structures, such as a rice bank or a PLWHA support group, or a funding proposal to the government.

Although AIDS Organisation started with three staff members, it grew quickly. By the late 1990s, AIDS Organisation had 16 people working with more than 20 PLWHA support groups in Chiang Mai Province. Their outreach area included districts within relatively close proximity to Chiang Mai City. AIDS Organisation's community health project, their longest running project, focuses on PLWHA as well as on community health approaches (i.e., community-centred outreach for PLWHA). The project was started with a small start-up grant from an international funding organisation and grew after receiving both a three-year grant from another international funding agency and several one-year grants from the Thai government.

The central focus of AIDS Organisation's project was (and continues to be) organising community-based efforts to assist PLWHA to meet their social welfare needs and broaden their healthcare options. Its goals and outreach approach have been influenced by PLWHA activists who organised themselves to lobby for their rights as healthcare consumers in the 1990s. In response to PLWHA's calls for more participation in government AIDS planning at all levels, AIDS Organisation began working with PLWHA in Chiang Mai at the *tambon*, district and provincial levels to organise support groups and develop a network among them. AIDS Organisation's staff helped to facilitate PLWHA group meetings, integrated new groups into the PLWHA network and its funding loop, and organised alternative economic projects so that PLWHA might have sustainable incomes. AIDS Organisation's sentiments are in line with the ideas echoed by PLWHA leaders themselves, as one AIDS Organisation staff member discussed:[2]

> "Right now NGOs go into communities to act as *phii liang* (advisors) to PLWHA support groups. There should be a day when these NGOs must pull out of their outreach areas. After that, other organisations (*ongkaan*, i.e. CBOs) in the area should be *phii liang* for their own community and *phii liang* for PLWHA support groups... The structure of the PLWHA support group should continue to change... Eventually, the PLWHA group should dissolve back into the community and there won't be issues of people speaking about discrimination" (PLWHA speaker at a meeting organised by the NGO-AIDS Network in the Upper North on the issue of *prachakom tambon*).

Even though AIDS Organisation has an international funding base and a similarly broad financial development approach, it has remained focused on

---

[2] I do not want to brush over differences in staff opinions regarding the goals of AIDS Organisation's outreach. Staff members have very different approaches to outreach and some were much more involved in the day-to-day activities of PLWHA support groups than others. In all sites, however, additional staff responsibilities, including developing outreach efforts at the district level and with *mor muang* (local village healers), *or bor tor* (sub-district councils), and district officials spread most staff quite thin. Moreover, in 1999 AIDS Organisation was in the midst of a funding crisis and much staff time was spent in the office writing grants.

local programming that targets specific groups and communities, including PLWHA. AIDS Organisation does not just target its activities at the local level, but is itself a product of a discourse of "localness" and local knowledge. It is local not only because it is located in Northern Thailand and was formed by people from the region, but because the people who work at AIDS Organisation are locals themselves. One of the most important contributions AIDS Organisation claims to make to the AIDS movement and the development of Thai society more broadly is its staff's knowledge of the local culture, economy, politics and the upper north region. They represent this local knowledge in their literature and in their day-to-day speech through the use of Northern Thai in the office, at meetings, and in casual conversations among staff. They talk proudly about growing up in rural areas and their continued attachment to the upper north. They sing in Northern Thai, crack jokes in Northern Thai, and discuss organisational issues in Northern Thai. They eat Northern Thai food. They believe they can actualise the goals of a broader AIDS-related NGO movement in Chiang Mai because they can relate to the outreach population in ways that outsiders cannot.

> "To this date AIDS outreaches have been effective to varying degrees. However, their effectiveness has been limited because they are generally based on foreign approaches to the problem and typically follow an informational model whereby "dry facts," which from a village perspective seem unrelated to village life, are presented to community groups. *Unfortunately these programmes have failed to recognise the traditional problem solving structures that exist in each village and have not taken advantage of the fundamental beliefs, relationships and structures that are essential to everyday life in rural areas.* Consequently rural community members have not been given substantial opportunities for creating and implementing their own initiatives. Essentially, knowledge has remained based in *urban* areas and the *rural* populace has been expected to passively accept the knowledge and programmes implemented" (AIDS Organisation source document; original in English; emphasis mine).

Despite its relationships with extra-regional and international organisations, therefore, AIDS Organisation defines itself as a local organisation with a particular purchase on local knowledge. As such, AIDS Organisation claims to be in a better position than other organisations (specifically urban-based international NGOs and government agencies) to address the needs of PLWHA and their communities in the upper north. As such, their outreach is different because it is held in opposition to top-down (state-centred), urban-based, 'western-style' outreach organisations.

In developing their outreach, AIDS Organisation staff work on a day-to-day basis with target populations, such as PLWHA support groups, in order to extend the boundaries of health care and address the needs of PLWHA. While they rely on a discourse of "local knowledge" in their day-to-day rhetoric, their practices are organised around several key issues (e.g. community health for PLWHA, holistic health care, and children affected by AIDS) that are tied to the agendas of the Thai government, the international funding community, and the structures of PLWHA outreach. Thus, even though AIDS Organisation claims to work from the ground up, its agenda is actually tied to a number of other organisational actors and spaces. In this way, AIDS Organisation participates in the reinscription of an epidemiological narrative that sutures outreach efforts for PLWHA to the local rural home.

This can be seen in the meetings and trainings that AIDS Organisation developed in conjunction with their PLWHA outreach efforts. For example, at one meeting that AIDS Organisation organised to train people living with HIV and AIDS on home healthcare, a number of breakout groups were assigned to answer the question, "What is a PLWHA?" After they finished, one PLWHA volunteer from each group presented the group's answers. Their responses were telling. Some of these included:

(1) We are people who are discriminated against. We are the mothers of children. We are villagers and community members. We are volunteers who visit other people's homes.

(2) PLWHA are people who help society. PLWHA earn money to help themselves and their children. PLWHA work for the future of their children.

(3) Society discriminates. The biggest problem is the death of parents. People don't want to get close to PLWHA.

As the trainees were predominantly women (only one man was present), it is not surprising that they identified themselves as mothers. Being a mother remains an important identity marker for women in Thailand and being able to provide for one's child remains a key symbol of motherhood. Therefore, women were interested in any activity that would provide for their family or assist them in their healthcare regimen, as women also often volunteered for training seminars and tended to be more active in PLWHA support group meetings than men (Lyttleton, 2004). In addition, PLWHA identified themselves as key actors in *tambon* life, who could provide basic information on HIV and AIDS as well as techniques on living a healthy life. Training as a healthcare volunteer allowed PLWHA to increase their base of knowledge, their perceived self-value to the community as a care provider, and thus activities such as this had the potential to improve self-esteem. Despite the optimism, however, problems of discrimination and the future of their children remained important issues for participants. Such images of PLWHA frustrated some men who felt that they were marginalised from government projects and programmes, most of which flowed through support groups.

In this context, PLWHA support and outreach sutures HIV to healthcare in ways that are supportive of the local and reifies women's community roles as caretakers. In the same ways that national identities have been feminised, so too have discourses of the local in the context of the HIV epidemic. As Lyttleton (2004) argues, this gendering of outreach is also tied to cultural practices that discursively link support group activities with self-reflexive practices that women are supported to engage. In this way, "local narratives ... are anchored in moral and emotional terms" and have "tremendous consequences" (Lyttleton, 2004) for HIV outreach programmes. NGOs working in and through the PLWHA support groups enable a particular discourse of outreach that favours local over mobile identities, and thus in many ways marginalises the mobile subjectivities that are such a critical aspect of the HIV epidemic in Thailand such as men, single women and those subjects beyond the margins of a fixed village space.

Mobility, is in fact a part of the life course of many Thai men and women (e.g. Mills, 1999), as was described by the experiences of Porn at the beginning of this chapter. Targets of support programmes such as familial networks are not always locally situated. Yet, there is little attempt to provide net-working across distant families who have been impacted by HIV. As an example, another HIV positive woman described her in-laws as distant and uninterested in her life and the lives of their two grandchildren. She had married a man from a poor agricultural family in the Northeast of Thailand. Her in-laws were thus far away, and she had only visited them once or twice. After her husband's death, his family made no effort to contact her or offer their support to her and their grandchildren. She had not talked to her in-laws since her husband died. At the same time, NGO's, targeting outreach in this women's local village did not try to coordinate healthcare across regions and familial networks. Thus, while there are certainly chal-lenges to constructing such networks, including the ways in which poverty and gender relations mediate care, it might be important to rethink how the "family" is constituted as a site of social support and healthcare in a Thai context. This also suggests that in general, home-based care may not always take into account that the "home" stretches beyond the physical boundaries of one or two structures in a particular village. This particular women's experience of home was striated across a rather large physical and cultural divide, a product of her own mobility as a migrant labourer before she contracted HIV and now her relative immobility as a person living with HIV.

In addition to the mobile familial networks that mediate much of the experience of HIV and healthcare, the people who were present at the above mentioned training all defined physical location in a village and a clear citizenship as a Thai. They thus benefit from *tambon* and village programmes and have access to local health care and NGOs that organise the healthcare through government-run local health care centres and stations (Del Casino *et al.*, 2000). As one AIDS Organisation worker describes the practice of organising PLWHA support groups, one begins by coordinating with the local health station.

"The method in the past was to coordinate with the health station and collect information on PLWHA in the *tambon*. What problems do PLWHA have? What type of assistance do they receive? Or, what impacts have they felt? If the health station staff doesn't have

the ability to answer my questions, I ask for the name of a PLWHA
who has come out in the community and who uses the services
of the health station. I ask if they know of a PLWHA who would
want to come to a meeting at the health station? We talk about who
has been adversely impacted and what assistance they might need.
I then ask the health station staff, do you think it is a good idea to
start a group? Is there any funding to assist the development of a
group?"

In collecting such information, this particular NGO practice is dependent
on government surveillance and becomes focused on only one segment of
the PLWHA community, i.e. locally-based citizens. Without access to a
health station or to a community organising, which is sometimes impossible
in a Thai context where the health station is strongly tied to local power,
many people are marginalised by these practices and remain outside the outreach of NGOs and the government health sector. While such organising
might work to prevent and fight discrimination, a problem still clearly artic-
ulated by PLWHA in the North, it also might create new layers of stigma
around those who cannot gain access to such resources. The privileging of
HIV positive identities can thus result in the marginalisation of the mobile
subjectivities of itinerant labourers, hill tribe peoples, or illegal immigrants
as well as other mundane identities and subjectivities, such as those occupied
by husbands, fathers, single women, gay, bisexual, lesbian, or transgendered
individuals. In organising support groups, HIV positive group member identities, as Lyttleton (2004) suggested, may become exclusively tied to very
specific subjectivities such as heterosexual, married (or widowed) women.
NGO outreach that works through government spaces may also demand
the reification of the HIV positive body as such, reinforcing what Foucault (1997) called the "regimes of governmentality" over those who can
be mobilised through support group efforts.

Ultimately, PLWHA support groups in the upper north of Thailand are
partially sutured to immobile subjectivities, such as the poor and landless in
particular village contexts, who are dependent on governmental and non-
governmental subsidies for their basic necessities. Throughout the course
of the ethnographic project, there was a tension in communities between
those who had and those who had not "identified" as HIV positive. In

many cases, those who had yet to formally "come out" in the community were less dependent on the social services linked to these groups. Thus, support groups that were constructed as sites of social welfare development and home-based care did not appeal to middle class or relatively healthy HIV positive individuals. These groups could thus not act as sites of HIV prevention programmes — training those who were both HIV positive and negative on how to reduce the risk of HIV — because they were discursively and materially linked to distinct HIV positive bodies and subjectivities. Unintentionally, NGOs may reinforce this marginalisation by favouring HIV positive (community activist) identities over other identities, such as those that people might claim as healthcare volunteers. Therefore, it is not surprising, that some of the more progressive moments in the HIV positive support group movement have been tied to dismantling support groups. By dismantling these structures of support, it may be possible for HIV positive people to reconstitute their subjectivities as community members and *not* as HIV positive individuals. This is of course a complicated balancing act that may also serve to socially and spatially "re-closet" HIV positive individuals.

Conclusions

Lyttleton (2004) argued powerfully for the ways in which community-groups for PLWHA are gendered through the discourses of belonging. Another discourse operates through the spatial fixity of NGO outreach which situates outreach in the home and village (and the local) in Northern Thailand. The organisation of support groups and their activities, which target *chaaw baan* with HIV, partly follow a scripted epidemiological discourse in constituting and considering HIV/AIDS. This discourse emerges out of a biomedical compulsion of subscribing blame and fixing risk around particular groups and places. I argue that NGOs are sometimes complicit in the reproduction and representation of a hegemonic epidemiological story and as such they support its power to inscribe difference through their everyday outreach practices. The activities of many support groups are organised around a singular epidemiological story, which marginalises mobility in favour of a hegemonic reading of locality. Using the rural home (and the local) as the site of organisation limits those who do not live at home on a regular basis. This results in support groups in Northern Thailand targeting the very poorest sector of the population and often serving those who are out of work at home in the first place, missing the important mobile population that lives with HIV disease, but has little in the form of psychosocial support.

I therefore suggest that an epidemiological model is not merely a representation "out there." It has real spatial affects and can be deployed in ways that regulate the spaces of healthcare and outreach. As many feminists have argued about the epidemiology of HIV/AIDS in the United States, which marginalises women in favour of models more suited to gay men, the epidemics in Thailand is based on a presumptive heteronormativity about the family, the home, and the rural, which constitutes outreach around an "innocent victim," often rural women and their children. We need to question the efficacy of how terms such as the "rural," the "village," and the "local" are practised in Thailand. Where does the local begin and where does it end? In what ways is the local (and rural) defined not as a positive whole but as the constitutive outside a global (and urban) centre? NGOs may naively romanticise rural life (Delcore 2003), arguing that healthcare outreach is best suited to the home and the family, which places women at the centre of the caring process. This does little to empower Thailand's mobile and migrant populations, including those people who are not considered to be citizens (McKinnon, 2005). Moreover, this approach does not engage with the sexual politics that mediate care, health and risk in everyday practice.

Practically, what I am suggesting is that NGOs, the Thai government and PLWHA themselves need to rethink the presumptions of an epidemiological model that places ill health and the care of the sick in the rural home. Creating positive identities before people become gravely ill is one way to address this problem. Another approach is to create outreach programmes that address the inequities of locally-situated outreach and take into account the mobile nature of the Thai population. Outreach programmes are needed that are as mobile as HIV/AIDS and the population living with this illness. Not everyone spends time in their rural home, and more importantly, not everyone goes home to die. Addressing positive health for HIV positive people from the upper north living in Bangkok might not only extend their lives, it might also mitigate the burden on those who are still living in rural

Thailand. However, it appears that new programmes and initiatives such as the implementation of highly active anti-retroviral treatments, are following the same path and ending up in the same place, the rural home. As a result, AIDS programmes may not necessarily be addressing the problem of a rural AIDS crisis, but may instead be paradoxically helping to create that crisis as men and women, who have no recourse once they become extremely ill, return home to die.

References

Altman D. (1994) *Power and Community: Organizational and Cultural Responses to AIDS.* Routledge, London and New York.

Bebbington A. (1997) New States, New NGOs? Crises and transitions among rural development NGOs in the Andean region. *World Dev* **25**(11): 1755–1765.

Bebbington A. Thiele, G. (1993) *Non-Governmental Organizations and the State in Latin America : Rethinking Roles in Sustainable Agricultural Development.* Routledge, London and New York.

Beyrer C. (1998) *War in the Blood: Sex, Politics and AIDS in Southeast Asia.* Zed Books, London and New York.

Brown M. (1995) Ironies of distance: An ongoing critique of the geographies of AIDS. *Environment and Planning D: Soc Space* **13**: 159–183.

Brown M. (1997) *Replacing Citizenship: AIDS Activism and Radical Democracy.* The Guilford Press, London and New York.

Bryant R. (2002) Non-governmental organizations and governmentality: Gon-suming biodiversity and indigenous people in the Philippines. *Pol Studies* **50**(2): 268–292.

Chiotti QP, Joseph AE. (1995) Casey house: Interpreting the location of a toronto AIDS hospice. *Soc Sci Med* **41**(1): 131–140.

Cochrane M. (2000) The politics of AIDS surveillance. *The Professional Geographer* **52**(2): 205–218.

Commins S. (1999) NGOs: Ladles in the global soup kitchen? *World Dev* **9**(5): 619–622.

Craddock S. (2000) Disease, social identity, and risk: Rethinking the geography of AIDS. *Trans Inst Brit Geograph* **25**(2): 153–169.

Craddock S. (2004) Beyond Epidemiology: Locating AIDS in Africa, in E Kalipeni, J Oppong & Jayati Ghosh (eds.) *HIV and AIDS in Africa: Beyond Epidemiology,* pp. 1-14, Blackwell Press, Malden, MA.

Del Casino VJ, Jr. (2000) *HIV/AIDS and the Spaces of Health Care in Thailand.* Unpublished Ph.D. Dissertation, Geography, University of Kentucky, Lexington.

Del Casino VJ, Jr. (2001a) Enabling geographies?: NGOs and the empowerment of people living with HIV and AIDS. *Dis Studies Quart* **21**(4): 19–29.

Del Casino VJ, Jr. (2001b) Healthier geographies: Mediating the gaps between HIV/AIDS and health care in Chiang Mai, Thailand. *Prof Geograph* **53**(3): 407–421.

Del Casino VJ, Jr. (2004) (Re)placing health and healthcare: Mapping the competing discourses and practices of 'traditional' and 'modern' Thai medicine. *Health Place* **10**(1): 59–73.

Del Casino VJ, Jr., Grimes A, Hanna SP, John Paul Jones, JP, III (2000) Methodological frameworks for the geography of organizations. *Geoforum* **31**: 523–538.

Delcore H. (2003) Nongovernmental organizations and the work of memory in Northern Thailand. *Am Ethnolog* **30**(1): 61–84.

Farmer P. (1992) *AIDS and Accusation: Haiti and the Geography of Blame.* University of California Press, Berkeley.

Farmer P. (1999) *Infections and Inequalities: The Modern Plagues.* University of California Press, Berkeley.

Farmer P, Connors M, Simmons J (eds.) (1996) *Women, Poverty, and AIDS: Sex, Drugs, and Structural Violence,* Common Courage Press, Monroe, ME.

Foucault M. (1997) Governmentality, in C Gordon & P Miller (eds.), *The Foucault Effect: Studies in Governmentality*, pp. 87-104, University of Chicago Press, Chicago.

Gatter PN. (1995) Anthropology, HIV and contigent identities. *Soc Sci and Med* **41**(11): 1523–1533.

Gould P. (1993) *The Slow Plague: A Geography of the AIDS Pandemic.* Blackwell, Oxford.

Killewo J, Dahlgren L, Sandström A. (1994) Socio-geographical patterns of hiv-1 transmission in kagera region, Tanzania. *Soc Sci Med* **38**(1): 129–134.

Knodel J, Saengtienchai C, Im-Em W. (2001) The impact of AIDS on parents and families in Thailand: A key informant approach. *Res Aging* **6**: 233–270.

Lam N, Lui K. (1994) Spread of AIDS in Rural America, 1982–1990. *J Acq Immun Def Synd* **7**:485–490.

Lyttleton C. (2000) *Endangered Relations: Negotiating Sex and AIDS in Thailand.* Harwood Academic Publishers, Singapore.

Lyttleton C. (2004) Fleeing the fire: Transformation and gendered belonging in Thai HIV/AIDS support groups. *Med Anthrop* **23**(1): 1–40.

Lyttleton C, Amarapibal A. (2002) Sister cities and easy passage: HIV, mobility and economies of desire in a Thai/Lao Border Zone. *Soc Sci Med* **54**(4): 505–519.

McKinnon K. (2005) (Im)Mobilisation and hegemony: 'Hill Tribe' subjects and the 'Thai' state. *Soc Cult Geography* **6**(1): 31–44.

Mills MB. (1999) *Thai Women in the Global Labor Force: Consuming Desires, Contested Selves.* Rutgers University Press, New Brunswick.

Nelson K, Suriyanon V., Taylor, E., *et al.* (1994) The incidence of HIV-1 infections in village populations of Northern Thailand. *AIDS* 8:951–5.

Patton C. (1990) *Inventing AIDS.* Routledge, London and New York.

Patton C. (1994) *Last Served? Gendering the HIV Pandemic.* Taylor and Francis, London.

Pokapanichwong W, Douglas D, Wright NH, Vanichseni S, Choopanya K. (1991) AIDS beliefs and behaviors among intravenous drug users in Bangkok. *Intl J Addict* 26(12): 1333–1347.

Pothisiri P, Tangcharoensathien V, Lertiendumrong J, Kasemsup V, Hanvoravongchai P. (1998) Funding Priorities for HIV/AIDS Crisis in Thailand. Paper read at 12th World AIDS Conference, at Geneva, Switzerland.

Pramualratana A. (1998) HIV/AIDS in Thailand UNAIDS Position Paper. ftp://lists.inet.co.th/pub/sea-aids/plpub/plpub21.txt Accessed 1 October 2004.

Pyle GF, Gross WA. (1997) The diffusion of HIV/AIDS and HIV infection in an archetypal textile county. *Appl Geograph Studies* 1 (1):63–81.

Rigg J, Ritchie M. (2002) Production, consumption and imagination in rural Thailand. *J Rural Studies* 18(4): 359–371.

Rojanapithayakorn W, Cox P, Bennoun R, Natpratan C, Doungsaa U. (1998) *Governance and HIV: Decentralization: An Aspect of Governance Critical to an Effective Response, A Case Study from Northern Thailand.* UNDP Regional Project on HIV and Development, New Delhi.

Shannon GW, Pyle GF, Bashur RL. (1991) *The Geography of AIDS.* The Guildford Press, London and New York.

Smallman-Raynor M, Cliff A, Haggett P. (1992) *London International Atlas of AIDS.* Blackwell, Oxford.

Takahashi LM. (1998) Concepts of Difference in Community Health, in RA Kearns & WM Gesler (eds.) *Putting Health Into Place: Landscape, Identity, and Well-Being,* pp. 143–67, Syracuse University Press, Syracuse.

Takahashi LM. (2001) *Homelessness, AIDS, and Stigmatization.* Oxford University Press, Oxford.

Tanabe S. (1998) Suffering and negotiation: Spirit-mediumship and HIV/AIDS self-help groups in Northern Thailand. *Tai Cult* 4 (1):93–112.

Tanabe S. (1999) *Practice and Self-governance: HIV/AIDS Self-help Groups in Northern Thailand.* 7th International Thai Studies Conference, 3–7, July, Amsterdam.

Thongchai W. (1994) *Siam Mapped.* University of Hawaii Press, Honolulu.

Treichler PA. (1992) AIDS, HIV, and the cultural construction of reality, in G Herdt & S Lindenbaum (eds.) *The Time of AIDS: Social Analysis, Theory, and Method,* pp. 65–98, Sage Publications, Newbury Park, NJ.

Treichler PA. (1999) *How to Have Theory in an Epidemic: Cultural Chronicles of AIDS.* Duke University Press, Durham, N.C. and London.

Ulack R, Skinner W. (1991) *AIDS and the Social Sciences*. University of Kentucky Press, Lexington.

Watney S. (1989) The spectacle of AIDS, in D Crimp (ed.) *AIDS: Cultural Analysis, Cultural Activism*, pp. 71–86, MIT Press, Cambridge.

Whippen D. (1987) Science fictions: The making of a medical model for AIDS. *Rad Am* **20**(6): 39–53.

Whittaker A. (2000) *Intimate Knowledge: Women and Their Health in North-East Thailand*. Allen and Unwin, St. Leornards, NSW.

Wilton R. (1996) Diminishing worlds? The impact of HIV/AIDS on the geography of daily life. *J Health Place* **2**(2): 1–16.

Wilton R. (1999) Qualitative health research: Negotiating life with HIV/AIDS. *Prof Geograph* **51**(2): 254–264.

Wolch JR. (1990) *The Shadow State: Government and the Voluntary Sector in Transition*. The Foundation Center, New York.

10

HIV/AIDS in Singapore: State Policies, Social Norms and Civil Society Action

Shir Nee Ong and Brenda SA Yeoh

Introduction

The first case of HIV infection in Singapore was detected in 1985 (MOH, 1997). Since then, increasing numbers of new cases have been reported each year. According to MOH (2005), 2,508 Singaporeans were HIV-positive at the end of June 2005, amongst them, 957 are asymptomatic carriers, 621 have full-blown AIDS and 930 have died. The reported rates of HIV infection and AIDS in Singapore per year have increased steeply within two decades from 0.8 per million population in 1985 to 89.2 per million population in 2004.

Other estimates suggest differing figures which are more alarming. Medical doctor Roy Chan, President for Action of AIDS (AfA, a local non-governmental organisation) said that the actual total figure was nearer 5,000, whereas UNAIDS programme estimates 12,000 people living with HIV/AIDS (PLWHA) in Singapore by 2001 (*Agence France-Presse*, 26 November 2001). Many people have not been tested for the disease because of the stigma attached and the fear of losing employment (*Agence France-Presse*, 26 November 2001). Under-reporting is likely to be significant

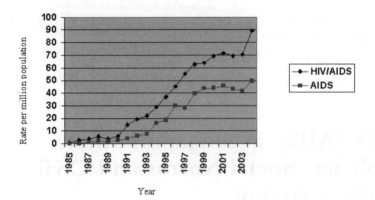

Fig. 1. Reported rates of HIV infection and AIDS in Singapore per year (1985–2004).

Source: Figure plotted with data from Ministry of Health MOH, 2005

and poses a major obstacle to a better understanding of the problem. MOH acknowledges the possibility that for every Singaporean detected with the AIDS virus, four others may have gone unreported (MOH, n.y.). Thus, the issue of HIV/AIDS in Singapore cannot be downplayed.

This chapter considers the dominant state and socio-cultural discourses that surround HIV/AIDS and PLWHA, and how these discourses attempt to discipline Singaporean bodies by encouraging 'safer sex' practices. Some discourses also (re)present HIV-positive bodies as 'deviant' bodies creating 'dis-ease' and therefore requiring regulation. This chapter also examines the extent of civil society activism and response through a consideration of how individuals and organisations help PLWHA in a number of ways, by providing 'space' for PLWHA to interact, by integrating them socio-spatially into the workplace, and through advocacy work in protecting their rights.[1]

---

[1] This study is based on in-depth interviews and archival research at Action for AIDS (AfA) and the Health Information Centre at the Health Promotion Board conducted in late 2002 and early 2003 (before the emergence of SARS outbreak in Singapore). People who help PLWHA were also interviewed to examine how non-state activism and response added another dimension to the dynamics of HIV/AIDS in Singapore. These consist of a medical staff from Communicable Disease Centre (CDC), two volunteers from Action for AIDS (AfA) who help PLWHA, and three employers and members of Business Coalition on AIDS Singapore (BCAS), who have employed/will employ PLWHA.

Spatial Patterns and Processes of HIV Seropositivity in Singapore

While HIV/AIDS poses a higher risk to the economically active and/or geographically mobile, the pattern of infection does cut across several boundaries — age, sexuality, ethnicity, gender, marital status and occupational status. Collectively, almost 90% of HIV-infected Singaporeans are aged 20 to 59, falling into the economically active group (MOH, 2005). Sexual transmission is the main mode of HIV infections among Singaporeans. Of the total 2,508 cases, about 74% of them were transmitted heterosexually, 15% homosexually, 8% bisexually and the remaining 3% through other modes such as intravenous drug use, perinatal (from mother to child), overseas renal transplant and blood transfusion (MOH, 2005). Heterosexual transmission has been the predominant mode since 1991, with most of these cases reported as contracted through casual sex and transactional sex with commercial sex workers (CSWs) in Singapore and overseas (MOH, 2005). However, it is possible that some infected homosexuals report themselves as heterosexual due to the stigma attached to homosexuality.

HIV infection cuts across ethnic boundaries where 84% infected are Chinese, 8% Malays, 5% Indians and 3% Others (MOH, 2003). However, when compared with the 2004 national-level ethnic composition of the country, i.e. 76% Chinese, 13.8% Malays, 8.4% Indians and 1.8% Others (Singstat, 2005), it is evident that Chinese and Others have a disproportionately larger representation in the HIV/AIDS figures. As the majority of HIV-infected Singaporeans are male, with 2,217 cases and female 291 cases, the sex ratio is very imbalanced at about eight males to one female, in a context where the national sex ratio is almost equal (MOH, 2005; Singstat, 2005). Among the males, 61% were single at the point of diagnosis, whereas 60% of the females were married (MOH, 2005). Married women are usually infected by their husbands.

HIV infection in Singapore also cuts across occupational boundaries. Service and sales workers account for 19.8%, while production craftsman/assemblers make up 18.4% (MOH, 2003). The disease does not only infect the low-skilled workers, but also semi-skilled workers in technical and clerical jobs (12.0%) and highly skilled managers and professionals

$(12.2\%)^2$ (MOH, 2003). Nevertheless, the health authorities announced in 2002 that the AIDS Education Programme would target men, especially blue-collar workers, since men aged between 20 to 59 accounted for nine in 10 HIV cases, with more than half holding blue-collar jobs (*The Straits Times*, 23 November 2002).

State Pragmatism, Control and Health Care Provision for HIV/AIDS

The Singapore government's pragmatic health care policies tend to approach AIDS in a single-sided manner, i.e. emphasising *preventive* measures through AIDS education, especially by disciplining bodies, rather than *restorative* health care like subsidising antiretrovirals or funding research in infectious and parasitic diseases (IPDs).[3] While comparable in many years to developed countries in terms of its advanced medical technology and services, Singapore tends to lack the political and social commitment to provide adequate restorative health care such as subsidised antiretrovirals, hence attracting the criticism of being 'a Third World country for HIV victims' (*Agence France-Presse*, 26 November 2001).

In response to increasing HIV/AIDS cases in Singapore, the government disseminates information on HIV/AIDS, encourages fidelity, abstinence and 'safer sex' practices (i.e. use of condoms). AIDS education advertisements in Singapore (MOH, 1988–1995) have adopted *behaviour-based* and/or *pro-family* approaches to discourage casual sex and to 'docilise' bodies to prevent familial disintegration since the early 1990s. Recently, 'scare tactics' of gory photographs of people with sexually transmitted diseases (STDs) are used to warn youths against pre-marital sex (*Agence France-Presse*, 12 December 2002). Here, the government's campaigns regulate Singaporeans by treating

---

[2]Ideally, it is important to compare the occupational statistics with national statistics to glean deeper insight. However the national statistics does not coincide with the categories used for HIV/AIDS statistics; the 2004 Population Census has consolidated certain categories like 'Sales & Services' with 'Clerical', as well as 'Professional' with 'Managerial' and 'Technical'.

[3]It was the outbreak of Severe Acute Respiratory Syndrome (SARS) in Singapore and worldwide in 2003 that led to a rethinking of existing policy. The Singapore government has since realised that infectious diseases cannot be overlooked and launched a joint research facility with the United States to research on SARS and other IPDs (*The Business Times*, 8 May 2003).

their bodies as tools to a 'Healthy Singapore'. The success of such an approach is however debatable.

In a recent survey conducted by the Singapore Press Holdings on 335 singles aged 25 to 49, 60% of the men have had multiple partners, compared with 40% of the women, and 30% of the men and 10% of the women have had one-night stands (*The Straits Times*, 29 September 2003). In a survey conducted by a tertiary research centre on undergraduates' sexual attitudes, about one in six has had pre-marital sex, only slightly more than a third (35.8%) among them use protection all the time (*The Straits Times*, 1 November 2003). A 2002 global sex survey revealed even more disturbing results with half of the 868 Singaporeans aged 16 to over 30 surveyed admitting to not practising safe sex (*The Straits Times*, 1 November 2003).

The healthcare delivery system in Singapore is based on personal responsibility, allied to government subsidies to maintain basic affordable healthcare, since '[w]hichever way we choose to finance the cost of healthcare, the burden ultimately falls on the people [either directly or through taxes]' (MOH, 1993:13). Patients are required to pay a portion of their medical expenditure, and expected to pay more when they demand better services. There are three general schemes, namely Medisave, Medishield and Medifund, to encourage Singaporeans to be responsible for their own health by saving for medical expenses (MOH, 2001–2003). In terms of specific health policies on HIV/AIDS, the government emphasises *prevention* and *education* (*The Straits Times*, 17 July 2001). In response to appeals from some members of the public and AfA for subsidisation of expensive antiretrovirals, the state has responded by citing *optimal* allocation for not subsidising, since HIV/AIDS (unlike cancer, heart disease, stroke and diabetes) is not among the top killers in Singapore; and antiretrovirals are considered *experimental* rather than *effective* drugs that allow recovery (*The Straits Times*, 9 December 1999).

PLWHA have to bear the full costs of antiretrovirals if they need the medication. However, like patients suffering from other diseases, PLWHA may withdraw up to S$550 a month from their Medisave accounts (provided there are sufficient funds). A 'cocktail' of imported AIDS drugs can prolong patients' lives for 10–15 years, but would cost S$1,200–S$1,500 a month (*Agence France-Presse*, 26 November 2001). The costs of antiretrovirals in Singapore are still the highest in the region, and some patients have gone to Thailand to buy cheaper drugs or have skipped medication altogether (*Agence France-Presse*, 26 November 2001). According to AfA, more than 70% of PLWHA in Singapore cannot afford any form of antiretrovirals, and fewer than ten percent are on optimum treatment (*Agence France-Presse*, 26 November 2001). Also, no government funds have been specifically allocated for AIDS research (*The Straits Times*, 24 May 1999).

Significant transmission of HIV infection occurs through the movement and interaction of people both domestically and internationally. Thus, countries often restrict the travel movement of PLWHA, hoping this would contain the diffusion. Singapore, like some other countries, requires mandatory HIV-antibody testing of *all* foreign students and employees, and deports HIV-infected foreigners. 'Safer sex' information and condoms are provided to Singapore national servicemen who go for overseas training; they have to undergo compulsory HIV-antibody medical examination upon their return. From 2003, Singapore men travelling alone overseas (to 'high risk countries') are given 'safe-sex' packs which include condoms, toiletries and information on the dangers of casual sex — a new approach adopted by the health authorities in collaboration with tour agencies (*The Straits Times*, 23 November 2002). AIDS is to some extent regarded as an imported or foreign disease which can be guarded against by careful policing of national borders.

Recently, a battery of new initiatives and tests for HIV were launched in Singapore. At the end of 2004, for example, HIV testing was made a standard of care during pregnancy. In 2005, an oral-based rapid HIV test kit has been made available, allowing non-invasive and quick testing for HIV without the need for a blood test.

Public (Mis)Conceptions and 'Dis-ease' Relating to HIV/AIDS Policies and PLWHA

In the research on the social aspects of HIV/AIDS, the common notion of stigma creating social boundaries, for example, in the form of an 'us'/'them' divide between PLWHA and non-PLWHA is widely acknowledged (Hull, n.y.; Crawford, 1994 cited in Green & Sobo, 2000). These boundaries are not fixed but nuanced and differentially experienced, varying with mode of infection and socio-cultural context. In Singapore, the structural conditions of an inherently heterosexist and family-oriented setting coupled with the lack of anti-discrimination laws (towards PLWHA, the disabled etc.) have aided in the (re)production of stigma towards PLWHA, as well as the exclusion of PLWHA from various social and economic spaces.

On the international stage, Nelson Mandela (*Third World Network*, 2000) had emphasised that "We need to break the silence, banish stigma and discrimination, and ensure total inclusiveness within the struggle against AIDS." (Third World Network, 2000). On World AIDS Day 2003, an unprecedented visit to PLWHA (with hand-shaking) at a Beijing hospital by Chinese Premier Wen Jiabao sent an important political and social message that China is determined to fight AIDS and stigma, and PLWHA are not to be feared (*South China Morning Post*, 2 December 2003). Indeed, it was argued in the Singapore press that 'gestures such as this break down prejudice better than a thousand appeals to see sufferers as victims, not enemies. Countries must seek to break the grip of stigma by providing the treatment that enables HIV sufferers to keep contributing to society. AIDS must be seen as a disease, not a curse' (*The Straits Times*, 4 December 2003).

However, in Singapore, World AIDS Day 2003 was quiet with no public display of the government's commitment to combat AIDS, whether in the form of symbolic visits to PLWHA or calls for increasing tolerance and socio-spatial integration of PLWHA. Public messages which aimed at increasing acceptance and integration of former criminals and mental patients in Singapore's society have been visible in the media and public spaces for some time now, such as in the newspapers, on television, at Mass Rapid Transit (MRT) stations, at bus stops and on buses. Yet, such messages were not extended to include the social integration of PLWHA. At least up to 2003, the elimination of stigma and the integration of PLWHA did not appear high on the state agenda in the fight against AIDS.

More recently, it is encouraging to note that the government has stepped up its fight against HIV/AIDS. During the biennial Fourth Singapore AIDS Conference in November 2004, the Senior Minister of State for Health Dr Balaji Sadasivan, reiterated that as a general principle, "Every AIDS patient must be treated with dignity and compassion. We must champion the right of AIDS patients not to be discriminated against". However, how this has been translated into specific policies is fraught terrain as some of the new initiatives and changes to health policies on HIV/AIDS invite controversy.

As mentioned earlier, while most of the cases by heterosexual transmission were contracted through casual sex and transactional sex with commercial sex workers (CSWs) in Singapore and overseas, there is a recent trend of increasing married women who have become infected with HIV, usually from their husbands. In response, a new rule has been recently implemented to inform spouses of HIV-positive patients of their partner's infection, regardless of whether the infected person agrees (*The Straits Times*, 15 July 2005). This is an unprecedented move and tantamount to official sanction to breach patient confidentiality to protect the vulnerable. MOH set up an HIV Prevention Unit with trained personnel to inform spouses in a sensitive way to reduce the possibility of doctors-patients' conflicts. Over the space of five months from July to December 2005, 41 women were informed of their husbands' HIV-positive status by hand-delivered letters and advised to get themselves tested for the virus (*The Straits Times*, 7 Dec 2005).

Recently, MOH has also introduced changes in the treatment of potential HIV/AIDS patients (*The Straits Times*, 15 July 2005). The previous requirement of a doctor getting a patient's consent and providing pre-test counselling before doing an HIV test is no longer necessary. Rather, the patient only needs to be 'appropriately kept informed' of the test. This implies that doctors are now expected to instruct a blood test if a patient shows HIV/AIDS symptoms, in a similar manner to instructing a chest X-ray if lung cancer is suspected. According to Dr Balaji, the logic here is that HIV patients, like people with other health issues, are entitled to early diagnosis and appropriate treatment.

Rather than attempt to take full responsibility for HIV/AIDS education, the state is conscious that it needs to strategically engage non-state actors and stakeholders to reach the wider community. MOH welcomes its citizenry and civil groups to contribute ideas to combat the illness. According to Dr Balaji, "My Ministry does not have a monopoly on ideas to stop AIDS. We will continue to engage and work with the community. We will periodically review our strategies and be ready to make changes as necessary. In other words, we will have an open mind to all suggestions even if we do not agree with them at this point in time" (4th Singapore AIDS Conference).

At the same time, the state takes a clear–cut stand in its policy approach to the disease. MOH has consolidated four HIV/AIDS education messages that it wants to communicate to the public. These are:

(1) Have only one sex partner and be faithful to that person.
(2) If a person is engaging in casual sex, the person should practise safe sex.
(3) If a person has multiple sex partners, and if there is unprotected sex, the person is at a high risk of contracting HIV/AIDS. Thus, we advise frequent testing for HIV.
(4) If a person is HIV positive, it is a criminal offence for that person not to inform his or her sex partner of the HIV status.

By and large, state-produced educational materials on HIV/AIDS are underwritten by the state's definition of what constitutes the sexual norm, i.e. responsible heterosexual behaviour towards one's spouse. Particularly with regard to AIDS prevention education for the young, the state stresses the importance of family and community values and the need to avoid casual sex. In Dr Balaji's words, "Young people need to be educated on the danger of AIDS and taught family values that promote abstinence and fidelity. We must discourage promiscuity and casual sex.... We must ensure that our AIDS prevention message does not give the impression that casual sex is OK so long as you use a condom' (*The Straits Times*, 7 Dec 2005). While safety within monogamous relationships form the foundation of the state approach to HIV/AIDS education, pragmatism dictates that the state also encourages safe sex practices in the case of 'high risk' groups (even as it continues to reiterate that casual sex is still risky even with condom use, as condoms do not reduce the health risk to zero). However, the state does not support a "stand-alone condom use" message for the general public, in order to prevent youths from thinking that causal sex is all right. Wary that HIV/AIDS prevention messages featuring condom use may inadvertently promote promiscuity or erode family values, MOH is careful to use more covert means of promoting condom use as opposed to explicit means such as 'condom parades' as used in some countries such as Thailand. Instead, the condom use message is targeted at 'high risk' groups such as homosexuals and people who visit red light districts in Singapore or overseas. For these 'high risk' groups, the state advocates frequent testing for HIV and emphasises personal responsibility by criminalising the failure to inform one's sex partner of one's HIV-positive status. This is in response to feedback received by MOH that some HIV-positive persons have been deliberately spreading the disease as a form of 'revenge' on society.

Civil Society Responses

Generally, the political climate in Singapore is quiescent with the government setting the tone of government-people relations through censorship and out-of-bounds (OB) markers. Thus, a rather depoliticised civil society exists alongside a paternalistic and omnipresent state. In a recent speech by former Deputy Prime Minister Lee Hsien Loong (*The Straits Times*, 7 January 2004), he outlined the future of Singapore politics and society by emphasising the government's continual efforts towards more openness and consultation, as well as building a civic society[4] and engendering civic participation, but within certain guidelines. For example, it was reiterated that criticism and actions should not be out to score political points and undermine the government, and 'crusading journalism' should be avoided. The speech sparked off both optimistic and cynical responses among Singaporeans; with some applauding the increasing opportunities for citizen participation in civic and political affairs, whilst others arguing that setting parameters around what constitutes openness is ridden with paradoxes and that more needs be done to stimulate a more active and independent civil society (*The Straits Times*, 10 January 2004a; 10 January 2004b; 13 January 2004).

Within such a socio-political context, individuals and non-governmental organisations tend to steer clear of politicising their agendas (especially given that some who appear to have crossed the OB markers were roundly chastised by the government). In terms of civil society responses towards helping PLWHA, most groups in Singapore (with some key exceptions as will be discussed later) take a non-confrontational approach, focusing primarily on

---

[4]The term 'civic society' has been the favoured term used by the Singapore government all along. 'Civic society implies groups with values of collaboration, personal responsibilities and courteous regard for others. Civil society, however, refers to groups of individuals concerned about rights and who keep a vigilant watch on a government that they view with suspicion. "The latter is political; the former is meant to be apolitical", says political scientist Kenneth Tan' (*The Straits Times*, 10 Jan 2004a).

providing material assistance (e.g. employment and financial help), creating 'space' for PLWHA, and changing mindsets regarding PLWHA and the disease through education.

As mentioned earlier, HIV/AIDS infects mostly people who fall into the economically active group (20–59 years old). It is thus very much a workplace issue and businesses have an important role to play. As the manager of a worldwide clothing brand explains,

> [HIV/AIDS] is not an issue that we can just rely on one government department or one organisation; ... it's a *collective responsibility*... [B]usinesses should take their own positions... [and] deal with HIV and the impact it'll have on the workplace....

PLWHA face barriers to employment as most businesses and organisations are reluctant to employ people with HIV. However, it is encouraging that some companies in Singapore such as The Body Shop, Levi Strauss and Porcupine (a local grocery company) have explicitly announced their willingness to employ them, if they have the right qualifications and experience, and have formed the Business Coalition on AIDS Singapore (BCAS) during the Singapore Business Forum (2002). According to its Executive Director, the Singapore National Employers' Federation (SNEF)[5] has been working with BCAS, AfA, Communicable Disease Centre (CDC), MOH, Ministry of Manpower (MOM) and other organisations to set employment guidelines to reduce prejudices against PLWHA and to handle HIV/AIDS in the workplace (Singapore Business Forum 2002).[6] This is a welcome change as SNEF currently permits termination of an HIV-positive employee if a large number of colleagues are unwilling to work with this person... [and] if employers construe AIDS as a disease contracted through 'misconduct', they need not bear the medical expenses for AIDS treatment for the worker (Leong, 1997).

---

[5]SNEF has 1,900 corporate members and represents employers at various national tripartite discussions, including those of the National Wage Council.

[6]Recently, the AIDS Business Alliance was launched to bring to the workplace "an AIDS education programme that will educate workers on AIDS prevention and fight discrimination against HIV-positive workers by teaching workers how to work with their HIV-positive co-workers" (*The Straits Times*, 7 Dec 2005).

These companies affiliated to BCAS provide their HIV-positive employees with regular medical benefits and do not impose compulsory HIV-antibody testing on their employees. If any employee declares his/her seropositivity, it will be kept confidential and only key managers need to know. In one company, the three PLWHA employed worked in the back office as the manager felt that they were better suited there and not in the frontline as sales personnel. The company also encourages ongoing AIDS education in response to the discomfort expressed by some co-workers who were uncomfortable when they get cuts, as they worry that the virus in the air would settle on the wound (even though HIV is not airborne). In another company, the manager has chosen to deploy the four or five PLWHA under her charge at the frontline as cashiers, as she does not believe in relegating them to back spaces and prefer to 'treat them as normal people'. At one point, this resulted in a 90% drop in sales, primarily because she was mis-quoted in the Chinese language press saying that 20 to 30 employees on her business premises were HIV-positive. Nevertheless, the manager continued with her policy of employing PLHWA as she felt that this provided them dignity and helped them see that 'life is worth living'.

Beyond the workplace, other organisations focus on providing spaces for social interaction and networking among PLWHA. A senior nurse who works in Patient Care Centre (PCC) in CDC believes in 'giving peo-ple [PLWHA] their space back'. PCC acts as a meeting place for inter-action among PLWHA, volunteers and medical staff and a safe haven for PLWHA. The well-being of PLWHA is improved in four ways: firstly, the PLWHA gather at the clinic and interact among themselves to share coping strategies; secondly, the PLWHA participate in normal socio-spatial interactions with volunteers and medical staff such as cooking, serving them meals and dining with them as a step towards integrating the PLWHA into society; thirdly, medical staff are better positioned to advise them on issues of health and welfare; and lastly, homeless PLWHA who are rejected by their families can stay in the CDC. Besides these 'formal' functions, PCC serves as a place to network with other PLWHA, e.g., in helping to locate someone going abroad (to India or Thailand, for instance) to pur-chase cheaper, generic drugs (although patients are not encouraged to do so).

PCC's 'Sponsor Workers Scheme' provides financial assistance for PLWHA from the lower socio-economic groups and employs patients for four hours each day on weekdays in return for a monthly stipend of $400, a food ration and daily lunch. The senior nurse at the PCC explained that this self-funded programme involves 23 patients who work on staggered shifts to make fabric roses and other handicrafts that are sold at the pushcart and at charity fundraisers alongside volunteers. She also remarked that the sale of handicrafts provides an opportunity to educate the public regarding AIDS, as more Singaporeans are open to this 'soft approach' and are thus more willing to help, in contrast to the 'hard approach' using activist demonstrations and the like, which she felt would not work in Singapore, given the socio-cultural and legal context.

Each year, several PLWHA face a homeless plight due to rejection from their families (*The Straits Times*, 30 Dec 2003). Although the PCC (Homeless) Fund was started in 2000 after homeless PLWHA were featured in the press, no more than S$3,000 of the collected S$20,000 has been used, as homeowners did not want to rent rooms or flats to PLWHA (*The Straits Times*, 30 Dec 2003). Since 2000, nursing homes, hospices and community hospitals have been permitted to receive PLWHA, but the CDC places only the terminally ill in nursing homes (*The Straits Times*, 30 Dec 2003). Other organisations which offer help include the AfA, which set up an HIV/AIDS halfway house[7] in 2002 to provide temporary lodging and the Beatitudes (part of the Catholic AIDS Response Effort), which rented an apartment in 2002 for 12 homeless PLWHA (*The Straits Times*, 30 Dec 2003). The CDC itself also houses a few of the homeless PLHWA.

Contrary to the PCC's 'soft approach', AfA takes a much stronger stand in advocating for the rights of PLWHA. In mid 2000, there was intense public discussion on the deportation of 12 foreign PLWHA (11 women and one man) in April 1999 and the potential deportation of nine foreign HIV-positive women, all of whom were married to Singaporeans (*The Straits Times*, 18 May 2000; 24 May 2000; 25 May 2000; *The Sunday Times*, 14 May 2000; 21 May 2000). AfA wrote a letter of appeal to President S R Nathan and hoped that the government would be humanitarian and flexible in enforcing these regulations, as these people have families in Singapore

---

[7] AfA had wanted to set up an AIDS hospice several years ago, but according to one of the committee members, the plan was not approved by the government and hence failed to materialise.

(*Inter Press Service*, 24 May 2000). Consequently, the government reversed the ban and allowed the foreign women to remain, promising to review the cases of the 12 who had left (*The Sunday Times*, 28 May 2000).

AfA was also at the forefront of advocacy work in appealing against the regulation which stated that deceased people with HIV had to be double-bagged and cremated within 24 hours. Initially, MOH 'claim[ed] that the HIV virus remains active for several days in the body of the deceased. As such, embalming is outlawed to minimise the risk of transmission...Without embalming, a body decomposes rapidly in Singapore's tropical heat, thus justifying the 24-hour cremation ruling'. AfA argued that such a rule is 'contrary to the norms of internationally accepted practices' and discriminatory towards PLWHA (*Inter Press Service*, 24 May 2000) and was eventually able to overturn the regulation (Chan, 2001).

In contrast to the state's approach to HIV/AIDS education which emphasises heterosexual monogamous relationships as its basic plank (while remaining silent on other sexualities), the AfA, along with some non-state actors such as Fridae.com (an online gay portal based in Hong Kong, www.fridae.com), have argued that as there are different modes of sexual behaviour, different target groups will require different messages or motivation to induce or sustain changes in sexual behaviour. Instead of one generalised approach to behavioural change as advocated by the state, they have favoured a more diversified approach including designing AIDS awareness materials tailored to their target groups such as men who have sexual intercourse with men (MSM). In promoting safer sex practices and HIV/AIDS education not only among heterosexuals, but also among those whose sexual behaviour falls outside the legal norm,[8] AfA exemplifies a rights-based, advocacy-oriented form of civil action not commonly found in Singapore's civil society landscape, which appears to be gathering strength despite the unfavourable political environment. In fact, Dr Balaji recently said that the government has now realised that AIDS education materials 'have to be customised for this high-risk group [gays]' and that MOH 'will work with

---

[8] In Singapore, under Section 377A of the Penal Code, there is a mandatory term of imprisonment for 'gross indecency' (i.e. oral sex, mutual masturbation or touching of genitals) between two males, either for committing or attempting to commit the act, and regardless of the location (private or public space). So far, only males have been criminalised for homosexual acts. However, in principle, certain lesbian acts can be charged under Section 20 of the Miscellaneous Offences (Public Order and Nuisance) Act (Cap. 184) (Leong, 1997: 130-131).

NGOs like AfA to develop these customised programmes' (*The Straits Times*, 7 December 2005). This is a heartening sign in view of the growing threat of HIV/AIDS in Singapore, for the state cannot afford to ignore it but will have to count on the help of businesses, religious groups and community organisations and activists of all stripes in its efforts to combat the disease.

Acknowledgements

We would like to thank the National University of Singapore for the financial support of the research upon which this paper is based. It is important to extend our heartfelt gratitude to the PLWHA, volunteers, caregivers, corporate personnel, and others who participated in this study by contributing their time and opinions generously. An earlier version of this paper was presented at the international workshop – *Social Science and AIDS in Southeast Asia: Inventory of Research Projects, Priorities and Prospects for the Future*, 10–12 November 2003, in Chiang Mai, Thailand. Responsibility for the paper, however, rests entirely with the authors.

References

4th Singapore AIDS Conference, 27 November 2004, Singapore International Convention and Exhibition Centre.

Agence France-Presse (26 November 2001) Singapore-AIDS: Singapore a Third World Country for HIV Victims: Activists. Available at http://www.aegis.com/news/afp/2001/AF011193.html

Agence France Presse (12 December 2002) *Singapore-AIDS: Singapore to Use Shock Tactics to Steer Teens Away from Sex*. Available at http://www.aegis.com/news/afp/2002/AF0212B2.html

Chan R. (2001) Editorial, *The Act*, issue 24. Available at http://afa.org.sg/issue/issue24/editorial.htm

Green G, Sobo E (eds.). (2000) Dangerous identities: Stigmas and stories, in *The Endangered Self: Managing the Social Risk of HIV*, pp. 10–30, Routledge, London.

Hull T. (n.y.) *HIV/AIDS in South East Asia: Stigma as a Barrier to Understanding*. Available at http://www.gaje.net.au/hivnotes.htm

Inter Press Service (24 May 2000) *Rights-Singapore: Deportation of People with HIV Stirs Row*. Available at http://www.aegis.com/news/ips/2000/IP000506.html

Leong W-T L. (1997) Singapore, in DJ West & R Green (eds.), *Sociolegal Control of Homosexuality: A Multi-nation Comparison*, pp. 127–144, Plenum Press, New York.

MITA (2003) *Severe Acute Respiratory Syndrome: Fighting SARS Together!* Available at http://www.sars.gov.sg

MOH (n.y.) *Health Educator: AIDS — What Is and What Is Not.* Available at http://www.gov.sg/moh/health/nhe/health_educator/vol19/aids.html

MOH (1988–95) *AIDS Television Commercials (1988–1995)* video tape, Singapore, AIDS Awareness Campaign, Training & Health Education Department.

MOH (1993) *Affordable Health Care: a White Paper.* Singapore National Printers.

MOH (1997) *HIV/AIDS Situation in Singapore, 28 November.* Available at http://www.gov.sg/ moh/health/releases/aids-edu.html

MOH (2001–3) *Your Health Dollar: Health Care Financing in Singapore.* Available at http://app.moh.gov.sg/you/you01.asp

MOH (2002) *Update on the HIV/AIDS Situation in Singapore,* Press Release, 22 November. Available at http://app.moh.gov.sg/new/new02.asp?id=1&mid= 5060

MOH (2003) *New Cases of HIV Infection Reported This Year,* Press Release, 24 November. Available at http://app.moh.gov.sg/new/new02.asp?id=1&mid= 8700

MOH (2005). *Update on Singaporeans Infected with AIDS,* Press Release, 1 December. Available at http://www.moh.gov.sg/corp/about/newsroom/ pressreleases/details .do?id=34963469

Singapore Business Forum (2002) *Managing HIV/AIDS in the Workplace,* 22 Nov, organised by AfA.

Singstat (2005) *Statistics on Singapore: Keystats — People.* Available at http://www. singstat. gov.sg/keystats/people.html#demo

South China Morning Post (2 December 2003) *Premier Brings the Fight Against Aids into the Open.*

The Business Times (8 May 2003) *Joint US-S'pore Facility to Study SARS, Other Diseases.*

The Straits Times (24 May 1999) *Cheaper HIV Treatment Needs Research.*

The Straits Times (9 December 1999) *HIV Treatment: No Govt Subsidies.*

The Straits Times (18 May 2000) *Let Women with HIV Stay On.*

The Straits Times (24 May 2000) *HIV Tests for Foreigners to Protect Public Health.*

The Straits Times (25 May 2000) *HIV-stricken Spouses Are Not a Risk to Public Health.*

The Straits Times (17 July 2001) *HIV/Aids Patients Receive Subsidised Care.*

The Straits Times (23 November 2002) *Soon, Safe-sex Packs for Male Travellers.*

The Straits Times (29 September 2003) *Sex and Singles.*

The Straits Times (1 November 2003) *Survey of NTU Undergrads: Protection During Sex? No Thanks.*

The Straits Times (4 December 2003) *Take AIDS Head-on.*

The Straits Times (7 January 2004) *DPM Lee Promises a More Open Singapore.*

The Straits Times (10 January 2004a) *Of OB Markers and Growing Open Spaces.*

The Straits Times (10 January 2004b) *A More Open Society, a More Exciting Singapore.*

The Straits Times (13 January 2004) *A Response to DPM Lee's Speech: Time to Do Some Crystal-ball Gazing.*

The Straits Times (15 July 2005) *HIV Patients' Spouses Will Now Be Told.*

The Straits Times (7 Dec 2005) *The Aids Battle: A Family Affair.*

The Sunday Times (14 May 2000) *Coping with AIDS in Family.*

The Sunday Times (21 May 2000) *No Room for Mercy?*

The Sunday Times (28 May 2000) *Repatriation Reversal: Govt Relents on Ban of HIV-infected Alien Spouses.*

Third World Network (2000) *Nelson Mandela Speaks Out Against AIDS*, December. Available at http://www.twnside.org.sg/title/2132.htm

SECTION 4
POPULATION MOBILITY AND
INFECTIOUS DISEASES IN ASIA

11

Cultivating the Market: Mobility, Labour and Sexual Exchange in Northwest Laos

Chris Lyttleton

Introduction

Development increases human movement; this is clear whether one considers trajectories of social change across time or analyses of human settlement across space. Not coincidentally, new infectious diseases are appearing regularly throughout the world. Their (re) emergence is often related to issues of development and mobile populations act as key vectors in their transmission (Morse, 1995; Wilson, 1995). Even as diseases such as Human Immunodeficiency Virus (HIV) and Severe Acute Respiratory Syndrome (SARS) have turned a glaring spotlight on links between migration and public health vulnerability, the specific dynamics underlying different forms of population movement that afford this connection are often ignored or taken for granted (Guest, 2000: 76). Quite reasonably, much attention has been on relatively overt forms of international labour migration and the attendant risks faced by migrants locked into social and economic relations over which they do not always have adequate control. We now have a far clearer sense of how HIV moves between certain populations through studies, for example, that expose how border dynamics transpose everyday sociality into risk and disease transmission or that examine how insidious forms of exploitation occurring within hierarchical structures of labour exchange both within and between nations create damaging impacts on migrant bodies.

More recently, it has been argued that we also need to consider "real dangers of infection through other forms of mobility that are inherent in the week-to-week, or even day-to-day behaviour of the population as a whole" (Skeldon, 2000). The logic behind this shift in focus is that while there are indeed hot spots where migrants are susceptible to (potentially) high levels of HIV infection, closer analysis shows that movement in a more generic sense is characteristic of huge numbers of people throughout the world. It is the very complexity of different movement dynamics that raises the need for more nuanced analysis if we are to appreciate the ongoing nexus of mobility and HIV risk. Not all movement can be categorised as migration. Furthermore, it is behaviours at key intersections of mobile and non-mobile groups that create the opportunity for increasing HIV transmission, and not movement per se. The pressing questions then become whether movement promotes new forms of behaviour at specific nodes where different populations conjoin (Skeldon, 2000); and if so, what are the underlying social, cultural and economic forces that foster these new forms of behaviour? It is to these questions that I turn in this chapter by looking at mobility and changing social interactions in one small mountain valley in Northwest Lao PDR (forthwith Laos).[1]

Infrastructure Development in Northwestern Laos

The upper Mekong region (UMR), has long been the focus of ambitious plans to promote transnational mobility. In the 19th century, British and French colonial powers explored the region in search of land-based trade routes linking mainland Southeast Asia to China. The French built a railway

---

[1]This chapter is based on ethnographic fieldwork conducted over six months in 2003 and 2004, in Sing and Long District, Luang Namtha Province, Laos (see Fig. 1). This study formed part of a larger project conducted in collaboration with the Lao Institute for Research on Culture, supported by Rockefeller Foundation and Macquarie University. Parts of this paper are excerpted from that project's research report 'Watermelons, Bars and Trucks: Dangerous Intersections in Northwest Laos' (Lyttleton et al., 2004).

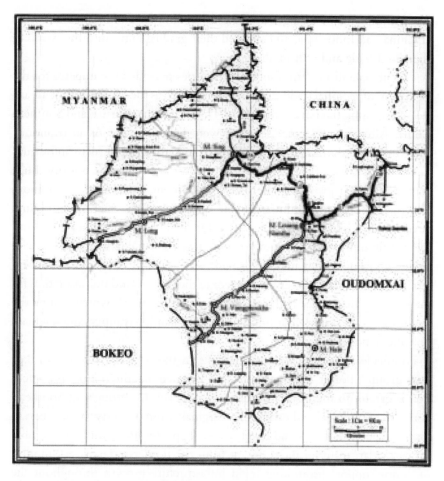

Fig. 1. The research site: Route 17 between M Sing and M Long
Source: Adapted from Chamberlain, 2000.

from Haiphong to Kunming (Yunnan) via the Red River and the British considered the construction of a railway from Northern Thailand. Prior to World War II, the Chinese acknowledged the importance of the resource-rich Yunnan province for trade between India and China, and built a road between Kunming and the frontier with Burma. Subsequent global and regional political events prevented the development of further cross-border transport and trade connections for more than 50 years. The breakup of the Soviet Union and its support to aligned countries in the late 1980s set the scene for major changes in economic policy in Communist countries of China and Indochina, and allowed their gradual entry into the world of liberalised trade and industrialisation.

This liberalisation within socialist countries provided the impetus for the formation of regional trading arrangements, such as the "economic quadrangle" comprising the border regions of Thailand, Laos, Burma, and Southern China. After private sector schemes were halted by the Asian economic crash in 1997, the Asian Development Bank took the lead in infrastructure development of the region. Transportation has been a priority; huge loans have been provided for road development, including an ambitious ring road linking the countries of the upper Mekong. Such infrastructure developments have major implications for the lives and livelihoods of both the people in existing proximity to the new thoroughfares and those who are drawn from further afield to provide services along these routes. Recent analyses suggest that Laos is set to become the hub of land transportation for the Greater Mekong Sub-region, especially in the north which will be the nexus of a road system that links China, Thailand, Myanmar and Vietnam (Chamberlain, 2000).

Foreshadowing the focus on migrants in the Mekong region as a key "risk group", Porter and Bennoun (1997) argued that the risk of HIV infection is greater in the case of border area populations throughout Southeast Asia, due to political and economic marginalisation, poverty, poor access to markets, public services and employment opportunities, and high mobility (in particular, from localities distant from the borders). The large amounts of donor support promoting rapid infrastructure growth throughout the region have drawn attention to high levels of mobility, but few studies have documented on-the-ground effects in northern Laos. In particular, the styles of engagement between mobile and non-mobile populations as Laos is criss-crossed by new transport channels have received little attention. Likewise, at the time of writing, there has been no effective HIV surveillance in Luang Namtha, a northern Lao province through which the economic quadrangle ring road passes. Levels of HIV infection (if any) in populations affected by these developments are simply unknown. In the absence of epidemiological data, it becomes necessary to consider corollary factors that might foreshadow or provide surrogate measures for vulnerability. There are no empirical figures that can enumerate precise risk quotients, but there are multiple behavioural contexts that are worthy of consideration. This chapter focuses on the conjunction of population movement and changing cultural norms to throw light on the severity of the current situation in northern Laos.

People and Place — The Road through Sing and Long

Sing and Long are two adjoining districts in Luang Namtha Province in Northwest Laos. They are cut by a valley that runs from the China border down to the Mekong River and Burma (and Thailand downriver). In the late 1990s, one million dollars from the World Bank upgraded a haphazard trail into an all-weather highway running through this valley. The completion of Route 17B, a small 80 km road bisecting the northwest corner of Laos where it joins China and Burma, parallels the bigger thoroughfares under construction: it provides a microcosm of the complex social interactions between local and transient populations. It also highlights that HIV risk emerges from a complicated mix of cultural, political and economic changes that accompany development.

The impact of Route 17B's completion in 2000 radiates in numerous directions. The road has and continues to play a key role in bringing development to the people of Sing and Long. It has concretely anchored a vast number of material and social forces that have an impact on almost every resident within the two districts. On the one hand, the road has played a significant role in promoting in-migration. Large numbers of Chinese now travel into or through Sing and Long. On the other hand, increased flows of goods, people and ideas have also transformed local social and demographic structures. Ethnic groups that lived in the mid and upper slopes of the mountains surrounding the valley for centuries are quickly moving down to be near the road and the market opportunities it represents. As large numbers of traditionally subsistent Akha relocate closer to paddy fields, traders and transport routes, the resulting articulation of social relations, bodies and minds requires new social competencies, in particular, with regard to wage labour. Recent developments have thus forged a crucible in the valleys where lowland residents, Chinese labourers and resettled Akha engage in forms of market-based economic and social relations that in turn have specific health consequences. One of these is the heightened potential for HIV to be rapidly spreading in Northern Laos.

The estimated population of Luang Namtha Province in 1998 was 124,600 (63,700 female), of which 97.7% are ethnic minorities (Chamberlain, 2000). The population of Muang Sing district in 2003 was 29,307 and 23,594 in Muang Long. The relatively small population in the two districts has fluctuated due to a long history of political upheavals ranging from the murderous incursions of invading armies from Thailand in the 19th Century, the influx of Tai Lue immigrants from Southern Sipsongpanna fleeing land collectivisation programmes and the turmoil created by the *Lao Issara* (Free Lao) uprising in 1962, where many locals were forcibly moved to other provinces. In recent decades, population numbers have grown gradually and steadily.

The lowlands of the Upper Mekong region have typically been settled by Tai people and the highlands by a diverse number of ethnic groups. This historical arrangement sets the stage for the intersection of different cultural beliefs and economic practices as cohabitation and in-migration increases in the regions serviced by the road. Despite different historical settlement patterns that highlight the dominance of the Tai Lue in the lowlands, both Sing and Long Districts are ethnically diverse. By far, the most populous ethnic group is the Akha, which constitutes 46% of the population of Muang Sing

Table 1. Ethnic diversity in Muang Sing (2003).

Ethnic group	Number of villages	Number of households	Population
Tai Lue	27	1,311	6,527
Tai Nuea	5	398	2,053
Khmu	1	39	236
Hmong	4	350	2,511
Yao	4	159	1,110
Akha	58	2,720	13,533
Mixed villages	4 villages in	556	3,337
Tai Lue, Tai Dam, Phu Noi	Muang Sing township		mainly Tai Lue

Source: Lyttleton et al., 2004.

Table 2. Ethnic diversity in Muang Long (2002).

Ethnic group	Villages	Households	Population
Lue	11	677	3,596
Lanten	2	74	434
Hmong	3	125	850
Kui	6	261	1,844
Doi	2	84	438
Akha	60	2,565	13,679
Muser	2	39	151
Yao (mixed with Lue)	1	77	419
Tai Khao, Tai Daeng, Kui	1	84	438
Tai Dam, Lue, Akha	1	84	503

Source: Lyttleton et al., 2004.

and 58% of Muang Long (Tables 1 and 2). In fact, the two districts have the highest concentration of Akha in Lao PDR, accounting for almost 50% of an estimated 60,000 Akha living in Lao PDR (Chazee, 1995).

Movement in Sing and Long

Two styles of population movement have set the stage for HIV to be potentially spreading in villages near the road and from there back and forth between the Laos highlands, other parts of Laos and home communities of Chinese labourers. The population dynamics are a recent phenomena, occurring only since the completion of the road in 2000. Firstly, there is rapidly increasing movement of highland villagers near the road. Secondly, there has been a simultaneous and expanding movement of Chinese traders and labourers into Sing and Long Districts. Most studies of mobility in Laos and its links to HIV vulnerability focus on the huge numbers of Lao crossing into Thailand in search of employment (Supang, 2000; Lyttleton and Amorntip, 2002). Far less attention has been directed at the growing number of Chinese coming into the country and accurate data are scarce. A recent summary reports that although there are only 6,889 registered foreign workers in Laos, Chinese authorities estimate 80,000 Chinese businessmen throughout the country engaging in various forms of mercantile and commercial trade (Asian Migration Centre, 2002). In addition, there are a large but unknown number of labourers, mostly construction workers, in projects concentrated in northern Laos.

It is equally hard to arrive at an accurate number of Chinese in the districts of Sing and Long. Arrivals first began when the Muang Sing border point was opened in 1962. The first Chinese workers officially arrived in the district in 1970 to construct the Muang Sing-Namtha road. All borders were closed with China from 1977–1983 during the Vietnamese-Chinese conflict. Most in-migration has occurred since 1992 as Lao and Chinese trade agreements were reached, opening up economic relations between the two countries. Since then, there has been a dramatic increase in the numbers of Chinese, some working legally, others operating clandestine trade beneath facades of legitimate businesses.

More transitory mobile groups include truck-drivers and day-trippers who come from nearby Chinese towns. Large ten-wheel trucks deliver and receive goods from large boats berthed at the port of Xiang Kok on the Mekong. Tables 3 and 4 show the number of people and vehicles coming through the two Muang Sing road border points. In comparison to nearby international border points (which allow foreigners entry) with China where the number of individuals entering Laos far overshadows the Lao leaving, the movement back and forth of Lao and Chinese at the Muang Sing border (which only allows local inhabitants to pass) is approximately equal, signalling casual passage back and forth. However, if we compare types of vehicles, the different types of mobility becomes clearer.

The unevenness of trade relations is evident in the styles of vehicles crossing the border. The majority of Lao vehicles crossing into China are

Table 3. Border crossings in Muang Sing.

People	2000	2001	2002	2003
Pangthong				
Entry (Chinese)	8,281	15,803	14,747	14,552
Exit (Lao)	10,352	7,924	11,696	15,035
Ban Mom				
Entry (Chinese)				2,067
Exit (Lao)				1,251

Table 4. Cross-border vehicle traffic: Phangthong border with China (near Muang Sing town) 2001–2002.

	Lao vehicles going to China	Chinese vehicles entering Muang Sing
Trucks	212	2,065
Buses	574	2,063
Motorcycles, tuk tuks	2,932	1,133

Source: Lyttleton et al., 2004.

motorcycles, i.e., local Muang Sing travellers visiting Chinese towns for shopping or visiting relatives. In marked contrast, Chinese buses and trucks are the predominant vehicles coming into Muang Sing at an average of 12 per day (an additional undocumented number also pass through the border of Ban Mom, 20 km to the north), which indicates that commercial and business trade brings the majority of Chinese into this area of Laos.

A growing number of Chinese seek forms of investment that allow longer term presence. This ranges from individual traders selling any number of items from vegetables to nail-clippers in the market, travelling medics selling injections and vitamins in the more remote villages, entrepreneurs who trek through the mountains collecting human hair for wigs and doll factories (or less scrupulous traders buying endangered turtles, orchids and perfumed wood), through to small factories producing animal feed, processing rice, liqueur or wood, and recently a larger copper mine. In total, the district governor estimated some 400–500 Chinese were resident in Muang Sing in 2003 conducting various kind of business, and official figures suggest another 100 in and around Muang Long. Their presence is most evident in the Chinese tea shops, bars, guesthouses, and the many appliance stores that they operate.

Outside of official businesses, large numbers of Chinese move into the plains of Muang Sing and Muang Long, either investing in or providing services (labour or advisory) for commercial crops such as sugar, watermelon, capsicum, rubber, corn and bananas. Some come individually with ten-day work permits; others come with agents who organise papers for them. It is estimated that during the dry season, there are several hundred agricultural labourers and advisors in both districts. They themselves are ethnically diverse, i.e. Chinese Akha, Chinese Lue and Chinese Haw, and this has significant implications for the differing styles of social interaction that emerge as a consequence of their presence.

This cross-border movement of Chinese into the valley is accompanied by another significant form of mobility. The boundary crossed here is not a national border, but one that is defined by elevation (Lyttleton, 2005). Many highland villages, in particular, the Akha and Kui, are relocating near the road. A complex mix of push-and-pull factors is at work. On the one hand, it is an undeniable attraction for highland villagers to exchange arduous subsistent swidden livelihood strategies for sedentary rice production and market opportunities. On the other hand, for those who may have been reticent about the move, the government prohibition of opium cultivation enacted in 2003 has forced many families to relocate due to immediate economic hardship.

Resettlement, the stabilisation of shifting cultivation and opium eradication are separate, but closely intertwined policies of the government of Lao PDR. The current Long District resettlement plan reportedly entails the displacement of 50% of upland villages by 2005 (Romagny and Daviau, 2003:7). Muang Sing authorities are less pro-active, as there has already been a far greater movement out of the highlands into the lower slopes over the past 15 years by villagers preferring sedentary styles of rice production and proximity to Muang Sing town and markets.

In both districts, the scale of movement has increased noticeably due to opium eradication policies. The enforced destruction of local poppy fields in 2003 imposed a heavy burden on highlanders, in particular, the sudden elimination of a major source of income. In a situation of declining swidden (dry) rice yields and government restrictions on shifting cultivation, opium was crucial to highlanders as a source of cash or item of barter to make up for rice shortfalls. These conditions have produced spontaneous and somewhat uncontrolled migrations of highland Akha down to the lower slopes of plain. As more and more villagers leave, the pressure on the remaining villagers to follow suit increases with the disruption of exchange and kinship ties.

Not surprisingly, this spontaneous exodus from the highlands has caused consternation among the Muang Sing officials as well as the disruption of district plans. This is aptly summarised in Muang Sing in the following report:

> It is estimated that about 15 villages with about 2000 people (300–400 families) from the mountains moved to lowland areas because their poppy fields were cleared. "We knew before the clearing of the poppy fields that villagers would move", the District Vice Governor informed the team. "On the one hand, it was good that they moved. For many years we had asked them to do so, but they did not. However, on the other hand, it made things more complicated because the district could not carry out the development as planned. Villages were messed up everywhere, it was not according to our plan". "We have to stop all development activities because of migration: everyday villagers ask the district authorities to find a new place for them to live", the Vice Governor added. (GTZ, 2003).

A UNDP document, *Basic Needs for Resettled Communities in the Lao PDR*, previously identified serious problems associated with relocation, including high mortality from disease epidemics (particularly malaria), loss of assets, debt accumulation, rice deficits, intensified competition for land, and the lack of government resources to provide assistance to relocated communities (Goudinaeu, 1997). These problems are clearly evident in recently resettled villages in Muang Sing and Muang Long (Gebert, 1995; Cohen, 2000; Romagny and Daviau, 2003; Alton and Houmpanh, 2004; Lyttleton, 2005). Despite a broad array of negative impacts implicit in the move into the lowlands (Evrard and Goudineau, 2004; Lyttleton 2004), my focus here is on a single element of the population dynamics in the area, that is the potential for HIV infection to be exacerbated by the intersection of the incoming Chinese and the relocating Akha and Kui villagers.

HIV in Northern Laos

At present, identified levels of HIV in Lao PDR are extremely low (Table 5), but there is abundant evidence of potential risks of increased

Table 5. HIV/AIDs situation in Lao PDR.

HIV/AIDS situation until mid 2005	
The first HIV identified	1990
The first AIDS identified	1992
Cumulative number of HIV/AIDS from 1990 to June 2005	
Number of provinces reported	15
Number of blood samples	117,531
Number of HIV positive	1,636
Number of AIDS cases	946
Number of deaths	584

levels of transmission. In particular, rates of certain sexually transmitted diseases (STDs) are worryingly high in some target groups, e.g. a national survey in 2001 and 2002 showed high sexually transmitted infections (STIs) prevalence among service women (a term common in Laos for commercial sex workers): 32% of chlamydia and 13.9% of gonorrhea (Family Health International, 2002).

The known cases of HIV in 2004 were distributed by province as shown in Table 6. Three provinces have had no testing done, while many of the provinces mentioned below have had only small ad hoc surveillance.

As can be seen, there is no detected presence of HIV in Luang Namtha. The forthcoming sentinel surveillance which was due in late 2005 includes

Table 6. Distribution on HIV cases by province in Lao PDR.

	HIV cases		HIV cases
Vientiane Municipality	358	Xayaboury	6
Vientiane Province	8	Khammouan	107
Borikhamxay	12	Savannakhet	602
Bokeo	79	Champasack	102
Luangrabang	21	Sekong	1
LuangNamtha	0	Salavan	29
Oudomxay	14	Attapeu	2

Source: NCCAB (National Committee for the Control of AIDS Bureau).
    : Center for HIV/AIDS/STI

Luang Namtha as one of five chosen provinces and may well show a different provincial distribution. This is not to say that HIV is not an issue. It is evident from numerous examples worldwide that levels of seroprevalence can escalate rapidly. There are a number of underlying variables that make the current combination of mobility and cultural intersections a potential tinderbox for HIV transmission. To date, there is no injecting drug use in the area. However, sexual contact between a broadened range of social groups is increasing. This is where we find the answer to the question of whether movement changes behaviour — it does and in specific ways.

Sexual Interactions along Route 17B

The number of nightclubs/bars and women selling sex in towns and villages along the road is growing steadily. In the recent past, commercial sex services were concentrated in the towns, in particular, at both ends of route 17B in Muang Sing and the small port town of Xiengkok (part of Muang Long District). However, in a significant departure from this pattern, more new bars have recently opened in Muang Long and in villages outside of Muang Sing along the road. At the start of 2000, there was only one nightclub in Muang Sing with five or six women (in the late 1990s, there had been several more locales, but they had been closed by the government decree), none in Muang Long and one in the port of Xiengkok. Three years later, this had grown to 16 venues where 60 women sell sex. While these numbers are small compared with regional hot-spots and transport hubs, it is the rapid growth that signals a trend towards commercialisation of sex and a growing number of local clients who previously had little access to such services.

Recently, two venues have opened several kilometres outside of Muang Sing on route 17B. This indicates an important transition to locales in immediate proximity of relocated Akha and other ethnic villages. The rationale is that men in the town will prefer more discreet venues some distance from their homes. However, it also places the form of social interaction right at many villagers' doorsteps. Increasingly, therefore, village men with money from various forms of market trade are engaging in new forms of social and sexual interactions with women from other parts of the country (CSWs almost inevitably move from other provinces). Whereas in the past, life in the mountains culturally and geographically circumscribed, to some extent, regular sexual interactions with women from other ethnic groups, these barriers are now disappearing for many Akha men and other relocated ethnic groups. This is not an issue of moral adjudication; cross-cultural sexual contact is nothing new anywhere in the world, but it warrants consideration if it increases the potential for HIV spread.

A number of economic, cultural and geographic variables have contributed to the low levels of HIV in Lao. Given the rampant epidemics in neighbouring countries, the concept of social and geographic boundaries are of particular salience. Remoteness and limited range of multi-partner sexuality coupled with the absence of needle-based drug abuse are key issues in the apparently low rates of HIV infection in most of Lao PDR. Route 17B represents the concrete dismantling of elements of these boundaries. Multi-partner sexuality is typically associated with the ethnic people living in and around Sing and Long. However, when sexual interactions create networks that extend beyond cultural groupings the potential for infection is broadened dramatically.

Women working in bars typically move widely and regularly throughout the country. A majority of women working in bars along Route 17B are young, from marginalised ethnic groups from other parts of the country (often Khmu), and have low levels of education. A significant number we spoke with indicated that they had been promised other forms of work only to find themselves trapped in prostitution. Generally, men frequenting these bars are a mixture of local townsfolk and visitors from other provinces. Assuming condoms are not always used in sexual interactions that take place (Lyttleton, 1999) the sexual networks that local Akha and other ethnic minority men connect themselves with are increased dramatically. These networks are not purely to the other parts of the country.

In Xiengkok, there has been a steady presence of Chinese women in one or two of the several desultory bars/restaurants that flank the road where the Chinese trucks come to park before loading or unloading goods. Sometimes, queues of eight to ten trucks[2] await the arriving boats and the

---

[2] The number of Chinese trucks arriving in Xiengkok lessened in 2004 due to changes in the Lao customs controls and an increase in Chinese cargo boats coming directly from Yunnan after rapids had been cleared in the Mekong but it may well increase again in the future.

service industry here is more geared to these clients or the timber labourers than the orientation of larger clubs to visiting government officials in the district towns. In Xiengkok, the majority of women work in small beer shops that have what are euphemistically called "emergency rooms" where clients can have sex.

Thus, the bars and nightclubs along Route 17B and their overlapping clientele are one very important nexus for possible HIV spread (and other STDs). In a marked change from the recent past, they provide opportunities for sexual exchanges between far more diverse groups of men and women in this area. Perhaps it does not need repeating that sexual customs of the local ethnic groups such as Akha and Kui provide minimal social constraints on multi-partner sexuality as this is often reiterated and sensationalised as the fundamental basis of ethnic vulnerability to STDs. Despite protestations to the contrary, multi-partner sexuality is also common amongst lowland Lao groups, in particular, in the context of men visiting bars and nightclubs. If HIV is transmitted in some of these interactions, then the potential for it to spread throughout ethnic group communities is raised exponentially.

One indication of the ability of infectious diseases to spread rapidly is the high levels of gonorrhoea noted in ethnic villages. Although, there exists no empirical evidence, there are numerous anecdotal accounts of widespread gonorrhoea (*nong nai*) from district and development agency health workers who indicate that many men from a number of their target villages have requested drugs for STD treatment.

The backgrounds of the women working in bars highlight very clearly the extent to which commercial sex and multiple partner sexuality is increasingly crossing ethnic divides. One very important corollary trend that is a direct consequence of the bars and economic transitions facilitated by the presence of the road is the increasing commodification of sexuality amongst local ethnic groups. While local Kui and Lanten women have occasionally worked in the bars of Xiengkok, there has been no evidence of Akha women selling sex in either Sing or Long districts in the past. However, in 2003, a notable trend has been observed for the first time. Several young Akha women from a village that has made itself well-known for its active embrace of the handicraft trade reportedly visit the Muang Sing nightclubs late in the evening soliciting male customers as they leave. The combination of a need or desire for money and the ongoing search for commodities that can introduce cash into the household follows a logical trajectory to the point that individual bodies become the commodity for sale. Women in this village have diversified from sale of opium and trinkets to other forms of commerce. The reports of young women capitalising on aspects of their sexuality outside the nightclubs signals a huge break with traditional customs and highlights the inroads that market commerce is making into traditional life-ways and understandings.

This form of an expanding realm of commercialised sexuality is not limited to a few fleeting encounters outside the bars of Muang Sing. It takes its place as one example of the ways in which market relations are increasingly impacting the life-ways of ethnic peoples as they move down to be near the road. Trade, commerce, labour, mobility, commodity exchange, tourism and resettlement are overt signs of rapid development along route 17B. While bars and nightclubs are an obvious site for the intersection of men and women from different geographic, ethnic and economic backgrounds, it is neither the only occasion where sexuality is commodified nor the only arena where HIV can spread. Due to a broad array of social changes in the lives of most people near the road, other forms of social and economic relationships taking place away from the bars are also a serious threat for HIV transmission that can take place in a rapidly expanding realm of sexual exchanges. They deserve attention precisely because they are more subtle and are less likely to be the target of specific health campaigns. They come as a direct product of the newly expanded mobility, economic practices and relationships.

Ethnic Sexual Customs and HIV Vulnerability

Much has been made of the traditional sexual customs of the Akha and Kui in the context of interventions targeting HIV transmission. While "free sex behaviours" are readily sensationalised and often form the basis for self-serving exoticisation of highland minorities by lowland men, I wish to focus on how HIV might enter a local ethnic community in the first place. This is precisely where population dynamics of the rapidly expanded social networks and shifting social consciousness implicit in resettlement coincide with and together provide social and sexual liaisons in situations apart from the bars and nightclubs.

Each of the local Akha villages has a youth group led by one man who makes important decisions concerning the application of village customs which in turn affect the ongoing reproduction of local social relations. In these communities, it is commonplace that young men and women congregate in the evenings in specially constructed sites usually with elevated rows of seating planks to exchange stories and songs. Some couples repair to designated sleeping huts and sexual unions between the young are commonplace. Such practices continue until marriage or the young woman becomes pregnant at which time she chooses which of the young men is her preferred husband. After marriage, older men can still sleep with the young women, but it occurs less often within the home village and more commonly on visits to other villages. Men visiting from other villages are customarily massaged by young women from this group of adolescents. If the visitor was so inclined, he could request that a young woman also has sex with him.

Such requests are typically accompanied by gifts of liquor and cigarettes to the young men within the youth groups as a form of recompense. It thus signals a nominal request for permission to access the sexuality of the young village women and rights of refusal lie with the head of the adolescent group who acts as a gatekeeper controlling the sexual contacts of the young women with outsiders (the young women also have some rights of refusal). Such exchanges have traditionally been predicated on the ability to talk with each other; one clear stipulation has been that the young Akha women will sleep with other Akha men because of cultural familiarity. Rights of access to men from other cultural groups are not always as forthcoming and sexual access to Akha women has been limited by local sanctions that are controlled and protected by the young men of the village, particularly their leader.

These cultural sanctions vary from village to village. In the past, the few Lao government officials working in the mountains could sleep with Akha women after a period of time as they became locally accepted, but this was not always assumed or always possible. These days, in some villages, Chinese Akha are allowed immediate access to sleep with local village women when they come to visit or work as they are considered to be of the same culture, whereas Lao government officials are not. In other villages, the reverse occurs; non-Lao nationality is a precluding criterion because local Akha men are concerned that allowing such liaisons with Chinese men would set in place an exodus of the young women who would be taken as wives across the border. These villages, on the other hand, voiced less concern with Lao men taking temporary sexual partners. All villagers suggested that non-Asian men would be denied sexual contact with local women.

In short, in many villages, there still exist some controls on men from outside the region accessing local Akha women's sexuality. The issue of concern is how these are rapidly changing. Increasing numbers of government staff are working in the mountains. Local Akha sexuality and customs are highly sensationalised in lowland understandings and the exotic "primitiveness" of the minority groups is heavily eroticised. Lowland Lao talk in glowing terms of the cultural stipulations that require young Akha women to massage visitors; those visiting the mountains often wish to experience local sexuality beyond just the massage, and the money, status and increasing familiarity they carry often allows such liaisons, to the extent that some NGOs have now officially prohibited local staff to have sex with local women. There are no such government policies in place, as remoteness and lack of government services reaching the mountains has in the past precluded high level contact. This is all changing as new roads are built and population movement directly facilitates new patterns of sexual interaction.

Labour Migrants and Sexual Commodification

Close to the road, the influx of Chinese workers has created nodes where social interactions are establishing sexual networks that extend beyond cultural and national boundaries. It is common for some Chinese agricultural labourers working in Sing and Long to visit nearby Akha villages and sleep with the women. It is commonplace because they are also Akha, albeit with Chinese nationality, and are thus familiar with the custom of hospitality in local villages. However, many of the advisors and traders who negotiate, supervise and assist in the cultivation of the sugar cane, capsicum and watermelon fields in Muang Sing and Muang Long are Haw Chinese. Nowadays, they accompany their Akha counterparts or employees to the nearby villages at night and the Chinese Akha introduce and facilitate sexual interactions for these men as well, gaining permission from the head of the adolescent group to sleep with the young women (if they are willing).

In Muang Long, where hundreds of hectares of watermelon have been planted using Chinese and local labour in 2004, the opportunities for sexual contact are rapidly diversifying. The Chinese prefer to hire female labour from the nearby villages, so there are often relationships born of this contact. The Chinese men will visit the villages of the labourers they hire and either take the women "out", that is to a nearby Lao village that might have a festival or a roadside stall with a TV or just simply back to their encampment. Other times, they will just stay in the village for shorter visits that include the provision of sex. Likewise, district and development staff also occasionally visit roadside villages. Usually, the cost of such liaisons is liquor and cigarettes for the young men of the village once approval has been gained from the head of this group and the young women.

In a telling departure from customary norms, forms of financial exchange are entering the picture. Money for service provision is now a logical accompaniment for any number of labour relationships that the Akha and Kui enter into as they become part of a market economy. It is becoming a key value that attaches to the assessment of the worth of everyday pursuits under the rubric of modernity. Following the arrival of watermelons, commodified sexuality has also entered the list of negotiable income-earning relationships in which the Akha can engage. Village men described how some of the more "modern" young Akha women will receive direct financial payment and gifts from visiting Chinese men for sexual services. This transition to commercialised sex has been taken further in some villages near the town. Here, Chinese and other workers appear regularly looking for sexual relations as they no longer have to get approval from the head of the adolescent group, but rather exchange money directly with the chosen girl.

Variations on this trend of money for sex are not only present in villages with women who provide labour or those located right on the road. Rather, we see far more widespread transformations in local sexual customs occurring in tandem with other forms of social change. For example, in a village about 12 km outside Muang Sing town that has had an actively entrepreneurial headman and regular visits from outside men for some years, the forms of sexuality are also evolving under the sway of the cash economy. Here, young women somewhat concerned about their lack of autonomy in receiving male guests have adopted a new strategy of negotiated compliance. Nowadays, it is no longer satisfactory that the leader of the youth group receives the whisky or cigarettes as coinage for sexual access. In order to keep the young women amenable within the culturally traditional form of hospitality, money must now be paid directly from the guest to the young woman who will receive him sexually. While the youth group still has rights to determine who has sexual access to young women, in order to cope both with increasing number of village visitors and the desires of the young women for some benefits in the exchange, the traditional system has changed to allow direct sex-for-cash transactions.

These new forms of commodified relationship and sexual opportunism signal profound transformations in the social relationships being constructed in the lowlands of Sing and Long and highlight the ways in which long-standing cultural formations adapt under new forces. In the absence of adequate HIV prevention activities reaching these populations they highlight the ongoing association of compensated sex and HIV vulnerability.

Ethnicity and sexual exploitation

The complicated ways that labour, markets, sexuality and disease transmission intertwine is not only an issue affecting Akha systems of cultural interaction and the men who engage in sexual commerce; other examples also show that exploitation readily accompanies ethnic difference and can exacerbate forms of sexual vulnerability. In a Kui village relocated near the road, money has not yet entered new forms of sexual contact, but the interactions between outside labourers and local women are nonetheless becoming part of a wider world of orchestrated relationships.

Kui customs encourage young women to build their own bedrooms separate from the main house once they reach puberty. They build small bamboo rooms high on stilts either completely by themselves or with the help of a friend. Once completed, they remove themselves from the main household each evening after dusk. At their discretion, young women are able to take regular partners into their rooms. This is how relationships are established, leading to marriage upon pregnancy.

The important distinction is that there are little in the way of controlling sanctions on outsiders coming in to sleep with the local women. In most Akha villages, the male head of the youth group has rights of refusal to visiting men who wish to sleep with one of the village women (he can also fine the woman if she takes a guest without his approval). In the Kui villages, it depends entirely on the young woman's inclination and Akha and other men have long visited Kui villages to avail themselves of the young women's sexuality. There is little in the way of any sort of recompense involved in these relations, although in the past, some level of courting was required before the girl would be compliant. The young women take multiple partners and it is a well established perception amongst local men that the young women can be fairly easily persuaded to her room. Sometimes, it appears that this persuasion is not far from coercion as the young women have little social support for any refusal.

During the period when this research was conducted, in one large Kui village (comprising five resettled villages) on some evenings, groups of up to 20 men would arrive looking for sex. Some of these men are local, for example, the neighbouring Akha; others come from further afield, for example, Lao (from distant provinces) and Chinese workers (from widely diverse locales in Southern China). While not all visitors gain sexual contact, this village is nonetheless providing sexual services for a wide range of men from nearby villages, township, and the nearby agricultural fields and is therefore acting as a sexual melting pot. In effect, it is almost a brothel for men who want "exotic" and free sex. The costs of these transactions have not been counted so far. A campaign had focused on this village for HIV awareness but achieved very little. Posters are used as wallpapers, and the use of condoms is entirely up to the male, with little understanding of the nature of STDs or HIV.

Conclusion

Resettled roadside villages in Muang Sing and Muang Long present a microcosm of larger changes taking place along new roads being built throughout the upper Mekong. Although one cannot pinpoint any particular road and the mobility it allows as solely responsible for the increase in sexual opportunism, the social and material relations that come as part of a wider parcel of changes typically termed "development" carry benefits and shortcomings including disease transmission directly related to the road's presence. Cultural intersections are inevitable when new thoroughfares allow movement within and between areas of ethnic diversity. At times, these cultural intersections merge seamlessly within a globalised world of myriad increasing flows. At other times, frictions and fissures emerge as cultural accommodation requires compromise and sacrifice. In certain instances, negative elements of mobility are clear for either the migrant or host community. In other examples, the complex mix of motivations and aspirations underpinning interactions between mobile and non-mobile populations shrouds public health threats. It is precisely the "less formal networks of ordinary people as they go about their everyday business" (Skeldon, 2000) that require attention in the resettled communities and the reconfigured relations that emerge as different populations interact.

Population dynamics in Muang Sing and Muang Long have brought into close social contact two groups of differently mobile people. In relocated villages, minority group labour is readily available in the fields along the road due to investment from migrant Chinese. Labour relations also bring outsiders into a geographic and social orbit that encourages increased sexual exchange. This is a significant facet of HIV vulnerability in the region. The Chinese labourers are supposedly subjected to rigorous health checks before they cross the border, including HIV tests; yet some of these labourers reported that some diagnostic tests are neither mandatory nor policed. In addition, the health certificates are valid for one year, which hardly provides an adequate assurance against the presence of STDs. In Laos, few individuals screen themselves for HIV. Nowadays, in bars and villages along Route 17B, individuals from widely diverse backgrounds interact socially and sexually. If HIV is introduced as part of the new forms of sexual exchange taking place in the roadside villages and bars, then the new parameters shaping everyday life including the commodification and exploitation of traditional sexual mores must be considered a serious threat to future livelihood of large number of people in Sing, Long and source communities of labourers and bar workers.

References

Alton C, Rattanavong H. (2004) *Service Delivery and Resettlement: Options for Development Planning.* Unpublished Report, Lao PDR, UNDP, Vientiane.
Asian migration centre (2002) *Migration: Needs, Issues and Responses in the Greater Mekong Subregion.* Mekong Migration Network, Bangkok.

Chamberlain J. (2000) *HIV Vulnerability and Population Mobility in Northern Provinces of Lao PDR*, UNDP, Bangkok.

Chantanavanich S, with Beesey A, Paul S. (2000) *Mobility and HIV/AIDS in the Greater Mekong SubRegion*. Bangkok Asian Development Bank.

Chazee L. (1995) *Atlas des Ethnies et des Sou-Ethnies du Lao PDR*, Chazee L, Bangkok.

Cohen P. (2000) Resettlement, opium and labour dependence: Akha-Tai relations in northern Laos. *Dev Change* **31**(1): 179–200.

Evrard O, Goudineau Y. (2004) Planned resettlement, unexpected migrations and cultural trauma: The political management of rural mobility and interethnic relationships in Laos. *Dev Change* **35**(4): 937–962.

Family Health International. (2001) *HIV Surveillance Survey and Sexually Transmitted Infection Periodic Prevalence Survey, Lao PDR, 2001*, Vientiane, Lao PDR.

Gebert R. (1995) *Socio-economic Baseline Survey*. Muang Sing: GTZ Integrated Food Security Programme.

Goudineau Y. (1997) *Resettlement and social Characteristics of New Villages: Basic Needs for Resettled Communities in the Lao PDR, Vientiane*, UNESCO-UNDP, 2 Vols.

GTZ. (2003) *Study Report of Drug Free Villages in Sing District, Luang Namtha Province*, Unpublished Report GTZ: Lao-German Program, Integrated Rural development in Mountainous Regions of Northern Lao PDR, Feb. 2003.

Guest P. (2000) Population mobility in Asia and the implications for HIV/AIDS, in Hsu LN (ed.) *Population Movement, Development and HIV/AIDS*, UNAIDS Report, Bangkok, April, pp. 76–87.

Lyttleton C. (1999) Any port in a storm: Coming to terms with HIV in Lao PDR. *Culture, Health and Sexuality* **1**(2): 115–130.

Lyttleton C, Amarapibul A. (2002) Sister cities and easy passage: HIV, mobility and economies of desire in a Thai/Lao border zone. *Soc Sci Med* **54**: 505–518.

Lyttleton C. (2004) Relative pleasures: Drugs, development and modern dependencies in Asia's golden triangle. *Dev Change* **35**(4): 909–935.

Lyttleton C. (2005) Market-bound: Relocation and disjunction in northwest Lao PDR, in M Toyota, S Jatrana and B Yeoh (eds.) *Migration and Health in Asia*. Routledge/Curzon, (forthcoming).

Lyttleton C, Cohen P, Rattanavong H, Tongkhamhan B, Sisaengrat S. (2004). *Watermelons, Bars and Trucks: Dangerous Intersections in Northwest Laos*. Vientiane: Institute for Research on Culture.

Morse S. (1995) Factors in the emergence of infectious diseases. *Emerg Infect Dis* **1**(1): 7–15.

Porter D, Bennoun R. (1997) On the borders of research, policy and practice: Outline of an agenda', in Linge G and Porter D. (eds.) *No Place for Borders: The HIV/AIDS Epidemic and Development in Asia and the Pacific*, pp. 149–163, Allen and Unwin, Sydney.

Romagny L, Daviau S. (2003) Synthesis of reports on resettlement. In *Long District, Luang Namtha Province, Lao PDR, Action Contre La Faim mission in Lao PDR.*

Skeldon R. (2000) *Population Mobility and HIV Vulnerability in South East Asia,* UNDP, Bangkok.

Wilson M. (1995) Travel and the emergence of new infectious diseases. *Emerg Infect Dis* 1(2): 39–46.

12

Household Poverty, Off-farm Migration and Pulmonary Tuberculosis in Rural Henan, China

Sukhan Jackson, Adrian C Sleigh, Guo-Jie Wang and Xi-Li Liu

Poverty and TB in China

Pulmonary tuberculosis is a disease of poverty. China is one of the 22 high TB-burdened countries which together account for 80% of the world's tuberculosis cases. Among China's 27 infectious diseases listed in the case report system for 2003, pulmonary tuberculosis had the second highest incidence rate (52.36/100,000) after viral hepatitis (China Statistical Yearbook, 2004: 868). Some 1.45 mil new TB cases are estimated each year (China Tuberculosis Control Collaboration, 2004). The Chinese Ministry of Health reports 4.5 mil TB patients, the second highest number in the world (World Health Organization, 2004: 29). About 130,000 people die from TB every year, the highest number among all the causes of deaths from infectious diseases in China, with 80% of TB occurring in rural households.

The post 1979 economic reforms and open-door policies have brought unprecedented socio-economic development in the past 25 years. The government is set on poverty reduction and the prevalence of poverty was reduced by 88% between 1978 and 2000. However, the high TB rates are a clear indication that poverty eradication is still an uphill task. Thus, despite an average annual economic growth of 9%, there were still 30 mil people whose annual per capita income was below China's official poverty line of 625 yuan or ~ US$80/year in 2003 (Alleviation Poverty Office of China State Council, 2004).

China's fast-tracked export-oriented industrialisation, economic disparity between interior and coastal provinces, and income gap between rural and urban areas are the main "pull" factors for the phenomenal out-migration of the rural poor to the cities. Farmers freely travel afar to seek employment. The 2000 Fifth National Census recorded China's internal migration at 121 mil, with 88.4 mil rural workers accounting for 73% of it (Zhang, 2004). At least 7 to 10 mil new migrants are estimated to leave the farm each year, a trend that is expected to continue. Authorities predict that the number will rise to 300 mil by 2020, and eventually to 500 mil. It is widely known that migrant workers are often exploited, having to work in harsh conditions and to endure long hours involving shift duties. Off-farm migration for work has reduced rural poverty to some extent, but it appears that TB incidence could be linked to this massive labour mobility.

In 2002–2004, we studied the socio-economic aspects of pulmonary tuberculosis in the rural areas of Henan Province and found that nearly half of our TB cases had out-migrated for work. Official statistics of 2003 showed that in Henan, a total of 3.07 mil farmers (compared with 2.52 mil in 2002) moved out of their villages for work in Henan itself or in the other provinces (Henan Province Statistical Yearbook, 2003). The nationwide random sample TB survey in 2000 showed that prevalence in Henan (population of 96 mil) was 497/100,000 and the prevalence of sputum-positive cases was 132/100,000.

Worldwide TB has re-emerged since the mid 1980s as a global health emergency and a major cause of death. Nearly two mil people died of TB in 2000 (Lee et al., 2002). In 1990, the Commission on Health Research for Development expressed concern for the neglect of TB disease by the international community (Hopewell, 2002). Consequently, the World Health Organization helped launch a new TB control strategy, the "Directly Observed Therapy Short-Course" (DOTS), including 6 months of treatment with four standard drugs.

The Chinese government in April 1991 adopted the DOTS strategy which provided patients with free DOTS supervision by health workers

(Chen *et al.*, 2002). Subsequently, the 4th national TB survey in 2000 found that the prevalence of smear-positive pulmonary TB in provinces using DOTS fell to 90/100,000, a decline of 36.7% since 1990, compared with a decline of only 3.2% in non-DOTS provinces. After 2002, the Chinese government greatly expanded the DOTS programme with a loan from the World Bank/UK DFID and the Japanese aid.

Tuberculosis has long been known to be an affliction of the poor (Long, 1941; Comstock and Cauthen, 1992; Floyd, 2003). A chronic and debilitating infectious illness such as TB imposes catastrophic costs on those who are already poor. In addition, the cost of a serious illness such as TB can lead to impoverishment of the entire household (Russell, 2004). Although the association of TB with poverty has been noted for China, direct evidence is lacking.

In 2002–2004, we collected direct evidence from individual TB cases and their households. As far as we know, this was the first use of community case-controls for TB research in China. We compared the TB cases and their controls for the association between household economic status (poverty), off-farm migration and TB incidence. Secondly, we calculated the economic costs of disease and looked into its impact on the households, where treatment costs were measured against annual household income.

Method

In October 2002, we began the study with three counties, Gongyi, Linying, Zhenping, where each had a different treatment and payment system as described below, and Yuzhou county was subsequently added to the study. At the start of our study, Gongyi and Yuzhou were under the World Bank TB project of free treatment. Linying was under the Henan Provincial TB Project where smear-positive patients paid half the price for diagnoses and TB medicines. In Zhenping, patients paid the full price for treatment. However, the Chinese government extended the World Bank TB project to all counties in Henan from January 2003 onwards; thus, Linying and Zhenping are now able to provide free TB treatment. The new policy did not seriously affect our results as it occurred only two months after our research began.

During 2002–2004, we prospectively gathered and studied 160 new TB cases and 320 neighbourhood controls of the same sex and 5-year age group. For each case, we had two matched controls without TB history, living in houses on the left and on the right. Investigated variables included marital status, education, smoking, financial burden, off-farm migration history, annual household income, and household assets.

We selected only those TB cases in the economically productive age group of 25–60 years. We included all eligible consecutive cases that occurred in the county until we reached our target of ∼ 40 patients in each county. Neither sex nor the age of our cases were pre-determined in our research design in order to capture the patients' characteristics. Re-treatment and non-pulmonary TB cases were excluded. All our cases conformed to the international case definition (World Health Organization, 2004) of two or more acid-fast bacilli positive (AFB+) sputum smears or one sputum smear AFB+ plus radiographic evidence of active pulmonary tuberculosis, as determined by the treating medical officer. All positive smears were validated by the Henan Provincial TB Institute.

TB cases and their controls were first interviewed in their homes between 1 to 3 months after patients registered as TB cases. We had follow-up interviews of the cases after 10–12 months; only 144 follow-up visits were done as 11 cases had died and 5 cases were missing.

Results and Discussion

Study Counties

All four counties have a large population of more than 700,000 and 80% were rural, representing the range of per capita GDP and per capita net income of farmers. They reported an incidence of active pulmonary TB between 26 and 75/100,000 and an incidence of smear-positive pulmonary TB between 9 and 36/100,000 (Table 1).

Characteristics of 160 TB cases

Among the 160 cases, we found that 77% were male, 38% (60/160) aged between 25 and 39 years old and the rest were between 40 and 60 years old. The sex distribution of our new cases conformed to that of TB in China

Table 1. Gongyi, Linying, Zhenping and Yuzhou Counties: Selected statistics, 2002–2003.

	Gongyi	Linying	Zhenping	Yuzhou
Population	790,000	710,000	950,000	1,190,000
Farmers as % of population	82	83	88	87
Average annual net income of rural residents (yuan)*	3,725	2,749	2,468	3,007
Per capita GDP (yuan)	15,602	8,212	8,888	8,958
Birth rate (/1000/year)	9.5	9.0	9.0	8.0
Death rate (/1000/year)	5.2	4.0	7.0	5.0
Male: Female ratio	103:100	117:100	131:100	137:100
Reported incidence of active pulmonary TB (/10^5 persons/year)	26	42	47	75
Reported incidence of smear-positive pulmonary TB (/10^5persons/year)	9	15	18	36

*US$1 = 8 yuan.
Sources: County Statistical Yearbooks and data from Henan Provincial TB Institute.

for the age group of 25–60 years, and reflected the sex ratio of out-migrants in Henan, among whom males were 2.5 times more frequent than females (Henan Province Statistical Yearbook, 2003). Among our 160 TB cases, 15% currently had no spouse (unmarried, widowed and divorced), 7% were illiterate and 47% had junior high school education, 72% were heads of household, 47% had out-migrated for work, and 71% had a smoking history (Table 2).

Household economic status (HES) of TB cases

We used three types of indicators to measure household economic status: (a) average annual household income (b) household assets and (c) relative wealth within village (Table 3). The HES of TB cases was substantially lower than that of the controls, as follows:

(a) Average annual household income of the 160 TB cases was 4,994 yuan, compared with 5,604 yuan for the 320 controls. Based on China's official

Table 2. Characteristics of 160 TB cases and 320 controls.

Characteristics	Cases (160)		Controls (320)	
	N	%	N	%
Sex				
Male	123	76.9	246	76.9
Female	37	23.1	74	23.1
Age (years)				
25–29	19	11.9	38	11.9
30–34	22	13.8	43	13.4
35–39	19	11.9	38	11.9
40–44	13	8.1	28	8.8
45–49	26	16.3	51	15.9
50–54	31	19.4	61	19.1
55–60	30	18.8	61	19.1
Marital status (current partner)				
No	24	15.0	19	5.9
Yes	136	85.0	301	94.1
Head of household				
Yes	115	71.9	242	75.6
No	45	28.1	78	24.4
Had out-migration work history				
No	85	53.1	226	70.6
Yes	75	46.9	94	29.4
Education				
Nil	11	6.9	17	5.3
Primary (6 years)	54	33.8	99	30.9
Junior high (3 years)	75	46.9	151	47.2
Senior high & above (3 years or more)	20	12.5	53	16.6
Smoking history				
No	47	29.4	145	45.3
Yes	113	70.6	175	54.7

poverty line of 625 yuan per person per year, we found that 29% of the cases were in absolute poverty compared with 23% of the controls ($z = 1.65$, $p = 0.05$).

(b) Household assets. Nearly one third of TB cases fell below the lowest asset quartile ($\leq 16,699$ yuan), but only one-fifth (20%) of controls did. The

Table 3. Household economic status of 160 cases (before TB illness) and 320 controls.

Annual household income (yuan — poverty line multiples)**	Case %	Control %	Adjusted OR* (95% CI)
< 2563 (below poverty line)	29.4	22.5	Reference
≥ 2563, < 5126 (1–2 times poverty line)	42.5	42.8	0.67 (0.39–1.14)
≥ 5126 (more than twice poverty line)	28.1	34.7	0.54 (0.26–1.12)
Household assets (yuan — quarters)***			
0–16699 (first quarter)	31.3	20.0	Reference
≥ 16700, < 21077 (second quarter)	26.9	25.9	0.74 (0.41–1.32)
≥ 21077, < 28780 (third quarter)	21.3	26.6	0.52 (0.28–0.94)
≥ 28780 (fourth quarter)	20.6	27.5	0.48 (0.25–0.92)
Relative wealth within village			
Lower third	46.3	19.7	Reference
Middle & upper thirds	53.8	80.3	0.2 (0.1–0.4)

*Matched analysis — two controls and one case in each matched set (see Methodology).
**Household poverty line (estimated to be 2,563 yuan/household/year based on average 4 persons per household and Chinese official poverty line of 625 yuan/person/year).
***Household assets were calculated from average market prices in study counties.

average value of household assets was 21,812 yuan for TB cases, significantly less than 24,489 yuan for controls ($t = 2.55$, $p = 0.01$).

(c) Relative wealth within village. Nearly half of our TB cases saw themselves belonging to the lowest third in the village, compared with one-fifth of the controls ($z = 6.08$, $p < 0.001$).

We further explored the relationship of TB to household economic status (HES) using multivariable analysis to adjust for potential confounding by other factors. Univariate conditional (matched) case–control logistic regression analyses found that all three household economic indicators were associated with TB. We then used a multivariable conditional logistic regression model and adjusted each HES odds ratio (OR) (with 95% CI) for the influence of other important variables (smoking history, marital status, previous out-migration for work). After adjustments, the household assets variable and "relative wealth within village" variable are still significantly correlated with TB incidence, whereas only the adjusted OR of the annual household income was not significantly different. For all indicators, the cases were substantially less likely to be in the upper HES categories than controls, indicating that cases were poorer than the neighbourhood matched controls.

Thus, we have evidence of a strong link between TB and poverty from our sample of 160 cases and 320 controls. Our results showed that the better the household economic status, the lesser the risk of TB. We also found that the costs associated with TB disease were high, even though the treatment was meant to be free in these counties (see below). Therefore, the poor were further impoverished by treatment costs.

Economic burden of TB disease

When TB symptoms appeared, individuals would normally consult doctors in private clinics or general hospitals; such expenditure in private clinics and hospitals averaged ~ 567 yuan. When suspected of TB, patients were transferred to the county's TB clinics and from the information provided by the TB cases, we calculated the average cost in the TB clinics to be 1,180 yuan (Table 4).

Direct costs refer to the cost of seeking diagnoses and treatment (Table 4, items 1–5). The average direct cost of treatment is 1,948 yuan, including

Table 4. Treatment costs of 144* TB cases within 10–12 months in four study counties.

		Average cost in yuan	Average cost in yuan	% of total average
	Cost items in County TB clinics			
	Drugs (HRZE**)	445.00		
	Other TB drugs	86.10		
	Other prescribed drugs	476.30		
	Sputum tests	18.90		
	X-rays	96.50		
	Blood tests	55.20		
	Urine tests	2.20		
1	Average total cost in County TB clinics		1180.10	16.0
2	Cost in general hospitals or private clinics		567.30	7.7
3	Cost in TB clinics above County level		75.50	1.0
4	Travel for tests/drugs: Patients & companions		92.90	1.3
5	Food during travel: Patients & companions		32.60	0.4
6	Self-medication (Chinese medicine)		117.30	
7	Nutritious foods		706.00	
8	Loss of income for patients		4559.40	
9	Loss of income for companions		36.00	
	Total average cost of illness for 144 TB cases		*7366.90*	*100*

*After 10–12 months 11 people had died and 5 went missing. US$1 = 8 yuan.
**HRZE = isoniazid, rifampicin, pyrazinamide and ethambutol — the 4 standard drugs for TB.

both medical costs and non-medical costs. Medical costs refer to expenses in county level TB clinics, in private clinics and in general hospitals relating to laboratory tests, clinical examinations, TB and non TB medicines. Direct non-medical costs refer to transport and food related expenses incurred while travelling to seek treatment. We also considered the indirect costs such as the opportunity costs of lost earnings of patients and their companions (Table 4, items 8 and 9) where the loss of earnings for individual patients averaged 4,559 yuan.

The average total cost of TB disease was high for the 144 patients at 7,367 yuan per patient. It was a huge burden upon a family with an average annual household income of 4,994 yuan. Excluding the income losses of patients and companions, the average cost was 2,772 yuan, accounting for 56% of annual household income. Some analysts have estimated that a cost-burden greater than 10% of household income is likely to be catastrophic for the family (Prescott, 1999). Thus, it was not surprising that most households in our study had little capacity to pay for the treatment. In our follow-up of 144 cases after 10–12 months, we found that 66% had borrowed from relatives or friends and 8% from banks; 96% of the borrowers could not repay or could only repay part of their loans. Of the follow-ups, 45% had to sell personal belongings and productive assets such as wheat, pigs, and cattle to defray the medical costs. Thus, TB often leads households to deep debts.

It is important to understand the high treatment cost illustrated in Table 4. In practice, the average total cost of treatment in the TB clinics amounted to 1,256 yuan (items 1 and 3 in Table 4). In our follow-up, we found that more than half of our cases (i.e. 54% or 77/144) exceeded the 6 months' standard DOTS treatment. Patients paid out-of-pocket in the extended period. This may be due to many doctors being too cautious to cease treatment, as there are no medical rules that stipulate the exact duration required for TB treatment.

Also, it was likely that the health providers were inclined to over-service with unnecessary examinations and tests, and over-prescribe drugs beyond the listed free items of the World Bank TB project. There is widespread criticism in the public media of supply-induced demand for health services and pharmaceuticals; an issue which was also raised in a recent report from China's State Council. Since the post 1978 market reforms, the government has been withdrawing its share in national health spending from nearly

100% to 16%. Most health providers rely on patients' medical bills to cover overheads, including wages and allowances for medical staff, new medical apparatus and hospital facilities (Lague, 2005). However, in the case of TB control, the central government and the Ministry of Health have stipulated that the local (county) government is expected to match the provincial government funding for TB, obtained as a World Bank loan. It is reasonable to expect that many local governments lacked the funds to do so, while others might have given TB a lower priority. We found that some local governments had been slow in releasing funds to the TB clinics, which were then forced to seek other alternatives to cover operating costs, salaries and so forth.

A few TB cases in our sample did not go for regular and proper treatment simply because they could not afford it. Sadly, ~ 50% of untreated TB patients would eventually die, thus rendering poverty a formidable problem for both TB mortality and TB control in China.

Poverty and out-migration for work

Among the 160 TB cases, nearly half reported off-farm migration and of these 75 cases, 51 had out-migrated in the last three years. Among the 320 TB-free controls, less than one third (94/320) had out-migrated for work and only 18% (57/320) did so in the last three years. The difference between the TB cases and their controls was significant ($p < 0.001$).

Of the 75 cases with out-migration work history (Table 5), 89% of them (67 cases) had annual incomes of $\leq 7,000$ yuan (US$847), falling below the international poverty line. Based on China's official poverty line of 625 yuan per person per year and the average rural household size of four, we estimated the household absolute poverty line to be 2,563 yuan per year, and 31% of out-migrants (23/75) belonged to the absolute poverty group according to this Chinese standard (Table 5).

In other forthcoming reports, we explored the harsh working conditions, excessively long working hours, and crowded dormitories of rural migrant workers, and found the influence of these factors on TB incidence to be significant. We emphasise that dire poverty would drive the rural poor to out-migrate for work in the cities. Crowded housing and the physical and mental stress from unpleasant workplaces, long working hours (> 8 hours

Table 5. Annual household income of 75 TB cases with out-migration work history.

Annual Household Income (yuan)*	County					
	Gongyi	Linying	Zhenping	Yuzhou	Total	%
0–2500	1	10	9	3	23	30.7
2501–7000	11	9	9	15	44	58.7
7001–10000	4	0	2	2	8	10.6
10001–25000	0	0	0	0	0	0
Total	16	19	20	20	75	100

*Note: International poverty line was 7,000 yuan; China's official poverty line was 2,563 yuan/ household/year (approximately 2,500 yuan). Categories chosen to reflect the two poverty lines. US$1 = 8 yuan.
Source: Field data for the case-control study.

per day), and the lack of rest days can increase the risk of TB transmission and infection to susceptible individuals.

Conclusions

In this chapter, we have focused on the poverty aspect of TB disease and found that a large proportion of our sampled TB cases had out-migrated for work. One-third of these off-farm migrants lived below the absolute poverty line, defined by the Chinese government. We also found that TB patients spent a large proportion of their household incomes seeking treatment. The majority borrowed money and resorted to selling household belongings and productive assets to defray costs. Thus, TB is not only a major public health problem, it is also a poverty indicator and an impoverishment factor.

We did not attempt to explain why migrant workers were more likely to contract active tuberculosis. It is reasonable to expect that crowded dormitories and the physical and mental stress that accompany working in suboptimal conditions, as well as poor nutrition increased the disease risk in vulnerable and poverty-stricken migrant workers.

The plight of migrant workers has been noted by the government in recent times (Yardley, 2004), yet the focus has been on unpaid wages and legal rights rather than health (*China Daily*, 8 August 2003). China has to impose stricter workplace regulations to prevent labour exploitation and sub-standard housing, which should assist in reducing the negative externalities of TB disease. As part of China's poverty reduction programme, adequate public health expenditure is needed in rural areas. Especially critical is the greater financial support for the poorer counties and the individual poverty-stricken TB sufferers who are further impoverished by income losses and the economic burden of the disease.

Acknowledgement

Research is funded by UNDP/World Bank/WHO Special Programme for Research and Training in Tropical Diseases (TDR) A10166.

References

Alleviation Poverty Office of China State Council. (2004) *Press Release*, 16 July, www.qianlong.com. Accessed March 2005.

Chen X, Zhao F, Duanmu H, Wan L, Wang L, Du X, Chin DP. (2002) The DOTS strategy in China: Results and lessons after 10 years. *Bull World Health Org* **80**(6): 430–436.

China Daily. (2003) Migrant Workers Invited To Join Unions, 8 August.

China Statistical Yearbook 2004. (2004) China Statistical Publishing House, Beijing.

China Tuberculosis Control Collaboration. (2004) The effect of tuberculosis control in China. *Lancet* **364**: 417–422.

Comstock GW, Cauthen GM. (1992) Epidemiology of tuberculosis, in LB Reichman & E Hershfield (eds.), *Tuberculosis: A Comprehensive International HPTB Approach*, pp. 23–48, Marcel Dekker, New York.

Floyd K. (2003) Costs and effectiveness — The impact of economic studies on TB control. *Tuberculosis* **83**(1–3): 187–200.

Henan Province Statistical Yearbook 2003. (2003) China Statistical Publishing House, Beijing.

Hopewell PC. (2002) Tuberculosis control: How the world has changed since 1990. *Bull World Health Org* **80**(6): 427.

Lague D. (2005) *Healthcare Falls Short, Chinese Tell Leaders. Asia-Pac Int Herald Tribune*, 20 August.

Lee JW, Loevinsohn E, Kumaresan JA. (2002) Response to a major disease of poverty: The global partnership to stop TB. *Bull World Health Org* **80**(6): 428.

Long ER. (1941) Constitution and related factors in resistance to tuberculosis. *Arch Pathol* **32**: 122–162.

Prescott N. (1999) Coping with catastrophic health shocks. *Conf Social Protection and Poverty*, Inter American Development Bank, Washington DC.

Russell S. (2004) The economic burden of illness for households in developing countries: A review of studies focusing on malaria, tuberculosis, and human immunodeficiency virus/acquired immunodeficiency syndrome. *Am J Trop Med Hyg* **71**(Suppl 2): 147–155.

World Health Organization. (2004) *Global Tuberculosis Control: Surveillance, Planning, Financing. WHO Report*, World Health Organization, Geneva, WHO/HTM/TB/2004.331

Yardley J. (2004) In a Tidal Wave, China's Masses Pour from Farm to City. *New York Times Weekly Rev*, 12 September.

Zhang XS. (2004) *China Newsnet Press Release*, 12 June. www.chinanews. com.cn.

13

Migration, Gender, and STD Risk: A Case Study of Female Temporary Migrants in Southwestern China*

Xiushi Yang

Introduction

After declaring its success in eradicating STDs in the 1960s, China has witnessed epidemic growth in STDs in the last two decades. The strong resurgence of STDs takes place in the context of widespread commercial sex and increasing sexual promiscuity (van den Hoek *et al.*, 2001; Parish *et al.*, 2003; Pan *et al.*, 2004), creating a serious public health challenge, as hundreds of thousands people are infected every year. In 2002 alone, 744,848 cases of STDs were officially reported nationwide, with the actual number perhaps many times larger (Parish *et al.*, 2003). While the cause of the STD epidemic is likely to be complex and multifaceted, increasing temporary migration has been portrayed by the media and implicated in the literature as the main catalyst in the spread of both commercial sex and STDs.

The growth of the temporary migrant population in China since the early 1980s has been truly phenomenal. Although varied by sources, the total number of temporary migrants was estimated to have grown from

*Funding for the research was provided through National Institutes of Health/National Institute on Drug Abuse Grant 1R01DA13145.

11 million in 1982 to 79 million in 2000 (Liang and Ma, 2004). Among the tidal waves of rural–urban labour migrants are hundreds of thousands of young women from poor rural villages (Roberts, 2002; Fan, 2003; Gaetano and Jacka, 2004). Living and working away from home and/or regular sexual partners, the uprooting of so many migrant men and women in their primary sexually active ages, have undoubtedly created conditions that are conducive to sexual promiscuity and commercial sex. In fact, residential immobility was considered the most important factor that explains the absence of commercial sex in pre-reform China (Troyer *et al.*, 1989).

However, while the link between migration, commercial sex and STDs has captured a great deal of research attention, the literature has not been very specific on whether there may be differences in the way that men and women experience behavioural change and STD risk as a result of migration. Similarly, while gender has become more explicit in the recent studies of labour migration in China, the increasing attention has been focused on the social, economic and cultural experiences of female migrants (Roberts, 2002; Fan, 2003; Gaetano and Jacka, 2004; Liang and Chen, 2004). Very little research has been done on the health consequences of migration, including HIV/STD risk, for female migrants. Completely lacking is our understanding of how the interplay between migration and gender may render female migrants particularly vulnerable to HIV/STDs.

Using data from a large population-based survey conducted in 2003, this paper examines the STD/HIV risk as a result of migration among female temporary migrants in China. The paper argues that given the gender inequality in education and occupational training, female migrants will experience greater difficulty in competing for mainstream employment in the city; many will end up working in the personal service or entertainment industry, where commercial sex is widely suspected. Economic hardship and competition may leave female migrants with little control in their commercial sex encounters; gendered moral and social values can further subject female migrants to a subordinate position in sexual relationships. Consequently, female migrants, particularly those working in the entertainment industry, are socio-economically highly marginalised, vulnerable to both economic and sexual exploitation and at high risk of STDs/HIV. The analysis will help shed light on the role that migration and gender play in female migrants' vulnerability to STDs. It will also provide important empirical data for the design of prevention intervention programs targeting female temporary migrants.

Migration and STD/HIV Risks

Numerous studies in China and other developing countries (Brockerhoff and Biddlecom, 1999; Skeldon, 2000; Wolffers *et al.*, 2002; Anderson *et al.*, 2003; Yang forthcoming) and the more developed countries (Organista and Organista, 1997; Gras *et al.*, 1999; Lansky *et al.*, 2000) have highlighted the vulnerability of migrants to HIV/STDs, and the subsequent spread of the disease through migrant travel.

At the aggregate level, migration brings more people into close contact and creates a greater mixing of population at places of destination, which provides the ready environment for disease transmission. Through the movement of infected persons, migration in turn offers a convenient vehicle to transport diseases to places where they are previously unknown. As such, prevalence rates of STDs/HIV tend to spread outward from its epicentres geographically along transport connections, trade routes, and migration systems, and socially along personal and social networks (Obbo, 1993; Wallace *et al.*, 1997; Wood *et al.*, 2000), and are positively correlated with the intensity of residential mobility (Yang, 2005).

At the individual level, migration is believed to actually create a sub-population (migrants) whose socio-economic contexts are conducive to STD/HIV risk sexual behaviours (Caldwell *et al.*, 1997; Wolffers *et al.*, 2002; Yang, forthcoming). In particular, separation from spouse or regular sexual partner and migrants' post migration milieus are encouraging risky sexual behaviour (Brockerhoff and Biddlecom, 1999; Yang, forthcoming). When separation from spouse is frequent and lengthy, it can disrupt migrants' regular sexual relationships. Together with post migration economic marginalisation and social isolation, this may lead to a more promiscuous life as a way to escape loneliness, bury anxieties about family and work, and release sexual frustration (Jochelson *et al.*, 1991; Caldwell *et al.*, 1997; Brockerhoff and Biddlecom, 1999). The separation from family and home community may also create some form of social control vacuum whereby migrants feel less constrained by social norms, since families and friends back home are unlikely to find out what they do while away from home (Maticha-Tyndale *et al.*, 1997; Yang, 2000a). Consequently, the anonymity of life and easier access to commercial sex in the city may help migrants to break away from social norms of morality and sexual fidelity, and to encourage them to seek casual sex.

Migration and Gender

The interplay between migration and gender has recently attracted attention from migration scholars both in and outside of China. Rural-urban labour migration in China, as in other developing countries (Chant, 1992), is increasingly recognised and studied as a gendered process (Davin, 1999; Fan, 2000; Roberts, 2002; Gaetano and Jacka, 2004). Due to and reflective of the deeply rooted gendered role expectations in the Chinese family and society, men and women often migrate at different rates and differ in both causes and consequences of their migration. There is mounting evidence in China that women are actively participating in labour migration and are doing so for economic reasons (Fan, 2000, 2004; Yan, 2000b; Liang and Chen, 2004; Liang and Ma, 2004). However, the conventional characterisation of male dominance in rural-urban labour migration and economic motives for male, as well as social and familial reasons for female migrants cannot be completely discarded.

For example, recent studies of migration continue to stress the sociocultural constraints facing rural women in China, which significantly limit women's participation in rural-urban labour migration (Fan, 2000, 2004; Gaetano, 2004). The structural forces unleashed by the economic reforms have not altered, and in some ways have actually reinforced patriarchal traditions in China that give the priority to "the social, economic and physical mobility of men and relegate women to secondary, supporting and care-giving roles" (Fan, 2000). When women migrate, they are usually for non-economic reasons such as marriage and accompanying family (Knight *et al.*, 1999; Yang and Guo, 1999). The most salient factor constraining women's participation in labour migration is marriage and its associated supporting and care-giving roles expected of married women from the family and society (Jacka, 1997; Davin, 1999; Yang and Guo, 1999; Fan, 2004). However, research has suggested that the situation may have changed; neither marriage nor having children seems to have deterred migration of women (Lou *et al.*, 2004).

More research has focused on the gendered consequences of migration in China (Fan, 2000, 2003, 2004; Roberts, 2002; Gaetano and Jacka, 2004; Liang and Chen, 2004). On the positive side, migration is seen to allow women to break away from traditional roles and help them to gain economic independence; the urban experience can empower woman migrants, change their views about gender roles, and enable them to benefit from development and to become potential agents for changing the socio-cultural norms that define women's roles and entitlements (Goldstein *et al.*, 2000; Fan, 2000, 2004; Lou *et al.*, 2004; Murphy, 2004).

On the other hand, migration may not be so positive for women. Due to gender inequalities in education and job training, female migrants are at a disadvantaged position in cities and do not do as well as their male counterparts (Huang, 2001; Fan, 2003; Liang and Chen, 2004). Furthermore, the market transition has weakened the institutional support for gender equality and increased gender segregation in the labour market. Consequently, female migrants are channelled mainly into low-status occupations, perpetuating and reinforcing women's inferior and subordinate status (Fan, 2000, 2003). Being heavily concentrated in labour-intensive assembly and personal service industries (Yang, 2000b; Roberts, 2002), where jobs are characterised by high turnover, low pay, long working hours and lax labour disciplines, female migrants are particularly economically marginalised and socially isolated, being vulnerable to economic and sexual exploitation in places of urban destination. While some may settle down in the city (Roberts, 2002; Tan and Short, 2004), many female migrants return to their rural villages when they reach marriageable age and face difficulties in readjusting to rural ways of life (Murphy, 2004). If gender segregation in the labour market and short duration in the city may have limited female migrants' positive experiences of labour migration, their potential roles as agents for social change may be further circumscribed by cultural and institutional constraints (Fan, 2004; Murphy, 2004).

Gender and HIV/STD Risk

Gender-related unequal power relationships and cultural norms about gender and sexuality are increasingly recognised as important determinants of risky sexual behaviour among women (Raffaelli and Pranke, 1995; Browning et al., 1999; Tang, Wong and Lee, 2001). According to the theory of gender and power (Connell, 1987; Wingood and DiClemente, 2002), women's heightened vulnerability to STDs, including HIV, is a function of gendered relationships between men and women that are rooted in the sexual divisions of labour and power and the gendered structure of social norms. The sexual division of labour limits women's equal access to the paid labour market and creates economic inequalities between men and women. This reinforces women's economic dependence on men and increases women's "economic exposure" to HIV/STDs. The sexual division of power leads to unequal power between men and women that results in men's control in relationships and renders women vulnerable to sexual or physical abuse. This limits women's ability to make decisions on sexual matters and increases their "physical exposure" to HIV/STD. The gendered structure of social norms generates gender-specific norms that restrict women's sexual expressions and submit women to men in sexual relationships. This discourages open discussion within relationships and limits women's access to information, thereby increasing women's "social exposure" to HIV/STDs.

Together, economic inequalities, unequal power and gender-specific cultural norms exert critical influences over women's sexual behaviour and render formidable barriers to women in exercising personal control in sexual and social relationships (Amaro and Raj, 2000). Research among Chinese women (Tang et al., 2001) suggests that the Confucian concept of model womanhood, which commands the submission of women to men, can significantly constrain women's ability to insist on condom use. In general, non-condom use among Chinese women is related to the lack of information, embarrassment in talking about condoms, and the fear of being perceived as sexually available as a result of conservative Confucian concepts regarding women and sexuality. Studies of women working in China's flourishing entertainment industry (Liao et al., 2003; Xia and Yang, 2005) have underscored the importance of cultural norms in understanding unprotected commercial sex. In general, women who felt guilty for their role in commercial sex, a social stigma deeply rooted in the Chinese culture and legal systems, were less likely to insist on the use of condom in commercial sex.

Despite mounting evidence that suggests interlinkages between migration, gender and STD/HIV risk, the literature on migration and STD/HIV risk has paid little attention to the issues of gender, while studies of migration and gender have largely bypassed the gendered health risk of migration. The lack of attention to the interplay between migration, gender and HIV/STD risk is particularly striking, given that a large proportion of female rural-urban migrants work in the personal service and entertainment industries, where commercial sex is widely suspected. This paper argues that female migrants in China are subjected to the influence of both migration and gender; any impact of migration and/or gender on sexual behaviour will be particularly pronounced among female migrants. Female migrants in general and those involved in commercial sex are particularly at high risk of acquiring STDs/HIV while in the cities; they may also act as a bridge population in the spread of the disease as infected women return to rural villages (as many of them do after a few years of working in the city) and unknowingly pass STDs/HIV to their marriage or sexual partners (Lau and Thomas, 2001; Hirsch *et al.*, 2002; Anderson *et al.*, 2003; Lurie *et al.*, 2003).

Data and Methods

Data used in the analysis are from a large population-based survey conducted in 2003, covering an entire province in Southwestern China. Sample selection followed a three-stage sampling procedure. Firstly, tabulations of known HIV/AIDS cases, drug users and migrants by counties were prepared with the data from the provincial public health and public security agencies and the 1995 mini-census. These tabulations were used to rank all counties and from the ranked list of counties, eight were selected, giving priority to counties with higher concentration of HIV, drug use and migrant population, and those geographically representing the province. Secondly, all rural townships and urban neighbourhoods in each of the eight selected counties were ranked according to estimates of HIV cases, drug users and temporary migrants, based on existing data from the same government agencies and the

1995 mini-census. From the ranked list of each county, five townships and neighbourhoods were selected from each list. Again, the selection was not random but priority is given to places with a combination of high prevalence of HIV, drug users and temporary migrants, and those geographically representing the varied parts of the county. This resulted in a total of 40 townships and neighbourhoods as the primary sampling units (PSUs).

Finally, in each PSU, all individuals 18 to 55 years of age were ordered in sequence in one of four categories: HIV positive, drug users, temporary migrants, and non-migrants. Information used to assign individuals to a category was based on household registration rosters (non-migrants) and confidential registrations of migrants, drug users and HIV/AIDS. They were cross-checked for multiple listings. If an individual appeared in more than one category, the individual was reassigned to only one category according to the following priority order: HIV, drug user, migrant and non-migrant. For example, a migrant who was also a drug user and was HIV positive, that individual was retained in the list of HIV positive persons and removed from the lists of migrants and drug users. Therefore, all individuals would appear in one and only one of the four lists, which were mutually exclusive.

In selecting individuals, disproportionate probability sampling (Bilsborrow *et al.*, 1997) was used to make sure that the resulting sample would contain sufficient numbers of rare populations, e.g., HIV positive and drug users, but not overwhelmed by non-migrants. A target random sample of ~ 150 individuals from each PSU was planned and distributed as follows: 20 HIV positive, 30 drug users, 40 temporary migrants and 60 non-migrants. In each category, sample selection began with randomly picking a person from the list and continued selecting at fixed intervals determined by the ratio between the total on the list and the target number for the category. If a list contains fewer than the target number, everyone on the list was selected. This is because not every PSU had the target number of subjects in all categories, and the actual sample size in a category varied across PSUs.

During the fieldwork, interviewers visited the sampled individuals, explained to them the purpose of the study, their right to refuse, the compensation for their time, and invited them to participate. If the respondent was absent, a second visit was scheduled. If a respondent could not be reached the second time or refused to participate, a replacement was selected randomly from the original sampling list containing the absent or refused respondent, unless there was no one left on the list. Participant refusal was low (3.3%). Of the original sample of 5,687, including 117 from the pilot testing town, 5,499 individuals consented to participate and completed a face-to-face interview, which took place in private at the respondents' home or elsewhere if they preferred. All interviews were conducted in Mandarin or the respondent's dialect, if the respondent could not communicate in Mandarin.

Version 7 of the STATA software is used to conduct statistical analyses, which will use the survey design-based "svy" methods in STATA to adjust for population weights and PSU design effects. The "svy" (survey-based) methods are a group of statistical analyses, including descriptive, linear and nonlinear logistic regression analysis in STATA. By specifying three variables representing sampling probabilities, strata (for stratified sampling) and PSU, respectively, the "svy" methods take into consideration different sampling probabilities and correct for the correlations among respondents from the same PSU, which violate independent observation assumption in standard regression analysis, thereby producing more reliable and accurate results in the analysis. Data analysis focuses on comparisons between temporary migrants and non-migrants in the prevalence of outcome variables, which are self-reports of (1) casual sex with non-stable partners and condom use in such casual sexual encounters, and (2) history of being STD or HIV positive. Temporary migrants are defined as respondents who were working and living in the place of interview at the time of survey, but without the official local household registration (or *hukou*). To highlight the increased STD risk associated with employment in the entertainment industry, female migrants who worked as dancers, singers, masseuses, or hairdressers in the entertainment industry (*fuwu xiaojie*) will be separated from other temporary migrants in the analysis.

To examine the impact of temporary migration on STD/HIV risk, the Pearson's chi-square test of difference in proportions further corrected for survey design and converted into F statistics in "svy" cross-tabulation analysis was used to test if migrants differ from non-migrants. However, when the variable of interest is continuous, the adjusted Wald test of difference in means was used. The analysis was conducted for males and females separately; differences between the male and female samples were examined to see if the impact of temporary migration is more pronounced among female than male migrants. Furthermore, similar statistical tests of difference in proportions or means were conducted between female migrant service and entertainment workers and other female migrants, but the test results will only be indicated where appropriate in the text but not shown in tables, in order to keep data presentation in the tables clear and easy to follow.

Logistic regression was then used to control for differences between migrants and non-migrants in individual characteristics that may confound the bivariate comparisons. Specifically, age, educational attainment, marital status, living arrangement, measures of economic marginalisation, social isolation, and lax social control, which are believed to also influence sexual behaviour, were controlled in the logistic regression analysis. All individual characteristics are self-explanatory.

The economic marginalisation index measures respondents' relative socioeconomic status. It was constructed by first dichotomising answers (1 *vs.* 0) to questions on employment (unemployed *vs.* employed), industry (agriculture, construction, and personal services *vs.* others), ownership of company (self/small privately owned *vs.* state/collectively owned), occupation (menial jobs, including farmers and personal service workers, *vs.* more prestigious ones), income (annual income below 600 yuan *vs.* 600 yuan or higher), perceived income level and working conditions (below average *vs.* average or better), and eight employment-related benefits (not having *vs.* having pension, health insurance, social security, unemployment benefit, paid holidays, paid sick leave, housing allowances, and on-job training). These 15 dichotomous answers were then summed to form the economic marginalisation index. The higher the score, the more economically marginalised is the respondent. Cronbach's alpha for the summative composite index with the data was 0.86, indicating high reliability.

Social isolation and lax social control were measured by a modified version of the UCLA Loneliness Scale (Russell and Cutrona, 1988) and a modified version of the Attitudes toward Authority Scale (Emler, 1999). The two English scales were translated and back translated, and thoroughly pretested before their actual use in the survey. In translating the scales, we paid particular attention to local cultural difference and sensitivity to make sure the original meanings of the scales were not lost in the course of translating. After passing a pretest, the Chinese version was back translated into English by a researcher who was not involved in the English-to-Chinese translation. Results of the back-translation were compared with the original English version for accuracy; adjustment and rewording of questions were made to insure that the Chinese version conveyed the same information intended in the English version.

For the social isolation (loneliness) scale, respondents reported on a four-point scale how lonely they felt on each of the 20 statements; answers to the 20 statements were summed to form the "loneliness" scale. For the lax social control scale, respondents reported 'yes' (1) or 'no' (0) on their personal experiences with nine events, indicating disrespect for laws or the use of "deviant" ways to achieve personal ends. Answers were then summed to create the lax social control scale. For both scales, the higher the score, the more likely the respondent was socially isolated and had behaved in disrespect for laws or deviant ways, indicating lax social control. Cronbach's alphas with the survey data were 0.80 and 0.71 for the loneliness and the lax social control scales, respectively, again indicating good internal reliability of the two scales.

Results

Overall, females made up 47% of the temporary migrant population in our weighted sample. Males had a slightly higher migration participation rate (9.7%) than females (9.1%), but the difference was statistically not significant. Among female temporary migrants, a majority (52.8%) worked in restaurants, hotels and entertainment establishments such as dancing/karaoke TV halls, hair/beauty salons, and massage parlors (*fuwu xiaojie*). By comparison, only 3.8% of female non-migrants were working as *fuwu xiaojie*. These statistics confirm that women are as actively participating in migration as men in contemporary China and female migrants are overwhelmingly channelled to the personal service and entertainment industry.

In terms of individual demographic and socioeconomic characteristics, female temporary migrants differed significantly from non-migrants; female migrant service/entertainment workers (FMSEWs) in turn differed from other temporary migrants in individual characteristics (Table 1). In particular, FMSEWs were on average more than ten years younger than

Table 1. Individual characteristics by migrant status among females 18 years or older.

Individual Characteristics	Unweighted sample size	Migrant status		
		Non migrants (n)	Temporary migrants (n)	FMSEWs (n)
Age (mean)	1,987	32.6 (1,301)	31.9 (360)	22.3 (326)**
Educational attainment (%) Illiterate	326	13.9 (239)	17.2 (66)**	6.6(21)**
Elementary school	584	23.6 (342)	38.5 (126)**	31.5 (116)**
Junior high school	776	38.9 (488)	33.8 (123)**	54.1 (165)**
Senior high school or higher	298	23.6 (228)	10.5 (45)**	7.9 (25)**
Married (%)	1,988	87.4 (1,302)	75.0 (360)**	19.7 (326)**
Live alone (%)	1,989	1.2 (1,302)	19.4 (360)**	23.9 (327)**
Econ. marginalisation index (mean)	1,989	10.1 (1,302)	11.1 (360)*	11.1 (327)**
Social isolation index (mean)	1,989	37.0 (1,302)	41.0 (360)**	41.6 (327)**
Lax social control index (mean)	1,989	0.2 (1,302)	0.4 (360)	0.5 (327)**

Note: Statistical significance tests presented are based on comparison to non-migrants.
$^*p < 0.05$; $^{**}p < 0.01$.

non-migrants, although other female migrants (excluding FMSEWs) did not differ significantly from non-migrants in age. Compared with non-migrants, both female migrant groups had significantly lower proportions of having a senior high school or higher education. Yet, FMSEWs had a higher proportion of junior high school education, while other female temporary migrants had a significantly higher proportion of elementary school education than non-migrants.

Non-migrant women 18 years of age or older were overwhelmingly married, and very few of them lived alone at the time of the survey. By contrast, both female migrant groups had significantly lower proportions that were married, but significantly higher proportions who lived alone. The discrepancies between FMSEWs and non-migrants were particularly striking with less than 20% of FMSEWs married and almost 24% of them living alone, compared with the corresponding proportions of 87% and 1.2%, respectively, for non-migrants.

On average, both female migrant groups scored significantly higher on the measures of economic marginalisation and social isolation than non-migrants. Similarly, while both female migrant groups also scored higher on the measure of lax social control than non-migrants, only the difference between FMSEWs and non-migrants was statistically significant. Clearly, FMSEWs in the sample were overwhelmingly young, single and living alone; they were also more likely to experience socioeconomic marginalisation, social isolation and lax social control than other female temporary migrants, although the difference in the three measures between the two migrant groups were statistically not significant (test results not shown but available upon request).

Table 2 presents prevalence rates of STD/HIV risk sexual behaviours and actual STDs/HIV prevalence by migrant status and by gender. Several generalisations can be made from the data. Firstly, for both males and females, temporary migrants had higher prevalence rates of risky sexual behaviours than non-migrants; FMSEWs in turn had significantly (significance tests not shown) higher prevalence rates of risky sexual behaviours and STDs/HIV than other female migrants. Secondly, differences in prevalence rates of risky sexual behaviours between migrants and non-migrants were more pronounced among females than males. In fact, male temporary migrants scored significantly higher only on three of the six measures, (only one at the 1% level) compared with their non-migrant counterparts. By comparison, both female migrant groups showed significantly higher prevalence rates of risky sexual behaviour in all but one measure in Table 2. This gender difference confirms the hypothesis that the impact of migration on STD/HIV risk sexual behaviour is significantly stronger on women than men.

Thirdly, except for female migrants with respect to involvement in commercial sex or casual sex in the 30 days prior to the survey, men in general had a sex life that was STD/HIV riskier than women, which is particularly apparent among the non-migrant population. However, regardless of migrant status, women had significantly higher prevalence rates of STDs/HIV than men (significance tests not shown), underscoring the increased vulnerability to STDs/HIV among women, which cannot be directly attributed to

Table 2. STD risk sexual behavior and stds by migrant status and by gender.

Risk behaviour/ STDs	Unweighted sample size	Migrant status		
		Non migrants (n)	Temporary migrants (n)	FMESWs (n)
Female sample:				
Ever had casual sex	1,931	4.5 (1,262)	16.2 (351)**	49.9 (318)**
Ever had unprotected casual sex	1,931	1.9 (1,262)	10.8 (351)**	31.6 (318)**
Ever taking alcohol/drugs having sex	1,647	2.7 (1,120)	7.4 (288)*	21.3 (239)**
Ever involved in commercial sex	1,748	0.3 (1,183)	9.3 (302)**	38.6 (263)**
Casual sex in prior 30 days	1,917	1.9 (1,254)	11.1 (347)**	38.0 (316)**
Unprotected casual sex in prior 30 days	1,917	1.0 (1,254)	2.2 (347)	6.5 (316)**
Ever had STDs or HIV positive	1,989	12.2 (1,302)	10.6 (360)	16.9 (327)
Male sample:				
Ever had casual sex	3,383	12.9 (2,470)	20.4 (913)*	
Ever had unprotected casual sex	3,383	6.2 (2,470)	13.2 (913)**	
Ever taking alcohol/drugs while having sex	2,748	16.1 (2,054)	16.2 (694)	
Ever involved in commercial sex	2,944	3.3 (2,209)	5.2 (735)	
Casual sex in prior 30 days	3,336	4.6 (2,434)	4.8 (902)*	
Unprotected casual sex in prior 30 days	3,336	3.0 (2,434)	2.3 (902)	
Ever had STDs or HIV positive	3.432	4.5 (2,504)	3.0 (928)	

Note: Statistical significance tests presented are based on comparison to non-migrants. $^*p < 0.05$; $^{**}p < 0.01$.

women's own sexual behaviour. FMSEWs in turn had a significantly higher prevalence of STDs/HIV (16.9%) than other female temporary migrants (significance tests not shown), who had the lowest prevalence rate (10.6%) among females.

Lastly, of the five migrant-by-gender groups in Table 2, FMSEWs had the highest prevalence rates of both risky sexual behaviours and actual STD/HIV infection. Clearly, the interplay of migration and gender had led to the concentration of female migrants in the personal service and entertainment industry, which in turn rendered them particularly vulnerable to risky sexual behaviours and STDs/HIV. In fact, FMSEWs had the highest prevalence rate of STDs/HIV, although the difference is statistically not significant between FMSEWs and non-migrants.

Recall that female migrants and non-migrants differed significantly in individual demographic and socioeconomic characteristics (Table 1), which may be correlated with risk sexual behaviour and thereby confounding any bivariate comparison between migrants and non-migrants. Multiple logistic regressions were therefore employed to control for potential confounding impacts of individual characteristics. Due to statistically insignificant difference between migrants and non-migrants in the prevalence rates of STDs or HIV (Table 2), the logistic regressions were focused on the two key measures of risky sexual behaviour, namely, the odds of having casual and unprotected casual sex.

Table 3 presents the bivariate (the unadjusted column) and multivariate (the adjusted column) logistic regression results for the lifetime measures of ever had casual sex with non-stable partner(s) and ever had unprotected casual sex. For both measures, the data suggest that a considerable amount of the observed differences in the likelihood of ever having casual and unprotected casual sex between migrants and non-migrants were indeed attributable to differences in their individual characteristics. However, migration status remained a significant and powerful predictor of the two lifetime risky sexual behaviours, even after differences in individual characteristics were accounted for in the multiple regressions. For example, the odds ratios between FMSEWs and non-migrants were more than halved in the multiple regression (from $\sim$ 21 to 10 and 25 to 12, respectively); those between other female temporary migrants and non-migrants were also considerably reduced when individual characteristics

Table 3. Logistic regression of impact of temporary migration on lifetime odds of having casual sex and unprotected casual sex among females.[a]

Explanatory Variables	Casual sex		Unprotected casual sex	
	Unadjusted	Adjusted	Unadjusted	Adjusted
Migrant status				
Non-migrants[b]	1.00	1.00	1.00	1.00
Other migrants	4.1(2.1–8.1)	2.2(1.3–4.0)	6.4(2.9–13.9)	4.1(2.1–7.9)
FMSEWs	21.4(11.3–40.6)	10.3(5.5–19.2)	24.5(12.8–46.9)	11.9(6.1–23.0)
Age (in five years)[c]	0.7(0.5–0.9)	0.9(0.7–1.2)	0.7(0.5–0.8)	0.9(0.7–1.2)
Educational attainment				
Illiterate[b]	1.00	1.00	1.00	1.00
Elementary school	1.8(0.9–3.4)	1.3(0.7–2.3)	2.6(0.9–7.7)	1.7(0.5–5.2)
Junior high school	1.5(0.8–3.1)	1.2(0.6–2.5)	1.9(0.7–5.5)	1.2(0.4–3.8)
Senior high school or higher	0.7(0.3–1.7)	0.8(0.3–2.6)	1.5(0.4–4.9)	1.0(0.2–5.3)
Marital status				
Single[b]	1.00	1.00	1.00	1.00
Married	0.2(0.1–0.4)	0.9(0.5–1.9)	0.2(0.1–0.3)	0.8(0.3–2.1)
Living arrangement				
Live with others[b]	1.00	1.00	1.00	1.00
Live alone	9.3(4.7–18.2)	2.4(1.1–5.0)	11.0(5.2–23.3)	2.2(1.1–4.4)
Economic marginalisation[c,d]	1.8(0.9–3.9)	1.0(0.4–2.6)	0.9(0.4–1.9)	0.3(0.1–1.2)
Social Isolation[c,d]	2.4(1.7–3.3)	1.7(1.2–2.3)	2.2(1.5–3.1)	1.5(1.0–2.2)
Lax social control[c]	3.0(2.3–3.9)	2.3(1.7–3.2)	2.8(1.9–4.1)	2.0(1.2–3.3)

[a]Results presented are odds ratios; numbers shown in parentheses are the 95% confidence intervals. [b]Reference category. [c]Continuous variables. [d]For ease of presentation, the odds ratios are presented with change of every 10 points in the scale.

were controlled for. However, the adjusted odds of ever having had casual sex and unprotected casual sex among FMSEWs remained at 10 and 12 times, respectively, that of the corresponding odds of non-migrants. Similarly, the adjusted odds of the two lifetime measures among other female migrants remained at two and four times those of non-migrants. The results indicate that migration and working in the personal service/entertainment industry exerted significant influence on Chinese women's HIV/STD risk sexual behaviours, independent of individual demographic and socioeconomic characteristics.

Among the individual characteristics included in the models, age and marital status were significant correlates of the two lifetime risky sexual behaviours among Chinese women at the bivariate level (unadjusted odds). Compared with the odds of younger and single women, older and married women's odds of having casual and unprotected casual sex were significantly reduced. However, both age and marital status lost statistical significance in the multiple regressions, indicating that their impacts on the two risky behaviours were mainly mediated by other variables in the model.

Living arrangement and measures of social isolation and lax social control were all significant factors influencing Chinese women's HIV/STD risk sexual behaviours at both the bivariate and the multivariate levels. Like those of the migration variables, the positive impact of living alone on risky sexual behaviours was significantly reduced, but remained significant with the adjusted odds of both lifetime measures more than doubled among women who lived alone than those living with others. Similarly, both social isolation and lax social control significantly increased Chinese women's odds of having ever had casual and unprotected casual sex with non-stable partner(s).

When the analysis was focused on the two risky sexual behaviours during the 30 days prior to the survey, data in Table 4 suggest very much the same pattern for the odds of having casual sex with non-stable partners. Both female migrant groups had significantly higher odds of having engaged in casual sex than non-migrants; in turn, FMSEWs had much higher odds of the risky sexual behaviour than other female migrants. However, the impacts of being a migrant and/or a FMSEW on risky behaviour were significantly reduced, once individual characteristics were controlled for in the multiple regressions. Both age and marital status reduced the odds of having casual sex

Table 4. Logistic regression of impact of temporary migration on 30-days-prior-to- survey odds of having casual sex and unprotected casual sex among females[a]

Explanatory Variables	Casual sex		Unprotected casual sex	
	Unadjusted	Adjusted	Unadjusted	Adjusted
Migrant status Non-migrants[b]	1.00	1.00	1.00	1.00
Other migrants	6.5(2.6–16.2)	3.2(1.4–7.2)	2.2(0.6–8.3)	1.6(0.4–5.6)
FMSEWs	31.9(14.3–70.9)	11.9(6.0–23.4)	6.6(2.4–18.5)	4.7(1.8–12.6)
Age (in five years)[c]	0.7(0.5–0.9)	1.0(0.9–1.1)	0.9(0.7–1.2)	1.1(1.0–1.1)
Educational attainment Illiterate[b]	1.00	1.00	1.00	1.00
Elementary school	2.6(1.1–6.3)	1.8(0.8–3.8)	3.2(0.7–13.4)	3.3(0.6–17.3)
Junior high school	1.8(0.8–4.5)	1.4(0.5–3.5)	2.4(0.4–14.2)	3.1(0.4–22.2)
Senior high school or higher	0.8(0.2–2.7)	1.0(0.1–7.2)	1.7(0.2–13.2)	4.2(0.3–51.9)
Marital status Single[b]	1.00	1.00	1.00	1.00
Married	0.1(0.1–0.3)	0.6(0.2–1.4)	0.3(0.1–1.0)	0.8(0.2–3.3)
Living arrangement Live with others[b]	1.00	1.00	1.00	1.00
Live alone	12.4(6.2–25.0)	2.3(1.2–4.2)	3.0(0.8–11.2)	1.0(0.2–4.0)
Economic marginalisation[c,d]	2.8(0.7–10.3)	1.2(0.1–9.4)	8.4(2.5–28.3)	10.0(2.9–34.2)
Social Isolation[c,d]	3.0(2.0–4.5)	1.8(1.3–2.5)	1.6(1.0–2.6)	1.3(0.8–2.1)
Lax social control[c]	3.2(2.3–4.5)	2.2(1.6–2.9)	1.6(1.0–2.6)	1.2(0.8–1.8)

Notes: [a]Results presented are odds ratios; numbers shown in parentheses are the 95% confidence intervals. [b]Reference category. [c]Continuous variables. [d]For ease of presentation, the odds ratios are presented with change of every 10 points in the scale.

in the 30 days prior to the survey significantly at the bivariate level, but lost their significance in the multivariate model. Living alone, social isolation and lax social control all predicted a significantly riskier sexual life at both the bivariate and multivariate levels.

However, the patterns for the likelihood of having unprotected casual sex in the 30 days prior to the survey differed in several ways. Firstly, the odds of having unprotected casual sex were no longer significant between other female migrants and non-migrants; while statistically significant differences in the odds between FMSEWs and non-migrants were also relatively more moderate at both the bivariate and multivariate levels. For example, instead of more than 10 times the odds of non-migrants for the two lifetime measures and the other monthly measure, the odds of having unprotected casual sex during the month prior to the survey among FMSEWs was less than five times that of non-migrants.

Secondly, while age was not a significant factor at the bivariate level, at the multivariate level, it significantly increased the odds of having unprotected casual sex during the 30 days prior to the survey among Chinese women. In other words, other things being equal, older women were more likely than their younger counterparts to have experienced unprotected sex with non-stable partners in the month prior to the survey. Thirdly, neither marital status nor living arrangement had a significant influence over women's likelihood of consistent condom use during casual sex during the 30-day period.

Fourthly, the measure of economic marginalisation turned out to be a significant predictor of the odds of unprotected casual sex among women during the 30-day period at both the bivariate and multivariate levels. Women who were economically more marginalised were more likely to have engaged in unprotected sex with non-stable partners, indicating that the cost of condoms might have deterred women with economic difficulties from purchasing and using condoms in casual sexual encounters. Lastly, once migration and other individual characteristics were controlled for in the multiple regression analysis, neither social isolation nor lax social control had significant power in predicting women's likelihood of consistent condom use in casual sex in the month before the survey.

Figure 1 presents the mean predicted probabilities of lifetime and 30-day measures of risky sexual behaviours by migrant status. Regardless of measure, FMSEWs had the highest probabilities of risky sexual behaviour, followed by other female migrants. Non-migrant women were the least likely to have had casual and unprotected casual sex with non-stable partners both in

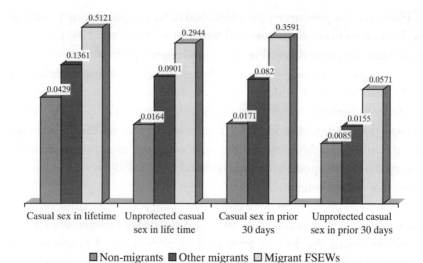

Fig. 1. Predicted mean probabilities of having casual and unprotected casual sex by migrant status among females age 18 or older.

Note: Results are based on the corresponding multiple logistic regression models in Tables 3 and 4. The bars are presented in a non-linear (logarithmic) scale. Mean probabilities are obtained by first predicting individual odds from the various models, using the "predict" option in the STATA software, and then calculating the mean odds by migrant status, which are then converted into corresponding mean probabilities.

their lifetime or during the 30-days prior to the survey. As a group, more than 51% of FMSEWs have had casual sex with non-stable partners and almost a third of them have engaged in such sexual relationship without the protection of condom in their lifetime; within the month prior to the survey, more than a third of FMSEWs had casual sexual encounters and almost 6% had unprotected casual sex with non-stable partners. Given that FMSEWs averaged only ∼ 22 years of age (Table 1) at the time of survey, for FMSWEs, what the predicted lifetime probabilities actually measured might not be so much of their "lifetime", but rather their recent experiences as migrants in cities. These statistics made it clear that young women who migrated from rural villages and worked in the personal service and entertainment industry in cities had experienced significant increases in their risk sexual behaviour and were consequently at higher risk of HIV/STDs.

Discussion and Conclusions

Despite growing recognition, few studies have actually addressed the interrelations between migration, gender and HIV/STD risk. Using data from a recent survey conducted in 2003 in China, this paper examines if and to what extent the interplay of migration and gender renders female migrants vulnerable to HIV/STD risk sexual behaviours. The results suggest that for the hundreds of thousands of young women from rural villages, life in a city is tough and does not offer many choices. While competition for mainstream jobs in cities has never been easy for rural-urban migrants, gender inequality in education and occupational training may cause the prospect for female migrants to be even more remote. With little education or occupational credentials, along with discrimination against women in workplace and an increasingly gender segregated job market (Fan, 2003), a majority of female migrants (52.8% in this study's weighted sample) resultingly worked in the personal service and entertainment industry.

While the interplay of migration and gender has undoubtedly contributed to the channelling of female migrants to jobs that increase their exposure to commercial sex, economic hardship and competition may have left female migrants with little control of their casual or commercial sex encounters and unable to resist the pressure for unprotected sex. Gendered moral and social values can further subject female migrants to a subordinate position in sexual relationships, which in turn limits their power in negotiating protective measures, makes them vulnerable to economic and sexual exploitation, and puts them at a high risk of acquiring and subsequently transmitting STDs/HIV.

Results presented in this paper show very clearly that female migrants, particularly those working in the personal service and entertainment industry, are much more likely than non-migrant women to have experienced casual sex, and to have engaged in such relationships without the protection of condoms. Both the lifetime and the 30-day measures suggest that the prevalence rates of having casual and unprotected casual sex among female migrants, FMSEWs in particular, are in most cases many times higher than the corresponding rates among non-migrant women. By contrast, male migrants do not always show higher prevalence rates of risk sexual behaviour than non–migrants, and when they do, the difference is not always statistically significant (Table 2). Multiple logistic regression of the same models in Tables 3 and 4, but including both males and females (results not shown but available upon request), revealed significant *negative* interactions between the migration and gender dummy (male = 1) variables, confirming that the impact of migration on risky sexual behaviour is more pronounced among female than male migrants.

However, migrants' increased risk of STDs/HIV do not seemed to have translated into a significantly higher prevalence rate of STDs/HIV, at least not statistically in the self-reported history of STDs or HIV positive. It is not clear and in fact surprising to find the comparably high proportion of non-migrant women, actually even higher than that among other female migrants, who reported a history of STDs or HIV positive. One possibility is that female migrants may have more limited access to health care services due to their marginal socioeconomic status, which may have under-diagnosed STDs among female migrants. On the other hand, the results may suggest that women's STD/HIV risk results not only from their own risk behaviour, but also and more importantly the risk behaviour of their trusted husbands or lovers (Aniekwu, 2002; Montgomery et al., 2002). More research is needed on the issue of gender and HIV/STD risk. The use of biomarkers and measures of relationship power and gendered cultural norms in sexual relationships may be particularly useful and highly recommended for future research.

Despite the absence of statistically significant increases in the self-reported STDs/HIV, the results make it clear that female migrants in general and FMSEWs in particular had experienced disproportionate increases in their risky sexual behaviour as a result of migration, which in turn puts them at increased risk of STDs/HIV. There are estimated several millions of FMSEWs at any point in time in China in recent years; the cumulative number could be many times larger since FMSEWs typically worked for only a few years on the service/entertainment job and the personal service/entertainment industry is characterised by quick rotations of workers. Furthermore, if the prevailing perception is correct, many FMSEWs would return to their home villages after a brief sojourn in the city, get married and settled there; the possibility of their becoming the unwitting source in the spread of STDs/HIV in China is real and serious. The potential human suffering and public health costs resulting from female migrants' increased risk sexual behaviour could be enormous in China in the coming decades.

References

Amaro H, Raj A. (2000) On the margin: Power and women's HIV risk reduction strategies. *Sex Roles* **42**(7/8): 723–49.

Anderson A, Qingsi Z, Hua X, Jianfeng B. (2003) China's floating population and the potential for HIV transmission: A social-behavioural perspective. *AIDS Care* **15**(2): 177–85.

Aniekwu NI. (2002) Gender and human rights dimensions of HIV/AIDS in nigeria. *African J Reprod Health* **16**(3): 30–7.

Bilsborrow RE, Hugo GJ, Oberai AS, Zlotnik H. (1997) *International Migration Statistics: Guidelines for the Improvement of Data Collection Systems.* International Labor Office, Geneva.

Brockerhoff M, Biddlecom AE. (1999) Migration, sexual behavior and the risk of HIV in Kenya. *Int Migration Rev* **33**(4): 833–56.

Browning J, Kessler D, Hatfield E, Choo P. (1999) Power, gender, and sexual behavior. *J Sex Res* **36**(4): 342–47.

Caldwell JC, Anarfi JK, Caldwell P. (1997) Mobility, migration, sex, STDs, and AIDS: An essay on sub-saharan Africa with other parallels, in G Herdt (ed.), *Sexual Cultures and Migration in the Era of AIDS: Anthropological and Demographic Perspectives*, pp. 41–54, Oxford University Press, New York.

Chant S (ed.). (1992). *Gender and Migration in Developing Countries.* Belhaven Press, New York.

Connell RW. (1987) *Gender and Power.* Stanford University Press, Stanford, CA.

Davin D. (1999) *Internal Migration in Contemporary China.* St. Martin's Press, New York.

Emler N. (1999) Moral character, in VJ Derlega, BA Winstead & WH Jones (eds.), *Personality: Contemporary Theory and Research*, Nelson-Hall, Chicago, IL.

Fan CC. (2000) Migration and gender in China, in CM Lau & J Shen (eds.), *China Review 2000*, pp. 423–54, Chinese University Press, Hong Kong.

Fan CC. (2003) Rural-urban migration and gender division of labor in transitional China. *Int J Urban Reg Res* **27**(1): 24–47.

Fan CC. (2004) Out to the city and back to the village: The experiences and contributions of rural women migration from Sichuan and Anhui, in AM Gaetano & T Jacka (eds.), *On the Move: Women in Rural-to-Urban Migration in Contemporary China*, pp. 177–206, Columbia University Press, New York.

Gaetano AM. (2004) Filial daughters, modern women: Migrant domestic workers in Post-Mao Beijing, in AM Gaetano & T Jacka (eds.), *On the Move: Women in Rural-to-Urban Migration in Contemporary China*, pp. 41–79, Columbia University Press, New York.

Gaetano AM, Jacka T. (eds.). (2004) *On the Move: Women in Rural-to-Urban Migration in Contemporary China.* Columbia University Press, New York.

Goldstein S, Liang Z, Goldstein A. (2000) Migration, gender, and labor force in Hubei province, 1985–90, in B Entwisle & G Henderson (eds.), *Re-Drawing Boundaries: Work, Household, and Gender in China*, pp. 214–230, University of California Press, Berkeley, CA.

Gras MJ, Weide JF, Langendam MW, Coutinho RA, van den Hoek A. (1999) HIV prevalence, sexual risk behaviour and sexual mixing patterns among migrants in Amsterdam, the Netherlands. *AIDS* **13**(14): 1953–62.

Hirsch JS, Higgins J, Bentley ME, Nathanson CA. (2002) The social constructions of sexuality: Marital infidelity and sexually transmitted disease — HIV risk in a Mexican Migrant Community. *Am J Public Health* **92**(8): 1227–37.

Huang Y. (2001) Gender, *hukou*, and the Occupational Attainment of Female Migrants in China (1985–90). *Environ Planning A* **33**: 257–79.

Jacka T. (1997) *Women's Work in Rural China: Change and Continuity in An Era of Reform.* Cambridge University Press, Cambridge.

Jochelson K, Mothibeli M, Leger JP. (1991) Human immunodeficiency virus and migrant labor in South Africa. *Int J Health Serv* **21**(1): 157–73.

Knight J, Song L, Jia H. (1999) Chinese rural migrants in urban enterprises: Three perspectives. *J Dev Studies* **35**(3): 73–104.

Lansky A, Nakashima AK, Diaz T, Fann SA, Conti L, Herr M, Smith D, Karon J, Jones JL, Ward JW. (2000) Human immunodeficiency virus infection in rural areas and small cities of the southeast: Contributions of migration and behavior. *J Rural Health* **16**(1): 20–30.

Lau J, Thomas J. (2001) Risk behaviors of Hong Kong male residents travelling to mainland China: A potential bridge population for HIV infection. *AIDS Care* **13**: 71–81.

Liang Z, Chen YP. (2004). Migration and gender in China: An origin-destination linked approach. *Econ Dev Cultural Change* **52**(2): 423–43.

Liang Z, Ma Z. (2004) China's floating population: New evidence from the 2000 census. *Population Dev Rev* **30**(3): 467–88.

Liao S, Schensul J, Wolffers I. (2003) Sex-related health risks and implications for interventions with hospitality women in Hainan, China. *AIDS Education Prevention* **15**(2): 109–21.

Lou B, Zheng Z, Connelly R, Roberts KD. (2004) The migration experiences of young women from four counties in Sichuan and Anhui, in AM Gaetano & T Jacka (eds.), *On the Move: Women in Rural-to-Urban Migration in Contemporary China*, pp. 207–42, Columbia University Press, New York.

Lurie M, Williams B, Suma K, Mkaya-Mwamburi D, Garnett G, Sturm A, Sweat M, Gittelsohn J, Karim S. (2003) The impact of migration on HIV-1 transmission in South Africa: A study of migrant and nonmigrant men and their partners. *Sex Trans Dis* **30**(2): 149–56.

Maticka-Tyndale E, Elkins D, Haswell-Elkins M, Rujkarakorn D, Kuyyakanond T, Stam K. (1997) Contexts and patterns of men's commercial sexual partnerships in Northeastern Thailand: Implications for AIDS prevention. *Soc Sci Med* **44**(2): 199–213.

Montgomery SB, Hyde J, De Rosa CJ, Rohrbach LA, Ennett S, Harvey SM, Clatts M, Iverson E, Kipke MD. (2002) Gender differences in HIV Risk behaviors among young injectors and their network members. *Health Wellness Res Center* **28**(3): 453–76.

Murphy R. (2004) The impact of labor migration on the well-being and agency of rural Chinese Women: Cultural and economic contexts and the life course, in AM Gaetano & T Jacka (eds.), *On the Move: Women in Rural-to-Urban Migration in Contemporary China*, pp. 243–76, Columbia University Press, New York.

Obbo C. (1993) HIV transmission through social and geographical networks in Uganda. *Soc Sci Med* **36**(7): 949–55.

Organista KC, Organista PB. (1997) Migrant laborers and AIDS in the United States: A review of the literature. *AIDS Edu Prev* **9**(1): 83–93.

Pan S, Parish W, Wang A, Laumann E. (2004). *Sexual Behaviors and Sexual Relationships in Contemporary China*. Social Science Manuscripts Publisher, Beijing.

Parish WL, Laumann EO, Cohen MS, Pan S, Zheng H, Hoffman I, Wang T, Ng KH. (2003) Population-based study of Chlamydial Infection in China. *J Am Med Assoc* **289**(10): 1265–73.

Raffaelli M, Pranke J. (1995) Women and AIDS in developing countries, in A O'Leary & LS Jemmott (eds.), *Women at Risk: Issues in the Primary Prevention of AIDS*, pp. 219–236, Plenum Press, New York.

Roberts K. (2002) Female labor migrants to Shanghai: Temporary "floaters" or potential settlers? *Int Migrat Rev* **36**(2): 492–519.

Russell DW, Cutrona CE. (1988) *Development and Evolution of the UCLA Loneliness Scale*. Unpublished manuscript, Center for Health Services Research, College of Medicine, University of Iowa.

Skeldon R. (2000) *Population Mobility and HIV Vulnerability in South East Asia: An Assessment and Analysis*. UNDP, Bangkok.

Tan L, Short SE. (2004) Living as double outsiders: Migrant women's experiences of marriage in a county-level city, in AM Gaetano & T Jacka (eds.), *On the Move: Women in Rural-to-Urban Migration in Contemporary China*, pp. 151–74, Columbia University Press, New York.

Tang CS, Wong C, Lee AM. (2001) Gender-related psychosocial and cultural factors associated with condom use among Chinese married women. *AIDS Edu Prev* **13**(4): 329–42.

Troyer R, Clark J, Rojek D. (1989) *Social Control in the People's Republic of China*. Praeger, New York.

van den Hoek A, Yuliang F, Dukers NH, Zhiheng C, Jiangtin F, Lina Z, Xiuxing Z. (2001) High prevalence of syphilis and other sexually transmitted diseases among sex workers in China: Potential for fast spread of HIV. *AIDS* **15**: 753–9.

Wallace R, Huang Y, Gould P, Wallace D. (1997) The hierarchical diffusion of AIDS and violent crime among U.S. metropolitan regions: Inner-city decay, stochastic resonance and reversal of the mortality transition. *Soc Sci Med* **44**(7): 935–47.

Wingood GM, DiClemente RJ. (2002) The theory of gender and power: A social structural theory for guiding public health interventions, in RJ DiClemente, RA Crosby, & MC Kegler (eds.), *Emerging Theories in Health Promotion Practice and Research: Strategies for Improving Public Health*, pp. 313–46, Jossey-Bass, San Francisco.

Wolffers I, Fernandez I, Verghis S, Vink M. (2002) Sexual behaviour and vulnerability of migrant workers for HIV infection. *Culture, Health Sexuality* **4**(4): 459–73.

Wood E, Chan K, Montaner JS, Schechter MT, Tyndall M, O'Shaughnessy MV, Hogg RS. (2000) The end of the line: Has rapid transit contributed to the spatial diffusion of HIV in one of Canada's largest metropolitan areas? *Soc Sci Med* **51**(5): 741–8.

Xia G, Yang X. (2005) Risky sexual behavior among female entertainment workers in China: Implications for HIV/STI prevention intervention. *AIDS Education Prevention* **17**(2): 143–56.

Yang X. (2000a) The fertility impact of temporary migration in China: A detachment hypothesis. *Eur J Population* **16**(2): 163–83.

Yang X. (2000b) Interconnections among gender, work, and migration: Evidence from Zhejiang Province, in B Entwisle & G Henderson (eds.), *Re-Drawing Boundaries: Work, Household, and Gender in China*, pp. 197–213, University of California Press, Berkeley.

Yang X. (2005) Does where we live matter? Community characteristics and HIV/STD prevalence in Southwestern China. *Int J STD AIDS* **16**(1): 31–7.

Yang X. (forthcoming) Temporary migration and HIV risk behaviors: A case study in Southwestern China. *Environment and Planning* A.

Yang X, Guo, F. (1999) Gender differences in determinants of temporary labor migration in China: A multilevel analysis. *Int Migrat Rev* **33**(4): 929–53.

14

The Hajj Pilgrimage: Public Health Consequences of the Largest People Mass Movement

Annelies Wilder-Smith

Introduction

The pilgrimage to Mecca (or Makkah in Arabic) is one of the five pillars of Islam and referred to as Hajj pilgrimage. This pilgrimage attracts more than two million Moslems every year and is therefore the largest people mass movement on earth. It is characterised by intense migration and religious rituals in overcrowded conditions and is associated with a number of medical hazards (Memish and Ahmed, 2002). This review describes the medical risks associated with the Hajj and their potential international public health consequences.

Background

Each Muslim has to perform one Hajj in his/her lifetime. For 14 centuries, countless mil of Muslims, men and women, from all over the world have made the pilgrimage to Makkah, the birthplace of Islam. Mecca today has a population of some 620,000 and is located in the south western region of the Kingdom of Saudi Arabia, about 80 km from the Red Sea coast. Saudi Arabia has a desert climate where heat can reach intense heights. The pilgrimage takes place each year between the eighth and the 13th days of Dhu al-Hijjah, the 12th month of the Muslim lunar calendar. The Islamic calender is based on lunar months, so the actual date moves forward about 11 days each year in relation to the western solar calendar (or Gregorian calender) (Esposito, 1999).

In the past decade, about two million pilgrims from 140 countries attend the Hajj annually. Breakdown of international pilgrims by country of origin is as follows: 63% from Arabic countries, 30% from Asian countries, 5% from African countries and 2% from Europe, Americas and Australia (Wilder-Smith and Memish, 2003). During the late 20th Century, the Kingdom of Saudi Arabia has developed the Al Haram Mosque to accommodate the colossal numbers of pilgrims now seen during the Hajj ceremony. The Al Haram is built on three levels covering an area of 356,000 square meters and has a capacity of one mil at any one time. The neighboring mosque at Madinah, which is often visited around the time of the Hajj, is also large with an approximate area of 165,000 square meters, easily accommodating 750,000 pilgrims at once.

At Mecca itself, the Kingdom provides free health care to all pilgrims. Seven modern, fully equipped hospitals, with a cumulative bed capacity of 2,070 are permanently located in the city. 73 medical centers providing 24-hour access are distributed throughout the pilgrimage route and operate without cost to the pilgrim patient. The medical centers work under the collaborative administration of the Ministry of Health, the Saudi National Guard, the Internal Security Forces and the Saudi Red Crescent Society. At the Hajj, accommodations range from the most basic to the most sophisticated, but most pilgrims have to share public facilities and live in semi-permanent tents. Inadequate storage, cooking or transportation, lack of refrigeration and lack of proper food handling all contribute to the risking of the pilgrim's health. Clean drinking water is readily available at most religious sites, provided for free by the Kingdom.

Although most pilgrims stay in Saudi Arabia for at least one month, the main rituals mandatory for the core of the Hajj are performed in eight days and include the circumambulation of the Ka'aba, standing at Arafat, three nights in the tents of the desert of Muzdalifah (Minah), stoning rituals, slaughtering of animals and shaving of the head for male pilgrims.

Non-communicable Diseases

The majority of Hajjis are adults and many are elderly, infirm Muslims (Memish and Ahmed, 2002). Heat exhaustion and heat stroke strike the pilgrims frequently, especially when the period of the Hajj falls in a very hot season (el-Bakry *et al.*, 1996).

Every year, increasing numbers of Muslims from all over the world pay pilgrimage. This creates a huge organisational burden for the Saudi authorities. As a result of overcrowding, accidents and stampede pose major problems and mass accidents (e.g. fires and stampedes) have been reported, sometimes involving thousands of individuals (Al-Harti, 2001). Burn injuries occurred in a fire in 1977 that destroyed many tents and led to considerable fatalities. The Kingdom has since replaced all the tents in the Mina area, where the pilgrims reside during most of their Hajj, with a variety of tents which are semi permanent and made of aluminium frames with fiber glass coated awnings (Memish and Ahmed, 2002). Pilgrims are barefoot in the holy areas. Standing on scorching marble of the mosques in the noonday sun can produce severe burns to the sole of the feet. Full thickness burns have been described (Fried *et al.*, 1996; Al-Qattan, 2000).

To celebrate the end of the Hajj (a celebration known as Eid), hundreds of thousands of sheep and cattle are slaughtered, often by pilgrims with no prior experience in butchering animals. As a result, accidental hand injuries are very common. Over a four-year period, 298 hand injuries related to animal slaughter were reported (Rahman, Al-Zahrani and Al-Qattan, 1999).

Communicable Diseases

Zoonoses

Large numbers of animals are imported to Saudi Arabia for the purposes of the Hajj, with a great potential for zoonotic diseases. For example in 2001, 603,393 sheep and 6,136 cows and camels were slaughtered (Memish, Venkatesh and Ahmed, 2003). Illegal slaughtering and inadequate disposal of animal remains are a potential hazard, and so is the butchering of thousands of cattle that occur during the end of the Hajj (Memish, Venkatesh and Ahmed, 2003). Saudi Arabia is highly endemic for brucellosis and imports animals for slaughter during the Hajj from brucella-endemic countries, with practically no quarantine or testing (Memish and Balkhy, 2004). Despite this, no study has documented brucellosis outbreaks during the Hajj. The Crimean-Congo hemorrhagic fever (CCHF) was reported in Mecca in 1990 (El Azazy, 1997). Exposure to animal blood or tissue in abattoirs was found to be a significant risk factor. It is possible that the CCHF virus was introduced to Saudi Arabia by infected ticks on imported sheep arriving at the Hajj from CCHF endemic countries in Africa (Memish, Venkatesh and Ahmed, 2003). In 2000 and 2001, Saudi Arabia had an outbreak of Rift Valley hemorrhagic fever (RVF), a cattle-borne zoonotic disease which resulted in more than 200 Saudi mortalities (Shawky, 2000; Ahmad, 2000). In response to this outbreak, the Ministry of Health of the Kingdom of Saudi Arabia banned the import of sheep from RVF endemic countries and launched education campaigns directed at the abattoir workers in Mecca, and enforced strict surveillance and supervision (Memish, Venkatesh and Ahmed, 2003). Orf, a viral disease of sheep and goats caused by a parapox virus, can result from direct contact with infected animals and manifests itself as a hand infection. Slaughtering of sheep during the Hajj has led to Orf infections of the hands (Hawary and Al-Rasheed, 1997).

Saudi Arabia is now a collaborator in the Mediterranean Zoonosis Control Program that aims to prevent, survey and control zoonoses and foodborne diseases due to animal products (Memish, Venkatesh and Ahmed, 2003).

Viral hepatitis

The Hajj also poses a unique risk of blood borne disease to male pilgrims, such as Hepatitis B and C. Most male pilgrims shave their heads at the completion of the Hajj in keeping with religious rituals. Barbers often re-use razors and grazes or abrasions from razor nicks are often seen on newly shorn pilgrims (Al Salamah, 1998). The prevalence of Hepatitis B carriers is reported to be high amongst Saudi barbers (Turkistani and Mustafa, 2000) Saudi Arabia now requires all barbers to be licensed and to use standardised shaving practices (Memish, Venkatesh and Ahmed, 2003).

Hepatitis A is highly endemic in Saudi Arabia (Memish and Ahmed, 2002). Although there are no published data on the incidence of Hepatitis A in pilgrims to Saudi Arabia, the incidence is likely to be high in accordance with other studies, suggesting that hepatitis A is one of the most frequent vaccine-preventable infectious diseases in travellers.

Respiratory infections

The severe congestion and proximity of pilgrims performing religious rites predispose to airborne infections (Wilder-Smith and Memish, 2003). Cough is a common complaint affecting more than 50% of the pilgrims (Wilder-Smith and Memish, 2003; Qureshi *et al.*, 2000; Wilder-Smith *et al.*, 2002). The commonest bacterial pathogen found in sputum cultures from pilgrims presenting with productive cough during the 1991 and 1992 Hajj were *H. influenzae, K. pneumoniae* and *S. pneumoniae* (El-Sheikh, El-Assouli, Mohammed and Albar, 1998).

Influenza

Influenza is a common problem during the Hajj (Balkhy, Memish, Bafaqeer and Almuneef, 2004). A large study on influenza-like illness (ILI) and medication use among Pakistani pilgrims to the Hajj found a high incidence of ILI (36%) and high medication use such as antibiotics and nonprescription cold medication (Qureshi *et al.*, 2000). Influenza vaccine was able to prevent 22 per 100 cases. To the extent that these results are generalisable to the broader population of pilgrims attending the Hajj, the public health consequence would be large. Applied to two million pilgrims, these data indicate that influenza vaccine could prevent approximately 440,000 cases of influenza and 340,000 courses of antibiotics (Qureshi *et al.*, 2000).

Pertussis

Pertussis is a frequent, but often underestimated cause of prolonged cough illness in adults and a highly communicable, vaccine-preventable respiratory disease (Senzilet *et al.*, 2001). Waning immunity plays a significant role in the occurrence of pertussis in adults and high attack rates of pertussis have been observed among adults in the setting of community outbreaks of pertussis, despite high childhood immunisation rates (Keitel, 1999). The overall incidence rate of pertussis (1.4%) we documented in our prospective seroepidemiological study related to the Hajj in 2002 (Wilder-Smith *et al.*, 2003) is higher than that of many other vaccine-preventable travel-related diseases (except influenza) and higher than the annual incidence rate reported in healthcare workers (Steffen and Willhelm, 1987; Wright *et al.*, 1999). This is not only of concern to the pilgrims, but also constitutes a public health problem as pilgrims may present a reservoir which may lead to secondary cases upon return to their countries of origin. Susceptible infants usually acquire pertussis from an infected adult, and many pilgrims return to countries where pertussis vaccination may not be part of the childhood immunisation programme.

Adult-type acellular pertussis vaccine confers safe and effective protection against pertussis (Keitel, 1999). The recent recommendations from the International Consensus Group on Pertussis Immunisation state that public health policy makers should target pertussis booster to adult risk groups (Campis-Marti *et al.*, 2001). Our findings suggest that departing Hajj pilgrims would be one risk group that would benefit from immunisation against pertussis.

Tuberculosis

The most common cause of pneumonia in hospitalised pilgrims during the Hajj is pulmonary TB (Alzeer, Mashlah, Fakim *et al.*, 1998). We did a prospective study amongst Singaporean Hajj pilgrims, using the QuantiFERON TB assay to determine the incidence of latent TB infection (Wilder-Smith *et al.*, 2005). We found a 10% incidence of *Mycobacterium tuberculosis* infection. These findings are consistent with the observation that the annual risk of TB infection is three times higher in Saudi Arabian cities hosting the pilgrims (Mecca, Jeddah and Medina) than the national average (Memish and Ahmed, 2002). This may have important international public health implications. Pilgrims who acquire TB infection during the Hajj may become a source of tuberculosis upon their return to the home countries. Given that nearly all Moslems go to the Hajj at least once in their lifetime, this could have a significant impact on TB incidence in countries with large Moslem populations. A policy of screening departing pilgrims from TB endemic countries may be justified to reduce the importation and subsequent dissemination of tuberculosis during the pilgrimage. Screening returning pilgrims for latent TB infection should be considered, especially

those returning to countries of low TB endemicity. In response to the outbreak of meningococcal disease among pilgrims, the Ministry of Health in
Saudi Arabia recently recommended the use of facemasks during the pilgrimage, although to date, compliance has reportedly been poor (Memish
and Ahmed, 2002). The findings of this study provide further rationale for
the use of protective masks.

Severe acute respiratory syndrome (SARS)

As the conditions during the Hajj pilgrimage amplify any infectious disease
with person-to-person transmission, the rapid spread of SARS, if imported
during the Hajj, is a major public health concern for Saudi Arabia (Wilder-
Smith and Freedman, 2003). Moreover, cough is a common complaint
during the Hajj and would lead to a delay in the diagnosis of SARS, potentially resulting in massive secondary transmission. With two million people
arriving around the same time for the Hajj, screening for SARS is a major
logistical challenge. If SARS had been imported and amplified during this
pilgrimage, an even worse international public health consequence would
have been the rapid dissemination of the disease around the world via pilgrims returning to their countries of origin. The control of SARS depends on
an efficient public health structure. Infection control measures within hospitals were strengthened, airport screening for fever was instituted at the entry
points, and pilgrims from SARS affected countries were banned from entry
(Memish and Wilder-Smith, 2004). Fortunately, no SARS was imported
during the early outbreak in the year 2003 which coincided with the Hajj,
and no cases were also detected upon airport screening, once screening
was instituted. This is most likely due to a combination of factors, such as
international travel restrictions on SARS-affected countries (Wilder-Smith,
Paton and Goh, 2003), the banning of pilgrims from SARS areas (Memish
and Wilder-Smith, 2004) and the exit screening done in many countries
worldwide.

Meningococcal disease

Of all the problems during the Hajj, meningococcal disease associated
with the Hajj has received most international and scientific attention.
Conditions of overcrowding during the Hajj facilitate person-to-person

transmission of meningococci (Wilder-Smith and Memish, 2003; Memish, 2002). Meningococcal carriage rates as high as 80% can be found in crowded areas around the holy mosque in Mecca (al-Gahtani *et al.*, 1995). In 1987, a major outbreak of group A meningococcal disease occurred during the Hajj, affecting 1,841 pilgrims (Wilder-Smith and Memish, 2003; Moore *et al.*, 1989). A high rate of nasopharyngeal carriage with serogroup A was documented in returning pilgrims (Moore *et al.*, 1988). Pilgrims who became group A carriers introduced this clonal group into sub-Saharan Africa on their return from the Hajj. The introduction of this clonal group into sub-Saharan Africa is thought to have been responsible for the subsequent epidemics in the meningitis belt in the 1980s and 1990s, and also for isolated cases in the Moslem populations worldwide (Wilder-Smith and Memish, 2003; Moore *et al.*, 1989). This outbreak led to the introduction of bivalent meningococcal vaccination (A,C) as a requirement for entry into the kingdom to perform Hajj or Umrah (Memish, 2002). The above measure was partnered with mass administration of decolonising agents to pilgrims from the African meningitis belt. No outbreaks with serogroup A was seen since the introduction of these measures.

An international outbreak of meningococcal disease occurred again in association with the Hajj pilgrimage in the years 2000 and 2001 (Hahne *et al.*, 2002). This outbreak generated particular interest as the oubreak strain was W135, a serogroup which had only caused sporadic disease previously (Taha *et al.*, 2000). More than 400 of the meningococcal meningitis cases due to serogroup W135 were reported in pilgrims and their close contacts, making it the largest reported outbreak of meningococcal disease caused by *N. meningitidis* W135 (Mayer *et al.*, 2002). The attack rate among pilgrims was 30 per 100,000, and the case fatality rate for this outbreak strain was 20%, which is significantly higher than the ratio reported in the UK for other culture-confirmed meningococcal disease (Wilder-Smith *et al.*, 2003). We documented a high acquisition and persistence rate of W135 meningococcal carriage in Hajj pilgrims in the year 2001, although all of them were vaccinated with quadrivalent meningococcal vaccine (Wilder-Smith *et al.*, 2002; Wilder-Smith *et al.*, 2003). The high predominance of one single clone which we found, as opposed to the usually reported clonal diversity in carriers, was unique. Returning pilgrims therefore represent a sizeable and sustained reservoir of *N. meningitidis* W135. A high transmission rate of W135 carriage from returning pilgrims to their unvaccinated household contacts was documented, which would put them at risk of developing invasive meningococcal disease (Wilder-Smith *et al.*, 2002).

Although carriage rates are indicative of the potential for spread, occurrence of invasive disease is ultimately more informative and should be the foundation to guide public health interventions. Worldwide reports of cases of W135 disease mainly in Muslim communities in 2000 and 2001 substantiate that the introduction of W135 via returning pilgrims indeed took place (Wilder-Smith and Memish, 2003; Hahne *et al.*, 2002; Issack and Ragavoodoo, 2002; Fonkoua *et al.*, 2002; Doganci 2004). Large numbers of secondary cases in household contacts of returning pilgrims were reported in the UK (Hahne *et al.*, 2002). The estimated attack rate in Singaporean household contacts of returning pilgrims was 18 per 100,000 and 28 per 100,000 for the years 2000 and 2001, respectively (Wilder-Smith and Memish, 2003; Wilder-Smith *et al.*, 2003). This indicates a shift of the burden of disease from pilgrims to household contacts. Based on transmission rates of W135 carriage and national epidemiological data, the risk of an unvaccinated household contact (who had acquired W135 carriage) developing invasive meningococcal disease was estimated to be 1: 70 (Wilder-Smith *et al.*, 2003; Wilder-Smith, 2003). This and the high risk of a carrier developing invasive disease indicates the virulence of this strain and/or the lack of acquired immunity to this strain.

The discussion of the origin of the W135 outbreak clone has generated particular interest. Mayer *et al.* suggest that small, short-term changes in meningococcal carriage during a period of intense transmission might have contributed to the expansion of this clone (Mayer *et al.*, 2002). Our data on carriage rates would substantiate this suggestion. In addition to being a member of the ET–37 complex, other molecular and phenotypic markers of this clone are very similar to those of serogroup C strains of the ET37 complex, which have caused hyperendemic disease and raised the question of whether the outbreak clone was developed from serogroup C by a capsule-switching event (Taha *et al.*, 2000). Capsular switching has been described in closely related *N. meningitidis* strains. Capsular switching from serogroup C to W135 may have been selected by mass immunisation campaigns in which A & C bivalent vaccine was used (MacLennan *et al.*, 2000). Mandatory bivalent vaccination is indeed the only major difference introduced in the

1990s, compared with the earlier decades for this pilgrimage, and would underscore this hypothesis.

The high carriage rates, persistence and substantial transmissibility in combination with a high attack rate and case fatality of the Hajj-associated W135 outbreak clone certainly raise considerable concern regarding the public health consequences of widespread dissemination of this organism and the potential for future epidemics. Indeed, a major outbreak of W135 meningococcal disease occurred in predominantly Muslim countries in Africa, affecting far larger numbers than the one associated with the Hajj in Saudi Arabia. It started in Burkina Faso in early 2002 and then spread to the Greater Lake area (Burundi, Rwanda, Tanzania). Some 13,000 people were infected, of whom 2,000 died (Chonghaile, 2002). It is now difficult to ascertain how many returning pilgrims carrying W135 may have contributed to this epidemic.

Since the introduction of quadrivalent meningococcal vaccine as Hajj visa requirement since the Hajj 2002, no further outbreaks have occurred and the meningococcal carriage remained low (Balkhy *et al.*, 2004; Wilder-Smith *et al.*, 2003). Continued surveillance and rapid readjustment of policies is now paramount. Polyvalent conjugate vaccines will be the main strategy in the future. In contrast to the classical polysaccharide vaccines, conjugate vaccines are immunogenic in young infants, induce long-term protection and reduce nasopharyngeal carriage and transmission (Maiden and Spratt, 1999). Conjugate vaccines are currently awaiting FDA approval.

Conclusion

The Hajj pilgrimage presents a formidable challenge to public health physicians and authorities. There is a high risk of diseases associated with person-to-person transmission such as influenza, tuberculosis, meningococcal disease during the Hajj, as well as returning pilgrims who may disseminate these diseases worldwide. This has important international public health implications.

References

Ahmad K. (2000) More deaths from rift valley fever in Saudi Arabia and Yemen. *Lancet* **356**: 1422.

al-Gahtani YM, el Bushra HE, al-Qarawi SM, al-Zubaidi AA, Fontaine RE. (1995) Epidemiological investigation of an outbreak of meningococcal meningitis in Makkah (Mecca), Saudi Arabia, 1992. *Epidemiol Infect* **115**: 399–409.

Al-Harthi AS A-HM. (2001) Accidental injuries during muslim pilgrimage. *Saudi Med J* **22**: 523–525.

Al Salamah Aa EBH. (1998) Headshaving practices of barbers and pilgrims to makkah. *Saudi Epidemiol Bull* **5**: 3–4.

Al-Qattan MM. (2000) The "Friday mass" burns of the feet in Saudi Arabia. *Burns* **26**: 102–105.

Alzeer A, Mashlah A, Fakim N, *et al.* (1998) Tuberculosis is the commonest cause of pneumonia requiring hospitalization during Hajj (Pilgrimage to Makkah). *J Infect* **36**: 303–306.

Balkhy HH, Memish ZA, Almuneef MA, Osoba AO. (2004) Neisseria meningitidis W-135 carriage during the Hajj season 2003. *Scand J Infect Dis* **36**: 264–268.

Balkhy HH, Memish ZA, Bafaqeer S, Almuneef MA. (2004) Influenza a common viral infection among Hajj pilgrims: Time for routine surveillance and vaccination. *J Travel Med* **11**: 82–86.

Campins-Marti M, Cheng HK, Forsyth K, *et al.* (2001) Recommendations are needed for adolescent and adult pertussis immunisation: Rationale and strategies for consideration. *Vaccine* **20**: 641–646.

Chonghaile C. (2002) Meningitis in Africa — Tackling W135. *Lancet* **360**: 2054–2055.

Doganci L BM, Saracli MA, Hascelik G, Pahsa A. (2004) Neisseria meningitis W135, Turkey. *Emerg Infect Dis* **10**: 936–937.

el-Bakry AK, Channa AB, Bakhamees H, Turkistani A, Seraj MA. (1996) Heat exhaustion during mass pilgrimage — Is there a diagnostic role for pulse oximetry? *Resuscitation* **31**: 121–126.

El Azazy OM SE. (1997) Crimean-Congo Haemorrhagic fever virus infection in the western province of Saudi Arabia. *Trans R Soc Trop Med Hyg* **91**: 275–278.

El-Sheikh SM, El-Assouli SM, Mohammed KA, Albar M. (1998) Bacteria and viruses that cause respiratory tract infections during the pilgrimage (Haj) season in Makkah, Saudi Arabia. *Trop Med Int Health* **3**: 205–209.

Esposito J. (1999) *The Oxford History of Islam*. Oxford University Press.

Fonkoua MC, Taha MK, Nicolas P, *et al.* (2002) Recent increase in meningitis caused by neisseria meningitidis serogroups A and W135, Yaounde, Cameroon. *Emerg Infect Dis* **8**: 327–329.

Fried M, Kahanovitz S, Dagan R. (1996) Full-thickness foot burn of a pilgrim to mecca. *Burns* **22**: 644–645.

Hahne SJ, Gray SJ, Jean F, *et al.* (2002) W135 meningococcal disease in England and wales associated with Hajj 2000 and 2001. *Lancet* **359**: 582–583.

Hawary MB HJ, Al-Rasheed SK. (1997) The yearly outbreak of ORF infection of the hand in Saudi Arabia. *J Hand Surg* **4**: 550–551.

Issack MI, Ragavoodoo C. (2002) Hajj-related neisseria meningitidis serogroup W135 in Mauritius. *Emerg Infect Dis* **8**: 332–334.

Keitel WA. (1999) Cellular and acellular pertussis vaccines in adults. *Clin Infect Dis* **28**(Suppl 2): S118–S123.

MacLennan JM, Urwin R, Obaro S, Griffiths D, Greenwood B, Maiden MC. (2000) Carriage of serogroup W-135, ET-37 meningococci in the gambia: Implications for immunisation policy? *Lancet* **356**: 1078.

Maiden MC, Spratt BG. (1999) Meningococcal conjugate vaccines: New opportunities and new challenges. *Lancet* **354**: 615–616.

Mayer LW, Reeves MW, Al-Hamdan N, *et al.* (2002) Outbreak of W135 meningococcal disease in 2000: Not emergence of a new W135 strain but clonal expansion within the electophoretic type-37 complex. *J Infect Dis* **185**: 1596–1605.

Memish ZA. (2002) Infection control in Saudi Arabia: meeting the challenge. *Am J Infect Control* **30**: 57–65.

Memish ZA, Ahmed QA. (2002) Mecca bound: The challenges ahead. *J Travel Med* **9**: 202–210.

Memish Z AQ. (2002) Mecca bound: The challenges ahead. *J. Travel Medicine* **9**: 202–210.

Memish ZA, Balkhy HH. (2004) Brucellosis and international travel. *J Travel Med* **11**: 49–55.

Memish ZA, Venkatesh S, Ahmed QA. (2003) Travel epidemiology: The Saudi perspective. *Int J Antimicrob Agents* **21**: 96–101.

Memish ZA, Wilder-Smith A. (2004) Global impact of severe acute respiratory syndrome: Measures to prevent importation into Saudi Arabia. *J Travel Med* **11**: 127–129.

Moore PS, Reeves MW, Schwartz B, Gellin BG, Broome CV. (1989) Intercontinental spread of an epidemic group A neisseria meningitidis strain. *Lancet* **2**: 260–263.

Moore PS, Harrison LH, Telzak EE, Ajello GW, Broome CV. (1988) Group A meningococcal carriage in travelers returning from Saudi Arabia. *Jama* **260**: 2686–2689.

Qureshi H, Gessner BD, Leboulleux D, Hasan H, Alam SE, Moulton LH. (2000) The incidence of vaccine preventable influenza-like illness and medication use among Pakistani pilgrims to the Hajj in Saudi Arabia. *Vaccine* **18**: 2956–2962.

Rahman MM, Al-Zahrani S, Al-Qattan MM. (1999) "Outbreak" of hand injuries during Hajj festivities in Saudi Arabia. *Ann Plast Surg* **43**: 154–155.

Senzilet LD, Halperin SA, Spika JS, Alagaratnam M, Morris A, Smith B. (2001) Pertussis is a frequent cause of prolonged cough illness in adults and adolescents. *Clin Infect Dis* **32**: 1691–1697.

Shawky S. (2000) Rift valley fever. *Saudi Med J* **21**: 1109–1115.

(2000) Rift Valley Fever, Saudi Arabia, August–October 2000. *Wkly Epidemiol Rec* **75**: 370–371.

Steffen R RM, Willhelm U. (1987) Health problems after travel to developing countries. *J Infect Dis* **156**: 84–91.

Taha MK, Achtman M, Alonso JM, *et al.* (2000) Serogroup W135 meningococcal disease in Hajj pilgrims. *Lancet* **356**:2159.

Turkistani A ARA, Mustafa T. (2000) Blood-borne diseases among barbers during Hajj, 1419H (1999). *Saudi Epidemiol Bull* **7**: 1–2.

Wilder-Smith A. (2003) W135 meningococcal carriage in association with the Hajj pilgrimage 2001: The Singapore experience. *Int J Antimicrob Agents* **21**: 112–115.

Wilder-Smith A, Barkham TM, Chew SK, Paton NI. (2003) Absence of neisseria meningitidis W-135 electrophoretic type 37 during the Hajj, 2002. *Emerg Infect Dis* **9**: 734–737.

Wilder-Smith A, Barkham TM, Earnest A, Paton NI. (2002) Acquisition of W135 meningococcal carriage in Hajj pilgrims and transmission to household contacts: Prospective study. *BMJ* **325**: 365–366.

Wilder-Smith A, Barkham TM, Ravindran S, Earnest A, Paton NI. (2003) Persistence of W135 neisseria meningitidis carriage in returning Hajj pilgrims: Risk for early and late transmission to household contacts. *Emerg Infect Dis* **9**: 123–126.

Wilder-Smith A, Earnest A, Ravindran S, Paton NI. (2003) High incidence of pertussis among Hajj pilgrims. *Clin Infect Dis* **37**: 1270–1272.

Wilder-Smith A FW, Earnest A, Paton NI. (2005) High risk of M. tuberculosis infection during the Hajj pilgrimage. *Trop Med Int Health* **10**(4): 336–339.

Wilder-Smith A, Freedman DO. (2003) Confronting the new challenge in travel medicine: SARS. *J Travel Med* **10**: 257–258.

Wilder-Smith A, Goh KT, Barkham T, Paton NI. (2003) Hajj-associated outbreak strain of neisseria meningitidis serogroup W135: Estimates of the attack rate in a defined population and the risk of invasive disease developing in carriers. *Clin Infect Dis* **36**: 679–683.

Wilder-Smith A, Memish Z. (2003) Meningococcal disease and travel. *Int J Antimicrob Agents* **21**: 102–106.

Wilder-Smith A, Paton NI, Goh KT. (2003) Experience of severe acute respiratory syndrome in Singapore: Importation of cases, and defense strategies at the airport. *J Travel Med* **10**: 259–262.

Wilder-Smith A. TBT, A. Earnest A, NI Paton. (2002) Acquisition of meningococcal carriage in Hajj pilgrims and transmission to their household contacts: Prospective study. *BMJ* **325**: 365–366.

Wright SW, Decker MD, Edwards KM. (1999) Incidence of pertussis infection in healthcare workers. *Infect Control Hosp Epidemiol* **20**: 120–123.

COMPARATIVE PERSPECTIVES ON SARS IN ASIA

15

Epidemiology of Emerging Infectious Diseases in Singapore, with Special Reference to SARS

Kee Tai Goh and Suok Kai Chew

Introduction

Emerging infections include new, re-emerging or drug-resistant infections whose incidence in humans has increased or threatens to increase during the last two to three decades. The emergence of more than 30 new infectious disease-causing microbial pathogens and re-emergence of some infectious diseases, previously thought to have been brought under control, have been attributed to a number of biological, ecological, demographic and socio-economic factors such as the development of antimicrobial resistance, the spread of known diseases to new geographical areas or new human populations, breakdown in public health measures, international travel and human migration, exposure to insects, animals or environmental sources that may harbour new or unusual infectious agents through deforestation or reforestation (Wong and Goh, 1997).

In Singapore, infectious diseases are controlled through a high standard of environmental sanitation, strict control on the import of food and livestock and a comprehensive childhood immunisation programme. With increasing trade and travel within and beyond the region, more infectious diseases are being imported into the country, and in some cases, this resulted in local transmission (Goh and Sng, 1987).

Bengal Cholera (*Vibrio cholerae* 0139)

In October 1992, a new cholera biotype, *Vibrio cholerae* 0139, emerged in the Indian subcontinent. There were massive outbreaks in Madras, Calcutta and Bangladesh, and soon spread to neighbouring countries such as Thailand, with imported cases reported in United States and United Kingdom (World Health Organization, 1993). Between March and May 1993, four Indian tourists from Madras and one local Indian resident who had recently visited the city were admitted to hospital with severe diarrhoea, and were subsequently diagnosed to be infected with this new biotype. No secondary transmission occurred in Singapore (Tay *et al.*, 1994). There is currently no vaccine against this new strain.

Campylobacter Enteritis

Campylobacteriosis, a zoonotic disease, has emerged as one of the most common human bacterial enteric diseases in developed countries, especially in young children. Since the first case was detected in Singapore in 1980, the incidence has increased to 10.6 per 100,000 in 1999. Majority of the infection was caused by *C. jejuni*. The incidence rate was highest in pre-school children below five years of age (Committee on Epidemic Diseases, 1999). In Singapore, the contamination rate of poultry was found to be 19.7% for imported chicken, 58% for imported chilled chicken, and 54% for chicken carcass and viscera from local abattoirs (Committee on Epidemic Diseases, 1999). Epidemiological investigations showed that the single risk factor significantly associated with acquisition of infection was the failure of caregivers to wash their hands after handling raw poultry and before preparing milk for infants and toddlers (Committee on Epidemic Diseases, 2001). A common source outbreak 93 cases of gastroenteritis in a secondary school, possibly due to campylobacter enteritis, was epidemiologically linked to the consumption of undercooked barbecued chicken (Committee on Epidemic Diseases, 2002).

Salmonellosis caused by Multi-drug-resistant *Salmonella* Typhimurium

Multidrug-resistant *Salmonella enterica* subsp. *enterica* serotype Typhimurium definitive type (DT) 104 first emerged in the United Kingdom in 1984 and soon became the second most prevalent type of salmonella isolated in humans there. It has also been isolated in increasing frequency in other European countries, United State and Japan. In Singapore, an unusual increase in the isolation of multidrug-resistant *S.* Typhimurium DT 104L was noted in July 2000. A total of 33 cases involving predominantly infants and toddlers were detected in the three-month period from July to October. Based on the case-control study using step-wise logistic regression, consumption of imported dried anchovy which was ground and sprinkled on to cooked porridge, was found to be the vehicle of transmission after adjusting for all confounding variables (Ling *et al.*, 2002).

Norovirus Gastroenteritis

Norovirus accounted for between 43% and 96% of outbreaks of non-bacterial gastroenteritis in North America and Western Europe. In Singapore, a total of 305 cases of gastroenteritis significantly associated with the consumption of imported oysters from Shandong, China were reported in 14 different outbreaks from 16 December 2003 to 4 January 2004. The oysters (*Crassostrea virginica*) were imported in a frozen state, thawed and subsequently served raw on the buffet table to customers in hotels, clubs and restaurants. Samples of stool and implicated oysters were tested positive for norovirus (genogroup II) by real-time reverse transcriptase-polymerase chain reaction (RT-PCR). Electron microscopic examination also indicated the presence of norovirus-like particles in the oyster samples. The implicated consignments of oysters were recalled from distribution and steps taken to ensure that food outlets do not thaw frozen oysters and serve them raw to consumers (Ministry of Health, 2004).

Nipah Virus Encephalitis/Pneumonia

Nipah virus is a new paramyxovirus which was responsible for 257 febrile encephalitis cases, including 100 deaths in Malaysia in 1998 and 1999 (Centers for Disease Control and Prevention, 1999). The virus was introduced into Singapore through the import and slaughter of infected pigs from Malaysia. A total of 11 abattoir workers, including one death, were reported between 10 March and 19 March 1999. The nucleotide sequences of RT-PCR products isolated from the Singapore cases were identical to Nipah virus sequences from Malaysian cases and pigs. Direct contact with the urine or faeces of live pigs appeared to be the most important risk factor for human Nipah virus infection (Chew *et al.*, 2000). The outbreak was rapidly brought under control by banning the import of Malaysian pigs and closing the abattoirs. In a serological survey conducted on 1,469 persons potentially exposed to Nipah virus, all 22 abattoir workers (1.2%), were tested positive for Nipah virus antibodies. Of the seropositive individuals, 12 (54.6%) were symptomatic and the remaining were clinically well and had no past history compatible with neurological or pulmonary disease. Three had been infected before the outbreak was recognised in March 1999. There was no evidence of human–to–human transmission (Chan *et al.*, 2002).

Meningococcal Disease caused by *Neisseria meningitidis* serogroup W135

An outbreak of meningococcal disease caused by a previously rare *Neisseria meningitidis* strain, W135, occurred among returning Hajj pilgrims and their contacts in Singapore in 2000 and 2001. The case fatality rate was 37% for the Hajj-related cases. This was part of an international outbreak. The outbreak in Singapore was contained after the introduction of quadrivalent meningococcal vaccine containing the W135 serogroup for the Hajj in 2001. No pilgrims developed W135 disease in 2001, compared with an attack rate of 25 cases per 100,000 pilgrims in the previous year. However, as vaccination does not prevent acquisition of nasopharyngeal carriage, transmission of infection could continue to occur among household contacts of returning pilgrims. The estimated attack rates were 18 and 28 cases per

100,000 household contacts in 2000 and 2001, respectively (Wilder-Smith *et al.*, 2003).

Enterovirus 71 Encephalitis

Epidemics of hand, foot and mouth disease (HFMD) associated with the complications of encephalitis, myocarditis and death were reported in Sarawak in 1997 (Cardosa *et al.*, 1999) and Taiwan in 1998 (Ho *et al.*, 1999). A nationwide outbreak of 3,790 cases of HFMD caused by enterovirus (EV) 71 occurred from September to October 2000, with majority of the cases among preschool children aged below four years old. EV 71 was isolated from four of the five children who died from encephalitis/myocarditis. The post-mortem findings were encephalitis, interstitial pneumonitis and myocarditis. Based on a preparedness plan for severe HFMD outbreak, all preschool centres were closed on 1 October and reopened on 16 October, when the disease incidence showed a rapid decline and no severe cases were reported (Chan *et al.*, 2003).

Severe Acute Respiratory Syndrome (SARS)

Singapore's outbreak of SARS started with a 22 year-old female local resident who reported ill on her way home from a holiday in Hong Kong on 26 February 2003. She was admitted to Ward 5A, Tan Tock Seng Hospital on 1 March and diagnosed to have atypical pneumonia. Another two Singaporeans, who were in Hong Kong at the same time and staying in the same hotel (Hotel Metropole), were also admitted to Tan Tock Seng Hospital and Singapore General Hospital (SGH) for atypical pneumonia. When the Ministry of Health (MOH) was notified of these cases on 6 March 2003, the hospitals were directed to isolate the patients as a precautionary measure.

Chain of transmission at healthcare institutions

Before the index case A was isolated and subsequently diagnosed to have probable SARS, she had already infected 22 persons, including 10 healthcare workers. One of the infected healthcare workers, provisionally diagnosed to have dengue fever, was later admitted on 10 March to Ward 8A of Tan Tock Seng Hospital where she in turn infected 21 persons, including an inpatient with ischemic heart disease and diabetes mellitus, before she was isolated on 13 March. The inpatient developed heart failure on 12 March, transferred to Ward 6A and isolated on 20 March when SARS was suspected. By that time, 21 healthcare workers and five family members had become infected. A total of 109 cases were epidemiologically linked to the index case A before intra-hospital transmission was interrupted on 5 April. On 22 March, Tan Tock Seng Hospital was designated as the SARS hospital for the treatment of all suspected and probable cases (Gopalakrishna et al., 2004). Despite the institution of very rigorous infection control measures, the disease spread to four other healthcare institutions and a vegetable wholesale market.

Index case B was a 60-year-old man who was a former patient of Tan Tock Seng Hospital with multiple medical problems, including chronic renal failure and diabetes mellitus. He was discharged from Ward 5A, Tan Tock Seng Hospital, on 20 March with no clinical manifestations of SARS, and admitted to Singapore General Hospital on 24 March for steroid-induced gastrointestinal bleeding. Although he had a low-grade fever since his admission to Singapore General Hospital, four consecutive chest x-rays were normal until 5 April, when he developed radiological evidence of pneumonia, and was clinically diagnosed as a probable SARS case. He started a cluster of 51 cases linked to Singapore General Hospital with the date of onset of the last probable case on 17 April. All the exposed health care workers and inpatients were transferred to Tan Tock Seng Hospital (Chow et al., 2004). Index case C at the National University Hospital worked as a vegetable seller at the Pasir Panjang wholesale market. He was infected when he visited his brother, the index case B at Singapore General Hospital, on 31 March. He developed a fever five days later and was admitted on 8 April to NUH. Index case C started a cluster of 12 cases, including seven in a family linked to this centre. The market was closed for 14 days from 19 April, and a total of 2,007 workers and regular visitors to the market were put on mandatory home quarantine. Teams of nurses visited all those under quarantine to check their temperatures and to ensure that they were well.

The outbreak at the Changi General Hospital was linked to a 90-year-old woman who had been warded next to a SARS patient in Ward 7D in Tan Tock Seng Hospital on 16 and 17 March. She was discharged to a private nursing home (Orange Valley Nursing Home) and then admitted to Changi General Hospital on 25 March when she subsequently fell ill again. This led to a small cluster of nine cases linked to the nursing home and Changi General Hospital. The date of onset of the last case at the nursing home and Changi General Hospital was 2 April and 4 April, respectively. Another outbreak in the community was linked to a healthcare worker at Singapore General Hospital who was given medical leave to stay at home, but had participated in a card game, leading to a cluster of eight new cases.

A total of 206 probable SARS cases, including seven imported cases, were diagnosed from March to May 2003. The majority (81%) were Singaporeans and 65.5% were females. Approximately half (45.7%) of the cases were in the 25 to 44 years age group. The ethnic distribution among the Singaporean cases was proportionate to that of the population of Singapore. Healthcare workers constituted 41%; family members, friends, social contacts and visitors constituted 43%, and inpatients, 13%. Transmission within healthcare and household settings accounted for >90% of the cases. The median incubation period was five days (range of one to 10 days). Of 1,300 clinically suspected and probable cases tested for SARS-coronavirus (SARS-CoV) antibodies, an additional 32 probable cases were picked up, giving the final figure of 238 cases and 33 deaths. The case-fatality rate was 14%.

A laboratory-acquired case

A probable case of SARS was diagnosed by Singapore General Hospital on 8 September 2003, after Singapore was removed from the WHO's list of areas with local SARS transmission on 31 May. The patient was a 27-year-old Chinese Singaporean in his third year of doctoral programme in microbiology at the National University of Singapore (NUS). He was working on the West Nile virus at a microbiology laboratory at NUS. He also did some work at the Environmental Health Institute (EHI) laboratory of the National Environment Agency. He last visited the EHI laboratory on 23 August. He had no history of travel to previously SARS-affected areas and had no known contact with SARS patients.

His onset of illness was on 26 August. When he was admitted to Singapore General Hospital on 3 September, he complained of fever, muscle aches and joint pains, but he did not have any significant respiratory symptoms.

He developed a dry cough after admission, but his fever resolved two days later. Three serial chest x-rays done at SGH were all normal. On 8 September, his stool and sputum specimens were tested positive for SARS-CoV by reverse-transcriptase polymerase chain reaction (RT-PCR). Three serial serological tests done on 3rd, 4th and 8 September showed a rising titre of SARS-CoV antibodies. He was immediately transferred to the Communicable Disease Centre, Tan Tock Seng Hospital, for further management.

A repeat of his PCR tests in two other laboratories in Singapore on 9 September was confirmed positive. Blood samples were also tested positive for antibodies to SARS-CoV in another laboratory in Singapore. The results from the Centers for Disease Control, Atlanta, corroborated with Singapore's PCR and serological results. Subsequent investigations of the chest on 13 September showed that he had evidence of pneumonic changes in his left lung. Tests for a whole range of other pathogens, including two human coronaviruses (OC 43, 229 E), were negative. The patient was discharged on 16 September and placed on a 14-day home quarantine.

Investigations by an 11-member review panel, comprising local and international experts, showed that the patient worked in the EHI laboratory 3.5 days before his onset of illness. Although the patient reported only working on the West Nile virus, the laboratory was doing live SARS-CoV work around the time. Poor record keeping made it difficult to ascertain if there was live SARS-CoV in the laboratory on the day of his visit, but it was there two days before. Testing of the frozen specimens that the patient worked with on 23 August was positive by RT-PCR for the SARS-CoV and West Nile virus, suggesting contamination. The laboratory only worked on one strain of the SARS-CoV so the laboratory strain and the patient strain were sequenced for comparison. Approximately 91% of the genome was sequenced from the patient's strain and found to be the most closely related to the sequence of the laboratory strain. Minor differences are likely the results of the natural mutations of the virus (Lim et al., 2004).

Prevention and control

Keys measures to prevent and control SARS in Singapore were directed at prevention and control in the community, healthcare institutions and the borders.

Community

To prevent and control SARS within the community in Singapore, the key strategy was to detect persons with suspected or probable SARS as early as possible and isolate them in Tan Tock Seng Hospital, the designated SARS hospital. Early identification was done through several ways, including active contact tracing to identify all contacts within 24 hours of notification of a case, mandatory home quarantine enforced through the use of electronic cameras, and intensive education of healthcare professionals and public.

The effectiveness of these strategies was reflected in the fact that from 3 March to 9 March, the average interval between onset of symptoms and isolation in hospital was 6.8 days. The interval was reduced to 2.9 days for the week 31 March to 6 April and 1.3 days for the week 21 April to 27 April.

Healthcare institutions

The Ministry of Health implemented very stringent measures to prevent and contain outbreaks in hospitals and other healthcare institutions, including nursing homes. These included strict infection control procedures, twice-daily temperature checks for all healthcare workers and active surveillance for clusters of febrile patients and staff from the same work area. Through these measures, SARS was eventually brought under control in the healthcare sector.

Border checkpoints

The risk of imported cases was minimised through various measures. Health screening of all incoming air and sea passengers and crew from affected areas was carried out through temperature checks using thermal imaging scanners (Wilder–Smith *et al.*, 2003). Persons identified by the scanners had their temperature re-checked by nurses and referred for further examination by doctors at the air and sea terminals if they were found to have a fever. Persons who were suspected of having SARS were referred to Tan Tock Seng Hospital for further assessment, and admission for isolation and treatment if necessary. Incoming bus passengers at the land checkpoints were also screened with the thermal scanners. Screening was progressively extended to persons coming in via other vehicles at the land checkpoints. All visitors to Singapore through air, sea and land checkpoints were required to complete a health declaration card for SARS. All travellers who entered Singapore from affected areas were given a health alert notice to explain the symptoms of SARS and how they could get help if they fell ill with suspected SARS.

Very stringent steps are taken to minimise the possibility of exporting cases to other countries. These measures included rapid containment of outbreaks in Singapore, and mandatory temperature screening of all out-going travellers from Singapore. In addition, a special bilateral arrangement between Malaysia and Singapore and a multi-lateral agreement among the 10 member countries of ASEAN plus China, Japan and Republic of Korea (ASEAN + 3) were concluded on the exchange of information for the pur-pose of contact tracing and quarantine.

Lessons learnt

In the early phase of the outbreak, stringent infection control measures were not enforced. It was only on 8 April that full personal protective equipment (PPE) was implemented for all areas in healthcare institutions and the no visitation rule was imposed. It is now known that the earlier the patient was isolated, the fewer the number of secondary cases would be generated (Lipsitch et al., 2003). Several factors had contributed to the rapid transmission of SARS within hospitals and across healthcare institu-tions. Delay in recognition and isolation of the index cases in Tan Tock Seng Hospital, Singapore General Hospital and National University Hospi-tal was responsible for the intra-hospital transmission. When the index case in Tan Tock Seng Hospital was admitted on 1 March, it was thought to be a case of avian influenza, which was not known to be transmittable from person to person. By the time the term SARS was coined by the WHO on 15 March, the index case had already spread the infection to more than 69 contacts in the hospital. Patients with co-morbidity presenting with atyp-ical clinical manifestations were transferred from one ward to another, and by the time SARS was suspected and the patient isolated, transmission had already occurred to their close contacts (Tan et al., 2004; Tee et al., 2004). The index case of SGH was an ex-patient of Tan Tock Seng Hospital with co-morbidity. SARS was only suspected when a cluster of fever cases was detected among healthcare workers who had contact with the patient. The index case at National University Hospital did not give a contact history when seen at the Accident and Emergency (A&E) Department (Singh *et al.*, 2003; Fisher *et al.*, 2003). Super-spreading events by five patients, including the three index cases at Tan Tock Seng Hospital, SGH and NUH, accounted for a large proportion of the cases. Fortunately, 80% of the cases did not transmit the infection to others. The laboratory-acquired case of SARS was due to inappropriate laboratory standards, non-compliance in laboratory procedures and an accidental cross-contamination, which led to infection.

Operational readiness

Based on the lessons learnt and to maintain a high level of preparedness for SARS and other emerging infectious diseases, a number of measures have been put in place to strengthen Singapore's ability to prevent a SARS outbreak, to detect new cases early and to respond effectively to contain new clusters.

SARS response framework

A SARS response framework has been put in place to provide a clear command structure for decision-making. The SARS Ministerial Committee provides policy guidance and strategic decisions. Selected Permanent Secretaries lead Crisis Management Groups with distinct roles and responsibilities for the operational and tactical actions in the combat of SARS and they report to the SARS Executive Group. A three-level response system, which corresponds to the existing level of local transmission of SARS and the severity of threat to public health, is in place and serves as a platform for coordinating the response measures for the various agencies.

There are three colour-coded alert status, known as SARS condition (SARSCON): yellow is defined as no or sporadic imported cases but with no local transmission; orange is defined as local transmission confined to close contacts in healthcare settings or households; and red is defined as outbreak in the community where local transmissions are no longer confined to close contacts in healthcare settings or households. This SARSCON status correlates with the colour-coded alert status adopted by the hospitals.

Preventive strategy

A three-prong strategy is adopted to combat the spread of SARS through prevention, detection and effective response. Within this framework, the various measures to be implemented will be based on the SARSCON state.

At SARSCON yellow, the main focus is to prevent imported cases and detect SARS cases early. Active surveillance and enhanced protection at high-risk areas in the healthcare settings underpin the prevention strategy. At immigration checkpoints, temperature screening of inbound visitors will be instituted at all entry points. Within the healthcare setting, active surveillance of atypical pneumonia as well as fever clusters will be carried out. For prevention, healthcare workers in high-risk areas such as A&E departments, isolation facilities, intensive care units and triaging areas will be required to don full PPE (N95 masks, disposable gloves and gowns). Workflow changes to separate febrile and non-febrile patients at hospitals, step-down facilities and primary health care clinics will be enforced. Containment measures will be triggered if necessary.

Moving up to SARSCON orange, the focus is to contain. Measures that are implemented at SARSCON yellow will continue, but additional measures will be introduced with the aim to contain the spread of SARS in Singapore as well as to prevent export of cases. Infection control measures in healthcare institutions will be enhanced to break the local chain of transmission. This will include restriction of hospital visitation and movement of healthcare workers and patients between healthcare institutions. Contact tracing and quarantine efforts will be stepped up. Community surveillance through daily temperature taking at workplace and school will also be instituted. Outbound screening and 'not to depart' measures will be implemented at the border checkpoints to prevent the export of cases. Health declaration will also be implemented for inbound travellers.

At SARSCON red, the strategy is to suppress. More measures will be added with the aim to gain control of community spread in Singapore and prevent the export of cases. These could include selective closure of schools, foreign worker dormitories, factories, places of mass gathering and suspension of selected public events. Contact tracing and quarantine measures will be strictly enforced.

Healthcare workers and those travelling to temperate countries were encouraged to receive influenza vaccination. Mandatory influenza vaccination was given to long-staying patients in nursing homes.

Early detection

For the early detection of SARS cases, Singapore continues to strengthen the linkages with international health organisations and other health authorities, and has enhanced surveillance for SARS and other infectious disease outbreaks. For patients who contracted SARS at the hospitals, the strategy is to detect them early, isolate them from others to prevent the spread of the disease, and ensure that the disease is contained by protecting the healthcare workers who are caring for them. A revised fever cluster surveillance system for SARS was implemented in public and private acute hospitals, nursing homes, chronic sick hospitals, community hospitals and hospices since August 2003. This system comprises surveillance and investigations into inpatients with atypical pneumonia, unexplained fevers of more than 72 hours with relevant travel history, sudden unexplained deaths with acute respiratory symptoms, and fever clusters among healthcare staff and inpatients in hospitals.

Effective response

To ensure a high level of vigilance and an effective response system, all the healthcare institutions and agencies have put in place their own contingency plans. Regular exercises and audits have also been carried out to ensure a high level of preparedness at all times. Depending on the SARSCON level and threat assessment, additional manpower resources would be mobilised to meet a surge requirement. Likewise, the various Crisis Management Groups under the direction of the SARS Ministerial Committee and the SARS Executive Group will be able to provide directions at the national level. The critical factor in containing an outbreak is the early detection and isolation of the infected patients, and the generation of a complete list of close contacts who are then put on home quarantine. Extra precautions are applied to immuno-compromised patients who tend to have atypical presentations of the disease.

To contain a SARS outbreak in Singapore, three separate hospital containment strategies have been used successfully. These are hospital closure (as in the case of Tan Tock Seng Hospital), ring fencing and transfer of an exposed group to the designated SARS hospital (as in the case of SGH), and management of the exposed cohort *in situ* (as in the case of NUH) (Gopalakrishna *et al.*, 2004). Supporting this containment strategy are the strict enforcement of the proper use of PPE, the restriction of movements of healthcare workers and patients, and the close monitoring of discharged patients from SARS affected wards. In this way, intra-hospital transmission of SARS is contained and the risk of healthcare workers transmitting the infection to their family and the community is minimised.

Since the last outbreak, all hospitals have either built up or developed contingency plans for additional isolation rooms. At the national level, a new isolation centre, Communicable Disease Centre 2, with 39 isolation beds and 18 ICU beds has been built beside Tan Tock Seng Hospital. It has been designated as the SARS hospital to isolate and contain an outbreak when the situation requires.

Contact tracing centre

A system for contact tracing has been put in place through the establishment of a contact-tracing centre within Ministry of Health. The centre will undertake all community contact tracing and coordinate and assist in the contact tracing efforts undertaken by the hospitals and government bodies. It also informs foreign governments on the movement out of Singapore of their nationals who are possible close contacts.

Ministry of Health centrally manages all matters related to the conduct of quarantine operations which encompass the issues and enforcement of home quarantine order, phone surveillance, ambulance services, home quarantine order allowances, appeal board and alternate housing facilities for those on home quarantine. The home quarantine order is a measure to minimise the risk of spread of SARS to the community. Persons on home quarantine are well and therefore not infectious. They are however at risk of becoming ill with SARS, due to prior close contact with a SARS patient. Close monitoring of those on home quarantine order for early signs of SARS, including twice–daily temperature taking, is carried out by officers designated by MOH. If they develop a fever, an ambulance will be immediately sent to fetch them to Tan Tock Seng Hospital/Communicable Disease Centre for a medical evaluation and for treatment if necessary. This will break the chain of transmission and control the spread of SARS.

IT infrastructure

A new IT infrastructure has been rolled out to support the surveillance and management of SARS and other emerging diseases. The SARS IT infrastructure is intended to provide MOH and other agencies with the ability to access integrated information of all SARS cases in Singapore in a timely fashion. For medical surveillance, there is the Infectious Disease Alert and Clinical Database System, which integrate critical clinical, laboratory and contact tracing information on SARS. In addition, the Health Check System allows healthcare professionals in hospitals and clinics to identify patients who may have been exposed to SARS. It also provides customised advisories for precautionary measures as well as follow-up actions to be taken. For contact tracing and quarantine operations, the Contact Tracing System is in place to capture SARS cases, contact history and home quarantine order status. This in turn allows speedier generation of the home quarantine order report, contact listings, and listings for external agencies automatically. An e-Quarantine Management System (eQMS) has also been developed for the better management of processing and enforcement of home quarantine order by a Singapore security agency.

Medical and logistic resource

MOH has stockpiled up to six months of critical supplies such as PPE items. An emergency procurement system to support the preparedness for outbreaks of SARS and other new infectious diseases has been established.

Laboratory safety

Based on the recommendations of the review panel appointed by MOH to investigate the laboratory-acquired case of SARS, steps have been taken to ensure that the biosafety requirements and practices at the laboratories, including training, adoption of national standards, audit and accreditation for biosafety, are put in place.

Conclusion

The outbreak of SARS was unprecedented. It has exposed the weaknesses of the epidemiological surveillance and healthcare system for emerging diseases, which are spread from person to person via the respiratory route. Based on the lessons learnt, Singapore has further strengthened its operational readiness and laboratory safety to respond to SARS, avian flu and other emerging diseases.

References

Cardosa MJ, Krishnan S, Tio PH, *et al.* (1999) Isolation of subgenus B adenovirus during a fatal outbreak of enterovirus 71-associated hand, foot and mouth disease in Sibu, Sarawak. *Lancet* **354**: 987–991.

Centers for Disease Control and Prevention. (1999) Update: Outbreak of Nipah Virus — Malaysia and Singapore, 1999. *Morb Mortal Wkly Rec* **48**: 335–337.

Chan KP, Rollin PE, Ksiazek TG, Leo YS, Goh KT, *et al.* (2002) Survey of Nipah Virus infection among various risk groups in Singapore. *Epidemiol Infect* **128**: 93–98.

Chan KP, Goh KT, Chia YC, *et al.* (2003) Epidemic of hand, foot and mouth disease caused by human enterovirus 71, Singapore. *Emerg Infect Dis* **9**: 78–85.

Chew MHL, Arguin PM, Shay DK, Goh KT, *et al.* (2000) Risk factors for Nipah Virus infection among abattoir workers in Singapore. *J Infect Dis* **181**: 1760–1763.

Chow KY, Lee CE, Ling ML, *et al.* (2004) Outbreak of severe acute respiratory syndrome in a tertiary hospital in Singapore, linked to an index patient with atypical presentation: Epidemiological study. *BMJ* **328**: 195–198.

Committee on Epidemic Diseases. (1999) Epidemiology of campylobacter enteritis in Singapore. *Epidem News Bull* **25**: 33–35.

Committee on Epidemic Diseases. (1999) Campylobacter bacteria in animals. *Epidem News Bull* **25**: 36–37.

Committee on Epidemic Diseases. (2001) Risk factors for the transmission of campylobacter bacteria infection in Singapore. *Epidem News Bull* **27**: 29–31.

Committee on Epidemic Diseases. (2002) An outbreak of gastroenteritis linked to consumption of barbecued chickens. *Epidem News Bull* **28**: 19–21.

Fisher DA, Chew MH, Lim YT, *et al.* (2003) Preventing local transmission of SARS: Lessons from Singapore. *Med J Aust* **178**: 555–558.

Goh KT, Sng EH. (1987) Changing patterns of infectious diseases in Singapore. *Ann Aca Med Spore* **16**: 563–566.

Gopalakrishna G, Choo P, Leo YS, *et al.* (2004) SARS transmission and hospital containment. *Emerg Infect Dis* **10**: 395–400.

Ho M, Chen ER, Hsu KH, *et al.* (1999) An epidemic of enterovirus 71 infection in Taiwan. *N Engl J Med* **341**: 929–935.

Lim PL, Kurup A, Gopalakrishna G, *et al.* (2004) Laboratory-acquired severe acute respiratory syndrome. *N Engl J Med* **350**: 1740–1745.

Ling ML, Goh KT, Wang GCY, Neo KS, Chua LT. (2002) An outbreak of multidrug-resistant *Salmonella enterica* subsp. *enterica* serotype Typhimurium, DT 104 L linked to dried anchovy in Singapore. *Epidemiol Infect* **128**: 1–5.

Lipsitch M, Cohen T, Cooper B, *et al.* (2003) Transmission dynamics and control of severe acute respiratory syndrome. *Science* **300**: 1966–1970.

Ministry of Health. (2004) Oyster-associated outbreaks of gastroenteritis. *Epidem News Bull* **30**: 9–11.

Singh K, Hsu LY, Villacian JS, *et al.* (2003) Severe acute respiratory syndrome: lessons from Singapore. *Emerg Infect Dis* **9**: 1294–1298.

Tan TT, Tan BH, Kurup A, *et al.* (2004) Atypical SARS and *Escherichia coli* bacteremia. *Emerg Infect Dis* **10**: 349–352.

Tay L, Goh KT, Lim YS. (1994) *Vibrio cholerae* 139 'Bengal' in Singapore. *J Trop Med Hyg* **97**: 317–320.

Tee AK, Oh HM, Lien CT, *et al.* (2004) Atypical SARS in geriatric patient. *Emerg Infect Dis* **10**: 261–264.

Wilder-Smith A, Goh KT, Barkham T, *et al.* (2003) Hajj-associated outbreak strain of *Neisseria meningitidis* serogroup W 135: Estimates of the attack rate in a defined population and the risk of invasive disease developing in carriers. *Clin Infect Dis* **36**: 679–683.

Wilder-Smith A, Paton NI, Goh KT. (2003) Experience of severe acute respiratory syndrome in Singapore: Importation of cases, and defense strategies at the airport. *J Travel Med* **10**: 259–262.

Wong SY, Goh KT. (1997) Emerging infections: Why we must be concerned. *Ann Aca Med Spore* **26**: 535–537.

World Health Organization. (1993) Epidemic diarrhoea due to *Vibrio cholerae* non-01. *Wkly Epidemio Rec* **68**: 141–142.

## 16

Probable Roles of Bio-Aerosol Dispersion in the SARS Outbreak in Amoy Gardens, Hong Kong

Yuguo Li*, Hua Qian, Ignatius Tak Sun Yu and Tze Wai Wong

Introduction

We spend more than 90% of our time indoors, and modern indoor environments are often connected within large building complexes in large and crowded cities. The growth of many Asian mega-cities and the construction of many high-rise residential buildings may have significant implications to the health and safe living for billions of future city dwellers. One of the important issues is whether the current standard of mechanical systems such as air conditioning, plumbing and drainage, and fire safety can satisfy the needs of safety, health, comfort and the rising living standards of the occupants.

Located between hills and a harbour, Hong Kong is one of the most crowded cities in the world. Population densities in Hong Kong are nearly three times higher than that in Singapore (Karakiewicz, 2002), six times higher than those in European cities and 30 times higher than those in American cities (Jenks and Burgess, 2000). The 2003 SARS epidemic in Hong Kong revealed a need to examine the interaction between population density, built environment facilities and the potential spread of infectious diseases.

The first SARS cases occurred in mid November in Guangdong, China. The disease spread to the rest of the world by a Guangdong infected medical doctor visiting Hong Kong in February 2004. He stayed in a hotel and infected at least 14 hotel guests and visitors from various countries including Hong Kong, Canada, Vietnam and Singapore (WHO, 2003a). Most of these infected individuals sparked large outbreaks in hospitals after they returned home. In Hong Kong, the Amoy Gardens outbreak of SARS has provided a unique opportunity for investigating transmission issues related to mechanical and utility services in high-rise buildings. The Amoy Gardens outbreak between 21 March and mid April 2003 was the largest community cluster during the 2003 SARS epidemic outside of mainland China, with a total of 321 infected cases and 42 deaths (Tsang, 2003). The flats where the infection cases occurred were not randomly distributed. Most occurred in certain blocks and at certain levels, and evidently conformed to a directional spatial pattern. The epidemic curve, the analysis by Riley *et al.* (2003) and the mathematical and statistical analysis by Li *et al.* (2004) all showed that most infections in the Amoy Gardens outbreak probably arose due to a super-spreading transmission event over a short period at some time between the 19th and 20th of March, 2003. Interestingly, the number of infected cases per super spreading event in Hong Kong was one magnitude higher than the corresponding number in Singapore (Li *et al.*, 2004). It is unknown whether this difference was due to differences in the choice or effectiveness of disease control measures, or due to other environmental factors such as the higher population density in Hong Kong.

Although SARS virus was primarily transmitted by large droplets and close contact (WHO, 2003b), the studies by Yu *et al.* (2004) on the Amoy Gardens outbreak suggested the airborne transmission of the virus between flats and buildings. Various other possible transmission routes for this outbreak were suggested by the Department of Health, Hong Kong Government (2003), and a WHO team (2003c), and Ng (2003). There are a number of significant issues to be resolved in the reported environmental analysis of the airborne transmission hypothesis for the Amoy Gardens (Yu *et al.*, 2004). For example, what was the effect of unsteady state winds on the dispersion as the analysis reported in Yu *et al.* (2004) was steady state? Could the drainage pipe system act as an alternative transmission route for SARS virus?

We present the three-dimensional spatial distribution of the cases and compare that to the predicted three-dimensional distribution of the bio-aerosols in the Amoy Gardens housing estate under differing wind directions. Our new results provide further environmental evidence for the airborne transmission hypothesis. We also present information and analysis suggesting that the virus transmission by the drainage pipe system between buildings is very unlikely.

Data and Methods

Epidemiological data

We obtained the data for the date of onset of symptoms and the location of flats of the 187 persons with SARS virus infection in the initial phase of the Amoy Garden outbreak. Most infections were believed to be linked to one common source. The index patient visited Flat 7 on the 16th floor of Block E at Amoy Gardens on two nights during mid March 2003. Subsequent infections occurred in a number of housing blocks in late March, with four blocks (B, C, D and E) being severely affected. In Yu *et al.* (2004), the probability of infection in individual housing units (characterised by flat, floor and block) was analysed using a statistical method to explore how the location of residence relative to Flat 7 in Block E had affected the probability of infection. The method was useful for analysing the risk factors, but did not capture the relationship between infection risk and the complex wind flow behaviours. It was not the location of residence relative to Flat 7 in Block E that affected the probability of infection, but whether a residence was located downwind of the air plume flows coming from the index patient's flat in Block E. We herewith use the three-dimensional graphical analysis of the spatial distribution of the flats with SARS infected cases to illustrate this spatial pattern of the infection.

Building and weather data

Detailed site plan, floor plans, as well as drainage system design drawings for the Amoy Gardens were obtained from the Buildings Department and the on-site visits in late March and early April 2003 during the outbreak.

Field measurements were also carried out in toilets and re-entrants in other similar apartment buildings in Hong Kong during April 2003 to obtain field data such as typical air speeds in a re-entrant, air temperature and relative humidity in bathrooms. The hourly weather data during March close to the site (the Kai Tak automatic weather station) were obtained from the Hong Kong Observatory.

Environmental Investigations

We undertook a study of airflows in the drainage system using a simple air-flow model, and computational fluid dynamics (CFD) simulations (Ferziger and Peric, 2002) of air flows around the Amoy Gardens housing estate. As accurate modelling of the air flows and the dispersion of the virus-laden bio-aerosols is difficult, in particular when dealing with wind flows over a complex building estate, we adopted two different modelling approaches: (1) basic buoyant plume analysis, and (2) CFD analysis.

Air flow calculations for testing the drainage system transmission theory

Air flow calculations were carried out based on a simple *macroscopic* air flow approach to analyse the air flow rates through the drainage system and the floor drains into bathrooms of Flats 7 in Block E (Fig. 1) to iden-tify the putative association between the infection distribution pattern and the virus-laden bio-aerosol flow rate through the dried-out floor drains in Flats 7 and 8.

Testing the buoyant transmission theory

We test the buoyant plume transmission theory that virus-laden moist air exhausted from a bathroom flows upwards and is dispersed in the deep open air slit between the wings of the high-rise tower, a space known as the re-entrant or the external air shaft (Fig. 1). This airflow can be considered as a two-dimensional moist buoyant plume. The air speed, airflow rate as well as virus-laden particle concentration decay are calculated as a function of height by a simple two-dimensional plume theory (Etheridge and Sandberg, 1996). The two-dimensional plume model is a simplification of the very complicated turbulent flow process in the re-entrant. This plume approach

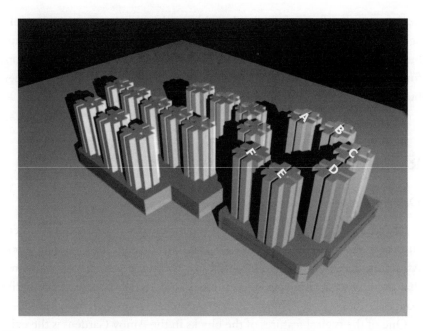

Fig. 1. Location of Blocks B, C, D and E in the Amoy Gardens housing estate (the 19th block is not shown).

has been widely used in the analysis of indoor air quality (Etheridge and Sandberg, 1996) and smoke flows (Klote and Milke, 2003) in buildings. The simple plume theory is used here to obtain the physical understanding of virus-laden bio-aerosol flows in the re-entrant.

Computational fluid dynamics (CFD) analysis

CFD allows detailed airflow pattern and the spread of virus-laden bio-aerosols in the re-entrant and around the buildings to be reasonably predicted. Two CFD software packages are used. "Fluent" is a three-dimensional general-purpose CFD package for modelling fluid flows. In this application, we used the basic RNG turbulence model and a Reynolds stress turbulence model for modelling turbulence affects. The simulated virus-laden bio-aerosols were found to evaporate rapidly in the air within a few seconds. In this paper, we neglected the particle settling and deposition effect of droplet nuclei, which are justifiable as the diameters of droplet nuclei are generally very small. "Airpak" is a three-dimensional CFD package, developed for modelling building ventilation flows, and the RNG turbulence model in "Airpak" is being used. We carried out CFD simulations for both the plume flow in the re-entrant and the bio-aerosol spread between building blocks for part of Amoy Gardens.

Results

Description of the buildings

There are a total of 19 high-rise housing blocks in the Amoy Gardens and each block has 33 floors. There are 264 housing units in each block. Assuming that the average household size was three persons, we estimated that there were 792 people in each block and 15,048 people in the entire housing estate.

One of the typical features of the blocks in the Amoy Gardens is the existence of four re-entrants in each block (Fig. 1). The re-entrant is a recessed space formed between two adjacent wings (Flats); which extends outward from a central core in a high-rise apartment building. This typical building feature in Hong Kong is essentially designed to maximise the availability of daylight and natural ventilation to the apartments to fulfil the building code requirements in Hong Kong. Lift lobbies, corridors as well as other public space are located in the central core. There are eight units on each floor and eight wings radiating out from the central core. The deep and narrow "I-shaped" re-entrant space allows the installation of the exhausts of kitchen, bathroom and gas heaters. The re-entrant between Flats 7 and 8 of Block E is 1.5 m wide and 6 m deep.

Figure 2 shows the hourly weather data between 8:00 am 19 March and 2:00 pm 20 March, the period of the second visit to the building by the index SARS case, who stayed in a middle level Flat in Flats 7 stack of Block E. During the 30-hour period, the wind direction fluctuated between northeasterly and southeasterly, and occasionally northerly. The wind speed ranged between 1.2 and 5.4 m/s, with a mean value of 3.0 m/s at the weather station. The outdoor temperature varied between 13.8°C and 16.5°C, with a mean of 15.2°C.

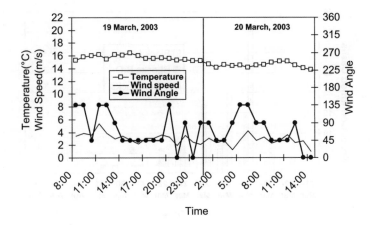

Fig. 2. Hourly temperature, wind speed and wind direction recorded at a weather station close to the Amoy Gardens housing estate during the suspected time of exposure, obtained from the Hong Kong Observatory.

Spatial distribution of infected flats

The first SARS case was confirmed in the Amoy Gardens on 21 March 2003. We have data for the first 187 confirmed cases (involving infected persons in 142 units up to 3 April 2003) of a total of 321 cases (up to 15 April 2003). The epidemic curve of confirmed SARS cases in Amoy Gardens as at 3 April 2003 is shown in Fig. 3. There is a tight clustering of cases in time with a sharp upslope leading to a peak on 24 March and a trailing down-slope until 1 April. This distribution suggests that a common source is responsible for the outbreak.

The flats with infected individuals located mostly in seven of the 19 blocks. All seven blocks with the majority of the cases are located at one end of the housing estate (Fig. 1). Block E had the most cases in all blocks (45% as of 11 April 2004, an unpublished report by the WHO investigation team, 2003), followed by Block B (13%), Block C (13%), Block D (12%), Block F (6%), Block A (4%) and Block G (3%). For all seven blocks (A–G), the middle level floors (15–25th floors) had the most cases. Figure 4 shows the distribution of infected flats where infection occurred. The spatial distribution of infected flats among the seven infected blocks is not random, but exhibits an obvious directional pattern. Examining the three-dimensional spatial distribution of infected flats in Fig. 4 revealed the same

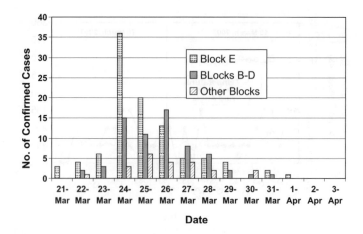

Fig. 3. Dates of onset of symptoms in different blocks in the Amoy Gardens between 21 March and 3 April.

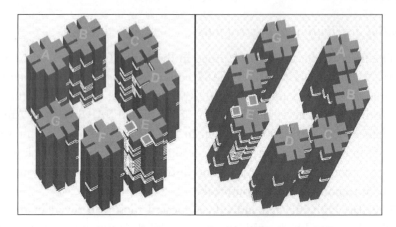

Fig. 4. A map of the three-dimensional spatial distribution of the infected flats in the Amoy Gardens between 21 March and 3 April. Two different perspectives are shown. Flats 7 and 8 in Block E were mostly infected. Flats 1–4 in Block E were moderately infected, while Flats 5 and 6 had fewer infections. Blocks B, C and D were infected in some concentrated areas. Most other Flats (wings) were not inflected.

conclusion as that from the statistical analysis in Yu *et al.* (2004). Through statistical analysis, Yu *et al.* (2004) found that the units in Blocks B, C and D that face Block E had the highest probability of being infected. The units between Blocks C and D also had a high risk of infection (Fig. 4).

Figure 4 also showed that the units in Blocks F, G and A that also faced Block E had a very low probability of being infected. This spatial distribution of infected flats agrees well with the three-dimensional spread pattern of the rising plume from the re-entrant between Flats 7 and 8 in Block E, shown in Yu *et al.* (2004). In Block E, most cases of infection were found in unit 7 (17% of all infected cases in Block E) and Flat 8 (43%), whereas units 5 and 6 had the least infections. This distribution correlates with the dispersion of virus-laden bio-aerosols between units in Block E, also discussed in details in Yu *et al.* (2004).

Drainage system as a possible transmission route

The Hong Kong SAR Government (2003) and the WHO team (2003c) suggested a possible transmission route by the drainage pipe system in the buildings. Most of the infected residents in Amoy Gardens showed diarrhoea symptoms. Many floor drains in the Amoy Gardens units were suspected to be dried-out, as most residents did not fill the floor drain with water to maintain the water seal in the U-traps. The dried-out floor drains could have enabled virus-laden bio-aerosols to leak back into flats. Among the various possible transmission routes, this transmission via the drainage system is the most difficult to prove or disprove. Both the HKSAR Government's and the WHO team's investigation were not fully supported by a detailed analysis or measurement of bio-aerosol generation and transport into the flats. Virus-laden bio-aerosol leaked back through the dried-out floor drain into at least one unit, most probably into the unit when the index patient stayed. The question is whether the spatial distribution of the putative leaked virus-laden bio-aerosol flow rates in the many different flats could explain the spatial distribution of infection risk, not only in Block E, but also for other Blocks. Such a study has not been presented elsewhere. We present below a preliminary calculation of leaked airflows in Flat 7 in Block E.

We studied airflow though pipe connections in the drainage system as a possible transmission route in Flat 7 of Block E. A sketch of the drainage pipe connection in the Amoy Gardens housing estate Blocks A–E is shown in Fig. 5. The main driving force for bio-aerosol movement in partially filled underground/above ground drainage pipes may be due to stack effects or waste water flows. In theory, the bio-aerosol movement through the entire drainage pipe system for the entire Amoy Gardens can be analysed using a

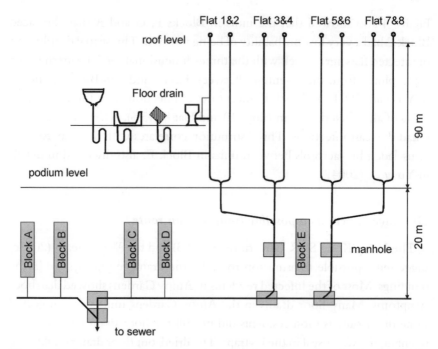

Fig. 5. A schematic diagram of the drainage pipe connections in Blocks A–E in the Amoy Gardens.

network air and water flow model, and by using a virus tracer measurement in the drainage system (Swaffield and Campwell, 1995). Such a model was not available to this project team. Instead, we made simple steady-state calculations of the airflows through the drainage pipes in unit 7 of Block E.

There are two possible major driving forces, i.e. the backpressure and the suction of exhaust fans. We first studied the airflows driven by the backpressure [see Fig. 6(a)]. The hypothesis was when the index patient used and flushed the toilet, the waste water flows in the vertical drainage stack caused a positive back pressure at the bottom of the stack for unit 7 only, which could "push" the air flows through each floor drain linked to the same vertical stack, i.e. Flat 7. The air flows in dried floor drains in Flats 8 induced by toilet flushing in the index patient's Flat 7 bathroom can be much more difficult to estimate. Based on our results, the lower floors of Flat 7 should be at a greater risk due to the action of backpressures in the drainage system. It is known that backpressure is higher in the lower floors

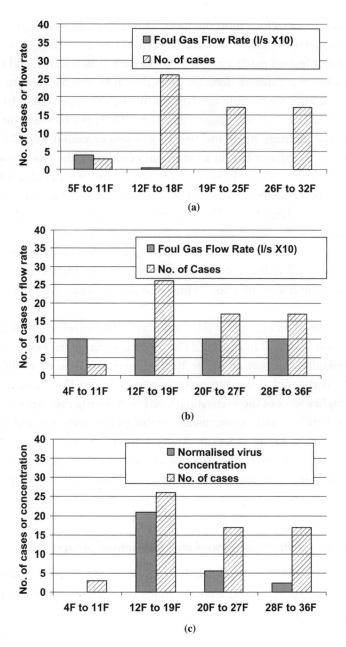

Fig. 6. Correlation between the number of the infected individuals and (a) the calculated foul gas flow rate through the floor drains by back pressure; (b) the calculated foul gas flow rate through the floor drains by exhaust fans; and (c) the calculated virus concentrations in the re-entrant at different stories for Flats 7 and 8.

and could only exit for a short duration. This analysis does not agree with the infection pattern in Flat 7 of Block E. It would be more difficult to explain the spatial infection pattern in other blocks such as Block B, C and D, if the transmission was through drainage pipes driven by this backpressure.

There is another possible mechanism for the drainage system to act as a transmission route. If we assume that the virus-laden bio-aerosols can be kept in the drainage pipes and vents for a longer period (e.g. 24 hours), the suction of exhaust fans in a bathroom could suck the bio-aerosols into a bathroom once the exhaust fan was on. Again, we calculated the air-flows through the floor drains in Flat 7's bathrooms due to exhaust fans in each bathroom [Fig. 6(b)]. The bottleneck of the flows is found to be the branch pipe with a small diameter (32 mm) and the floor drain entry. We found that the suction flow rates due to exhaust fans were approximately the same for all units. This means that all units in Flats 7 and 8 should have the same risk of infection, which also did not agree with the infection pattern.

Thus, our studies ruled out the possibility of transmission by the drainage pipe system for Flat 7 in Block E. The vertical drainage stacks of Flats 7 and 8 are linked at the bottom of the Block E and it will be more difficult to show how the virus-laden bio-aerosols travelled from Flat 7's vertical stack to the higher level of the vertical stack of Flat 8. Further studies can include a detailed analysis and on-site measurement of bio-aerosol transport in the drainage system for all blocks in Amoy Gardens. Examining the drainage system design drawings, we could not find any strong engineering evidence of the possible transmission routes that could explain the spatial pattern of the infected flats.

Drainage system as the virus-laden bio-aerosol source

Yu *et al.* (2004) suggested that large amounts of bio-aerosols were generated in the vertical stacks after the index patient used the toilet. It is not known how many bio-aerosols were generated or what the bio-aerosol concentrations and sizes were in the vertical stacks. The calculated average flow rate of foul gas through the floor drain by exhaust fans is 1 litre per second [Fig. 6(b)], which suggests the potential of a high influx of virus-laden bio-aerosols into the bathroom. It is also not known how many viruses could exist in one bio-aerosol. Further study is needed to estimate the number of droplet nuclei after these bio-aerosols were released into the re-entrant.

We also do not know the exact timing of the use of the toilet by the index patient, but it could be during the peak hours or non-peak hours late at night. The probability is small that two households used the bathrooms connected to the same vertical stack in Block E at the same time. Accordingly, the possibility of having two exhaust fans turned on is very small. The latter could be confirmed by further questionnaire studies. The concentration of the virus-laden bio-aerosols after the index patient used the toilet would be higher in the vertical stack close to the index patient's bathroom than other vertical stacks in Block E. We suspected that the bathroom on a middle level Flat 7 used by the index patient was the most likely source bathroom, which sucked in the virus-laden bio-aerosols and then exhausted them into the re-entrant. It was also possible that a bathroom located at the floors lower than 16th floor might also be the source bathroom. However, from the infection pattern, it is very unlikely that the source bathroom is located in floors lower than the 12th floor, as there were no infections in the lower floors in Block E.

A large amount of bio-aerosols could be generated within the drainage system due to hydraulic interactions after the index patient flushed the toilet (Yu *et al.*, 2004). The bio-aerosolisation process of water mixed with urine and/or faeces originating from the index patient is suggested as the source of the bio-aerosol generation in the Amoy Gardens outbreak. Obviously, much work is needed to confirm this hypothesis. The virus-laden bio-aerosols most likely entered one or two bathrooms at middle floors of Flat 7 in Block E through branch pipes and dried-out floor drains, then became airborne and were further extracted into the re-entrant between Flats 7 and 8, rising as a plume. It is also unknown as to how long that the virus-laden aerosols could exist in the vertical stack.

Transmission route by bio-aerosols for Flats 7 and 8 in Block E

Due to the narrow space, air conditioners are not located in the re-entrant in the Amoy Gardens buildings. The moist and warm air exhausted from the bathrooms into the re-entrant forms a thermal plume. One simple confirmatory test that we did was in a domestic bathroom of size 1.5 m by 2.2 m with the fittings arranged similar to those in Amoy Gardens on 9 April 2003 (Dr Dennis Leung, The University of Hong Kong, personal communication). The shower was turned on continuously for 12 minutes at a maximum flow with the thermostatic mixer set at 38°C for the hot water supply. The 150 mm diameter exhaust fan was also turned on at the same time. The initial bathroom air temperature and relative humidity were 22.6°C and 73.3% respectively. The final air temperature and relative humidity at the exhaust fan inlet were 24.7°C and 92.8% respectively.

The plume is developed after continuous supply of warm and moist air from the bathroom [see Fig. 7 for an illustration of the flow pattern of bio-aerosols based on the CFD predictions (Li et al., 2005)]. The resultant flow due to the exhaust of moist and warm air from a bathroom can also be modelled as a two-dimensional thermal plume. The similarity solutions of a two-dimensional turbulent plume are well established in the literature, including reports by Fisher et al. (1979) and Etheridge and Sandberg (1996).

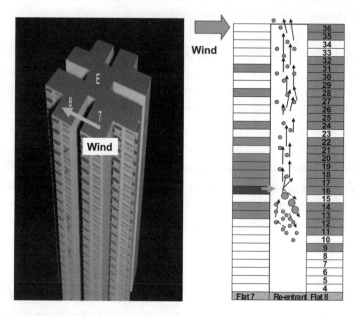

Fig. 7. Predicted buoyant plume in the re-entrant between Flats 7 and 8 in the Amoy Gardens Block E. The predicted concentration decay is only about 4 times when the plume reaches the top of the re-entrant when there is a north-easterly wind velocity of 2 m/s.

However, as the plume develops, it attaches to the end wall due to the negative pressure created by the plume entrainment. We are not aware of any existing study of the attachment of two-dimensional wall plumes. It might be reasonable to apply the two-dimensional jet theory to estimate the vertical distance when the 2D plume attaches to the end wall, which was found to be 13 m for the current study.

Based on our assumptions, the density difference due to air temperature alone between the exhaust air and the ambient air is 2.06% of the reference air density. Using the formulas presented in Etheridge and Sandberg (1996), the airflow rate of the plume, the decay of the virus concentration as well as the air speed in the plume are calculated and presented in Fig. 6(c). There seems to be a correlation between the predicted normalised virus concentration and the number of cases.

The plume centreline velocity does not depend on the plume height. With a density difference of 2% and an initial airflow rate of 0.18 cubic metre per second, the plume velocity is 0.8 metre per second. The plume flow rate grows linearly along the height. This has resulted in a linear decay of the virus particle concentration in the plume as a function of height.

The virus-laden buoyant moist air can find its way into bathrooms or living rooms of upper floors due to negative pressure created by exhaust fans or the action of wind flows around the building. Thus, buoyant moist and warm air plumes in the re-entrant is suggested to be responsible for the rapid virus spread in the Amoy Gardens Flats 7 and 8, Block E. There is still one problem with this hypothesis. How did the virus spread DOWN for flats between the 12th floor (the lowest infected) and 16th floor? There are at least three possibilities. The first possibility is a vent pipe leak on the 4th floor (Department of Health, 2003); the second possibility was the fall of large bio-aerosols from the 16th floor (see Fig. 7), while the third possibility was that someone in the lower floors in Flat 7, such as the 12th floor, used the toilet and turned on the exhaust fan while the index patient flushed his toilet.

Effect of fluctuating wind direction on wind spread from Block E to other Blocks

In Yu *et al.* (2004), we suggested that prevailing northeasterly wind flows were responsible for carrying the uprising plume from the Block E re-entrant

to downstream Blocks B, C and D. For a 45° wind, the wake flow of
the construction site created a negative pressure region in the open space
between Blocks E, C and D [Fig. 8(a)]. This negative pressure region caused
the plume to bend downwards, reaching the middle levels of Blocks C and
D (Yu et al. 2004). The negative pressure region between Blocks C and D
also sucked the plume into the narrow gap between Blocks C and D, causing
a relative high risk for infection for the nearby flats in both Blocks C and D
[Fig. 8(a)]. If we changed the wind direction slightly from 45° to 43°, we
found that the plume spread pattern changed sharply and the Blocks C and
D suction phenomenon disappeared. This wind direction change caused the
plume to reach Block B directly. In Figs. 8(a) and 8(b), we also plotted the
number of total infected persons in each Flat for comparison. We do not
know the exact duration of the infection nor how long the infection took
place. However, what we do know is that the wind direction fluctuated
between 19–20 March at a weather station close to the Amoy Gardens
(Fig. 2). Assuming that the wind direction was perfectly north-easterly as
simulated in Fig. 8(a), then the Block B infections might be much less
than those presented in Fig. 8(b). Our steady-state CFD simulations so far
demonstrated the importance of fluctuating wind direction. As we could not
determine the exact time when the exposure occurred, we could only base
on the statistical information of the wind direction to make a judgement
that the north-easterly wind is the most likely prevailing direction during
the exposure period. Wind fluctuations could introduce more flow mixing
and carry down the virus-laden bio-aerosols from Block E to other blocks,
but at a reduced level. The results presented in Figs. 8 seem to suggest the
need for unsteady-state simulations of wind flows in the Amoy Gardens,
which will be investigated in the near future.

Our CFD simulations also revealed that the virus concentration is 5,000
times diluted when the plumes from Block E reached Blocks B, C and D.
The virus bio-aerosols can enter into the nearby flats by the action of winds
or exhaust fans, i.e. infiltration and natural ventilation flows. There are
a lot of measured data on the correlation between the bio-aerosol levels
indoors and outdoors (Dockery and Spengler, 1981; Chao et al., 2002; Li
and Chen, 2003). The mechanisms of particle penetration and deposition
through the building envelope including windows have also been studied
(Chao et al., 2002). The reduced virus concentration levels in Blocks B, C

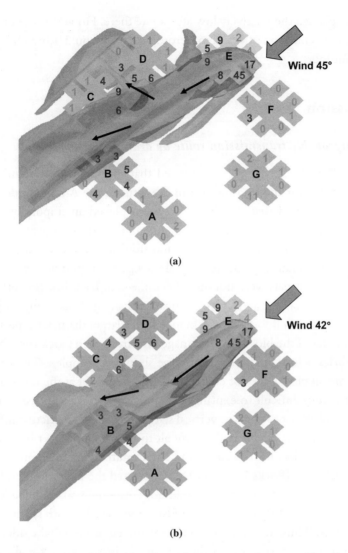

Fig. 8. The buoyant plume rising from the re-entrant between Flats 7 and 8 in Block E was carried downstream by a north-easterly wind, 45° from north for (a) and 42° from north for (b), reaching middle levels of Blocks C and D, where were mostly infected in the two blocks. The letters refer to the building block, and the numbers refer to the number of the infected people in each stack (wing) of flats for a block.

and D explained the relatively low attack rate there. However, it is expected that the concentration of virus bio-aerosols indoors would be much less than those outdoors.

Discussion

The improbable transmission route by drainage system pipes

The HKSAR Government suggested that the 'drainage system' might be responsible for the transmission of the virus in the Amoy Garden. Our findings confirmed that the drainage system played an important role in the Amoy Gardens outbreak, probably not as a transmission route, but as a generator of bio-aerosols from urine and stool of the index patient. After examining the drainage pipe network drawings, we found that the drainage pipes for various flats were not directly connected. Each Flat (tower) has its own drainage stack (pipe). Two vertical stacks (e.g. Flats 7 and 8) joined together at the 4th floor level as a branch into a larger diameter pipe around the perimeter of the block. The drainage pipe from each block runs through three stories below the blocks, in a large shopping complex. The drainage pipes from all blocks are not connected until they meet at the underground level. It is very difficult to explain how the virus was transmitted from one vertical stack of flat to another vertical stack and caused a particular infection pattern in Block E, and it is also difficult to find any engineering evidence to support the idea that the virus can be transmitted through drainage pipes from Block E to Blocks B, C and D, and created the pattern noted for the infected flat distribution. Also, it could not create the vertical infection risk distribution noted for Block E in the Flat 7 and 8 stacks, with sparing of the lower floors. Thus, we could not identify any environmental evidence for the transmission of SARS virus through the drainage system for all cases in the Amoy Garden outbreak.

Although the drainage pipe system was not identified as the transmission route for the entire Amoy Gardens outbreak, the roles played by the vertical drainage stack for Flat 7 in generating and keeping the suspended bio-aerosols in the stack for some time duration should not be under-estimated. As discussed, there were two possible escape routes of the virus-laden bio-aerosols into the bathrooms from the vertical drainage stack. The first escape route was through the index patient's bathroom floor drain on the 16th floor and the second was through the bathrooms on other floors. Thus, the vertical drainage stack for Flat 7 could be considered as a part of the SARS virus transmission route. It is not unexpected that bio-aerosols in a vertical drainage stack contain viruses and bacteria. The relevance to building drainage system and maintenance is that a building drainage system should not allow the foul gas to re-enter the indoor environment in any situation and this appears to be a problem in high-rise buildings such as Amoy Gardens, a very common design in Hong Kong.

Possible roles played by dried-out U-traps of floor drain

The number of bio-aerosols generated in the drainage stack and the number of bio-aerosols entering a flat are still unknown. The number of bio-aerosols generated in the drainage stack could be "huge" as evidenced by flow visualisation (Yu *et al.*, 2004). However, what percentage of these bio-aerosols could enter into a flat were a question of the relative negative pressure and the dryness of floor drains. All Amoy Gardens flats had a floor drain in the bathroom when the buildings were first built. Many of them were potentially dried out as the water seals were evaporated if they were not being used for more than two months. At the same time, when someone used the bathroom, closed the bathroom door and turned on the exhaust fan in the bathroom, negative pressure was established which could drive the bio-aerosols in the drainage stack to enter the bathroom.

We consider the issue of bio-aerosols generation and transport in the drainage system as a complex network flow problem. Both waste water flows and associated airflows in the drainage pipes are coupled. Drainage systems or traps (water seals) were one of the most important "old inventions" in buildings to keep the indoor environments hygienic. If our hypothesis is right, the incident of the Amoy Gardens outbreak shows the need for continuously improving hygienic design in modern buildings. Specifically, we need to design U-traps that always remain water sealed.

The size distribution of bio-aerosols generated in the drainage stack is also important. We noted in our simulations that the evaporation of bio-aerosols were rapid as bio-aerosols moved up in the re-entrant. In less than a few seconds, the bio-aerosols less than 100 μm in diameter became droplet nuclei. The droplet nuclei moved further up in the re-entrant to a height of more than 50 m (the total height of the block was 90 m, and our index patient's bathroom was on the 16th floor) and then carried away downstream for a further 60 m before arriving at the opposite blocks. There is a need for studying the bio-aerosol generation process in the vertical stack, as well as the "escaping" process of the bio-aerosols in the drainage system for preventing future outbreaks of infectious diseases.

Implications of the airborne transmission in the Amoy Gardens outbreak to hospital infection control

Most of the existing studies on SARS transmission suggested that SARS was mainly spread by large respiratory droplets (WHO, 2003b). The Amoy Gardens outbreak seems to be a unique one as its drainage system provided a bio-aerosol virus source from the urine and stool of the index patient, which allowed a large number of virus-laden bio-aerosols to be emitted into the environment. From the bio-aerosol flow and dispersion theory, it is known that as one moved away from the source, the bio-aerosol concentration decays. In this outbreak, we found 5,000 times dilution when it reaches the middle levels of Blocks B, C and D. Lower bio-aerosol concentrations correspond to lower attack rates. The airborne transmission and the mass infection in the Amoy Gardens outbreak could well be an isolated case. The present study may not establish the airborne transmission as a common transmission route for SARS virus, but the results justified the need for airborne precaution in hospitals for SARS virus.

Our CFD simulations in Fig. 8 well demonstrated that plumes from Flats 7 and 8 were carried downstream by the wind flows to reach the infected flats in Blocks B, C and D. There is a good correlation between the plume path and the spatial pattern of the infected flats. The wind flows are highly unsteady and are affected by the local terrain and surrounding buildings, large or small. An unsteady-state simulation of the airflows around the Amoy Gardens, taking into account the effects of the main upstream buildings, is needed. Ideally, the global wind flow pattern around the building blocks under the effect of the surrounding building developments and topographic features should also be taken into consideration. This could be studied with a small-scale wind tunnel model.

The possible faeco-respiratory airborne route for the Amoy Gardens outbreak

Various routes are possible for the airborne diseases such as the respiratory route in which the respiratory secretions are expelled into the air environment and inhaled by the susceptible persons. SARS virus infection in the Amoy Gardens seems to be of an unusual, perhaps even novel, faeco-respiratory airborne route. It is difficult to rule out the possibility of surface contamination by aerosols and subsequent mucous membrane infection, rather than necessarily respiratory inhalation. However, it is also difficult to imagine that residents in more than 142 flats for the first 187 cases were infected through surface contamination simultaneously. Faeco-aerosols as household toilet hazards were reported 30 years ago by Gerba et al. (1975); however, there are no studies on faeco-aerosols spread through the dried-out floor drains. In the Amoy Gardens outbreak, the hydraulic process in the vertical stack of the sanitary drainage system of Block E generated a large number of virus-laden faeco-aerosols, which were leaked back into the indoor environment of at least one flat through dried-out drains. The movement of faeco-aerosols in the sanitary drainage pipes has not been studied in detail, and questions to be answered include how long the aerosols would stay in the vertical stack, the sizes and concentration of aerosols, and effects of transient water flows on the movement of aerosols. The information we presented here clearly suggested that the leaked bio-aerosols were further spread by plumes and wind air flows through the large housing estate.

The faeco-respiratory airborne route in the Amoy Gardens outbreak involved a complex sequence of transmission components. For prevention purposes, the most effective engineering method is to control the source production of faeco-aerosols, which can be achieved by improving the sanitary drainage design and maintenance standards to avoid any potential leak of foul gas into the indoor environment. In buildings, effective and efficient ventilation should be provided. Airflow pattern in an apartment or in a building should also be controlled. Pollutants or infectious bio-aerosols should be controlled to prevent entry to occupied regions. Hygiene promotion in sanitary drainage systems is already known for preventing diarrhoeal diseases and other infectious diseases transmitted by the faeco-oral route. The probable faeco-respiratory route in the Amoy Gardens outbreak suggested the need of good practice in both sanitary facilities and building ventilation.

Acknowledgement

The work described in this paper was supported by a grant from the Research Grants Council of the Hong Kong Special Administrative Region, China (Project No. HKU 7020/02E). The first author also wishes to thank the Project Amoy team at the University of Hong Kong, Faculty of Engineering for many inspiring discussions about the Amoy Gardens outbreak. We also thank Adrian C. Sleigh, National Centre for Epidemiology and Population Health, Australian National University, Canberra, Australia for first suggesting the concept of faeco-respiratory airborne route.

References

Airpak (Computer Software). Fluent Inc., Lebanon, New Hampshire, USA. Available at http://www.fluent.com.

Chao CYH, Wong KK. (2002) Residential indoor PM10 and PM2.5 in Hong Kong and the elemental composition. *Atmos Environ* **36**: 265–277.

Department of Health, HKSAR. (2003) Outbreak of Severe Acute Respiratory Syndrome (SARS) at Amoy Gardens, Kowloon Bay, Hong Kong — Main Findings of Investigation, 17 Apr 2003. Available at http://www.info.gov.hk/info/ap/pdf/amoy_e.pdf, Accessed 25 October 2003.

Dockery DW, Spengler JD. (1981) Indoor–outdoor relationships of respirable sulfates and particles. *Atmos Environ* **15**: 335–343.

Etheridge D, Sandberg M. (1996) *Building Ventilation — Theory and Measurement*. John Wiley & Sons, Chichester.

Ferziger JH, Peric M. (2002) *Computational Methods for Fluid Dynamics*. Springer, Berlin.

Fisher HB, List JE, Koh RCY, Imberger I, Brooks NH. (1979) *Mixing in Inland and Coastal Waters*. Academic Press, New York.

Fluent (Computer Software). Fluent Inc., Lebanon, New Hampshire, USA. Available at http://www.fluent.com.

Gerba CP, Wallis C, Melnick JL. (1975) Microbiological hazards of household toilets: Droplet production and the fate of residual organisms. *Appl Microbiol* **30**(2): 229–237.

Jenks M, Burgess R. (2000) *Compact Cities: Sustainable Urban Forms for Developing Countries*. Spon Press, London.

Karakiewicz J. (2002) *Exploring the Dimensions of Urban Densities*. PhD Thesis, Department of Architecture, the University of Hong Kong.

Klote JH, Milke JA. (2002) *Principles of Smoke Management*. ASHRAE.

Li Y, Chen ZD. (2003) A balance-point method for assessing the effect of natural ventilation on indoor particle concentrations. *Atmos Environ* **37**: 4277–4285.

Li Y, Yu ITS, Xu P, Lee JHW, Wong TW, Ooi PP, Sleigh A. (2004) Predicting super spreading events during the 2003 SARS epidemics in Hong Kong and Singapore. *Am J Epidemiol* **160**: 719–728.

Li Y, Duan S, Yu ITS, Wong TW. (2005) Multi-zone modeling of probable SARS virus transmission by airflow between flats in block E, Amoy Gardens. *Indoor Air* **15**: 96–111.

Ng SKC. (2003) Possible Role of an Animal Vector in the SARS Outbreak at Amoy Gardens. *Lancet* **362**: 570–572.

Riley S, Fraser C, Donnelly CA, Ghani AC, Abu–Raddad LJ, Hedley AJ *et al.* (2003) Transmission dynamics of the etiological agent of severe acute respiratory syndrome (SARS) in Hong Kong: The impact of public health interventions. *Science* **300**: 1961–1966.

Swaffield JA, Campbell DP. (1995) The simulation of air pressure propagation in building drainage and vent systems. *Building Environ* **30**: 115–127.

Tsang T. (2003) SARS-Environmental Issues. Presentation in WHO Global Conference on Severe Acute Respiratory Syndrome (SARS), 17–18 June 2003, Kuala Lumpur, Malaysia. Available at http://www.who.int/csr/sars/conference/june_2003/en/, Accessed 1 May 2005.

WHO (2003a) Final Report — Metripole Hotel by the WHO Environmental Investigation. Available at http://www.iapmo.com/common/pdf/ISS-Rome/SARS_Metropole_Hotel_HK.pdf, Accessed on 20 May 2004.

WHO (2003b) Consensus Document on the Epidemiology of Severe Acute Respiratory Syndrome (SARS). Available at http://www.who.int/csr/sars/en/WHOconsensus.pdf, Accessed 12 February 2004.

WHO (2003c) Environmental Health Team Reports on Amoy Gardens. Available at http://www.info.gov.hk/info/ap/who-amoye.pdf, Accessed 25 October 2003.

Yu ITS, Li YG, Wong TW, Tam W, Chan A, Lee JHW, Leung DYC, Ho T. (2004) Evidence of airborne transmission of the severe acute respiratory syndrome virus. *New Eng J Med* **350**: 1731–1739.

17

Discourse of "Othering" During the SARS Outbreak in Taiwan: A News Analysis

Mei-Ling Hsu and Ching-I Liu

SARS Outbreak in Taiwan

The emerging epidemic known as Severe Acute Respiratory Syndrome (SARS) took many regions and countries such as China, Hong Kong, Vietnam, Singapore, Canada, the U.S., and Taiwan by storm in the spring of 2003. The World Health Organization (WHO) issued a global alert on the outbreak of SARS on 12 March 2003 (Koh, Plant and Lee, 2003), but the outbreak in Taiwan occurred at a relatively late phase of the global SARS epidemic. The first suspected case was diagnosed on 14 March when a Taiwanese businessman who had been infected with SARS in Guangdong, China, returned to Taiwan. By mid April, there had been sporadic cases of SARS in persons coming back from China, but the health authorities stated that Taiwan still maintained a spotless record of "three zeros": zero deaths, zero community transmissions, and zero cases of Taiwanese taking the disease abroad. As such, WHO classified Taiwan as an "area with limited local transmission" (Chen *et al.*, 2003). The health authorities remained in a state of blissful optimism, even though such optimism did not last long.

A large-scale outbreak of SARS infection soon occurred in Taipei and then spread throughout Taiwan. On 24 April, a local hospital in

Taipei was contained and all patients, visitors and staff were quarantined within the building. SARS later extended to multiple cities and regions of Taiwan. It was not until 5 July 2003 that Taiwan was removed from the WHO list of SARS-affected countries.Taiwan was also the last country to be taken off the WHO list (Center for Disease Control, Taiwan, 2003).

According to the official statistics, there were 664 probable cases of SARS by September 2003 in Taiwan. The Taiwanese Center for Disease Control re-analysed the 356 probable SARS cases that were positive when tested with the antibody [SARS CoV(+)]. Among them, 20.5% ($n = 73$) were deceased with 10.4% ($n = 37$) directly due to SARS and 10.1% ($n = 36$) indirectly related. Further epidemiological investigation indicated that as high as 40.4% ($n = 144$) were hospitalised patients, 29.5% ($n = 105$) were health workers, 11.8% ($n = 42$) were infected by family members, and 6.2% ($n = 22$) were imported cases (Center for Disease Control, Taiwan, 2004).

Before the epidemic grew rapidly in mid April, the local health authorities had initiated efforts to control SARS, including the isolation of suspected and probable case-patients, the use of personal protective equipment for healthcare workers and visitors, and the quarantine of contacts of known SARS patients. Beginning in mid April, more widespread quarantine measures were used (Lee et al., 2003a). By the end of the epidemic, more than 150,000 persons had been in contact with probable case-patients or returned from an affected area. All of them required quarantine, either in negative-pressure rooms or at home (Chen et al., 2004). While these procedures were considered necessary public health measures to handle this type of emerging infectious disease, news reports and portrayals of how SARS-related people were traced and treated have posed an intriguing question of concern.

Although this was not the first time that Taiwan was struck by an epidemic, the impact that SARS brought to the society appeared to be tremendous. Aided by globalisation and the ease of modern air travel, this emerging infectious disease spread throughout the nation at a speed faster than anyone could imagine. Public panic triggered by the mass media, amplified the human fear of the disease and infected people. This became particularly salient when a kind of social reality was constructed in the media discourse to dichotomise people into "healthy" versus "unhealthy" and "safe" versus "dangerous."

Media Effects on Public Perception

Mass media uses a mode of address which constructs receivers of the messages as a unified "general public" with shared values and characteristics (Watney, 1987). They are also important sources of health information for both private individuals (Freimuth *et al.*, 1984; Simpkins and Brenner, 1984; Wallack, 1990) and policy-makers (Weiss, 1974). Deviant or marginal groups are sometimes made to stand outside the general public, inevitably assuming the appearance of a threat to its internal cohesion. News media in particular tend to shape an ideal audience of a national mainstream group, surrounded by threatening "others." For a society such as Taiwan where the mass media have been a major conduit through which public perceptions of emerging infectious diseases are formed, the negative impact of the SARS outbreak seemed to be unduly amplified (Lin and Chen, 2003; Lu, 2004; Liu, 2004).

The news media continued to be the major source for the public to obtain SARS information, but a surprisingly large proportion of the Taiwanese were in fact critical of the role that the media had played during the peak period of the outbreak. According to a national telephone survey conducted on 2 May 2003 by the Taiwanese Broadcasting Developing Fund, nearly 40% of the 1,093 adults surveyed were dissatisfied with the news, as high as 65% of them considered SARS coverage too sensational, 29% thought it was too negative, 17% did not think the news media had provided necessary information, and 16% mentioned there were too many inaccurate reports in the news (Lin, 2003). Similarly, in a comparative study of public opinion on SARS between Taiwan and Hong Kong conducted in late May by Academia Sinica, the most prestigious research institute in Taiwan, of the 1,730 Taiwanese respondents, as high as 44.4% attributed the seriousness of the infectious disease to the sensationalism of the news, while only 18.6% of the 1,018 respondents in Hong Kong said likewise (Chu *et al.*, 2003).

Such strong criticisms from the public resulted in many letters to news editors, calling for more efforts to improve the medical and social condition of people in the lower social strata (Yang, 2003). Discontent over media performance even triggered various groups and individuals, such as medical workers and SARS patients (with some quarantined in the hospitals), schol- ars and local non-profit organisations to disseminate SARS information on their own or to monitor SARS-related news reports by way of e-mails and websites (Lu, 2004). There seemed to be a consensus among the public that SARS-related news reports had not done much other than labelled infected persons and frightened other people.

These public reactions were also supported by various news analyses on SARS in Taiwan. For example, the Foundation for the Advancement of Media Excellence (FAME), a local non-profit media-watch organisation, conducted a content analysis of SARS coverage in seven Taiwanese news-papers from March to May 2003. The study found that three types of poor news performance could be identified: false reports, sensational and exag-gerated news, and violation of SARS patients' human rights (Lu, 2004). Other studies found that political forces, rather than medical and scientific ones, dominated in framing the news discourse on SARS (Yang, 2003) and that marginal social groups such as the homeless, working class (e.g. Liu, 2004), and foreign labourers (e.g. Lin and Chen, 2003) were stigmatised in the local news.

Instead of asking whether the epidemic was handled well or poorly in the nation, the current study will examine how various groups had been stigmatised as the others in the SARS public discourse in Taiwan's soci-ety. Specifically, we will use news as a site to observe the power struggle and dynamics of positioning within it. Social, cultural, and political forces that had been involved in the othering processes will also be discussed. As previous research findings have documented that various deviant groups have been constructed in the discourse on the AIDS epidemic throughout the world (Bardhan, 1996), including Taiwan (Hsu *et al.*, 2004), the study will compare the othering process between the discourse on SARS and the discourse on HIV/AIDS.

Conceptual Framework: Othering and Stigma

The social construction of disease-related groups or individuals, or the othering process discussed above, is closely tied to the human psychology of stigma formation. The term "stigma" originally referred to a sign or mark, cut or burned into the body, that designated the bearer as a person who was morally defective and was to be avoided (Goffman, 1963). In modern society, a stigma can be seen as an identity that is socially constructed (Archer, 1985). It can also be perceived as a type of social identity that is devalued in a particular context (Crocker *et al.*, 1998).

According to Goffman (1963), stigmatising conditions can be categorised into the following three types:

1. Tribal stigmas, which are passed from generation to generation, and include membership in devalued racial, ethnic, or religious groups;
2. Abominations of the body, which are not inherited physical characteristics that convey a devalued social identity such as being physically disadvantaged; and
3. Blemishes of individual character, which are devalued social identities related to one's personality or behaviour.

It should be noted that some stigmatising conditions might fit into two or more types. In relation to infectious diseases, the stigmatisation of the associated risk groups is due to the fear that the social barriers for protection will be breached, leaving the general population open to the infections (Albert, 1986). Thus, maintenance of a social distance is crucial, which results in blaming an individual as being responsible for his own disability. Taking HIV/AIDS for example, it has shown that news reports often carry accusations that gay men are justifiable objects of the righteous punishment of God for sinful behaviour (see Hsu *et al.*, 2004).

Link and Phelan (2001) went further to define stigma as the co–occurrence of its components — labelling, stereotyping, separation, status loss, and discrimination. They further indicated that for stigmatisation to occur, power must be exercised. The convergence of the interrelated components occurs as follows:

1. On distinguishing and labelling human differences: Why is it that some human differences are singled out and deemed salient, while others are ignored? What are the social, economic, and cultural forces that maintain the focus on a particular human difference?
2. On associating human differences with negative attributes: Dominant cultural beliefs link labelled persons to undesirable characteristics, i.e. negative stereotypes.

3. On separating the us from them: Labelled persons are placed in distinct categories so as to accomplish some degree of separation of us from them.
4. Status loss and discrimination: Labelled persons are set apart and linked to undesirable characteristics that lead them to experience discrimination and loss of status.
5. Dependence of stigma on power: Stigmatisation is entirely contingent on access to social, economic, and political power that allows the identification of differences, the construction of stereotypes, the separation of labelled persons into distinct categories, and the full execution of disapproval, rejection, exclusion and discrimination.

Link and Phelan's conceptualisation of stigma has a dramatic bearing on the distribution of many of life chances, such as earnings, housing, criminal involvement, and of course, health and life itself. It should also be noted that stigma associated with certain social groups is not fixed. The stigmatising process is dynamic, depending on how the groups or individuals are positioned or repositioned by the social, cultural, or political forces at a particular time (Davies and Harré, 1990).

This study intends to observe how the stigmatising conditions dominated in the news discourse of SARS. The language mechanisms used in the discourse to facilitate such othering processes will also be discussed.

Method: A Qualitative Textual Analysis of News

The news texts for the SARS discourse analysis were examined from the first reported local case on 1 March to 5 July 2003, the date when Taiwan was removed from the SARS list of the WHO. A specific sample was selected based on the key events or issues within the above time frame. By using "SARS" as a keyword, we first conducted a news text search on two major on-line database systems: one from the United Daily News and the other from China Times. Specifically, we selected three mainstream newspapers for this purpose, *China Times*, *United Daily News*, and *Min Seng Daily*. The first two papers have the largest circulation, whereas the third is the only paper in Taiwan that has a full-page health section targeted at medical care workers.

We then narrowed down the number of articles by focusing on those that deal with specific individuals or groups related to the disease. After collecting the relevant news articles, we looked into the texts to identify the patterns and changes in the discourse in relation to our research questions. As the major purpose of our study is to decode the meanings underlying the news texts, instead of analysing all the articles in detail, we will focus on certain selected texts that can help illustrate and interpret the major findings. Furthermore, as the study aims to examine the patterns and changes of the discourse in the mainstream news media as a whole, we will not compare the differences in news reporting among the three newspapers.

Othering Processes in the News on SARS

Our database news search generated 536 articles that may be considered as discourse on othering in SARS. They include 74 articles on probable-case patients, 163 on those quarantined, 148 on healthcare workers, and 151 on the homeless and blue-collar workers (both local and foreign). In the following section, we analyse this discourse in the news texts by these categories.

Probable-case patients and the quarantined as emerging others

Imagining the scary other

Before the name SARS was given to the disease by WHO, this emerging infectious disease was labelled by various mysterious or horrifying terms such as "unknown pneumonia," "scary pneumonia," "bizarre, fierce disease," "bizarre disease of the 21st century," "mysterious fatal disease," and so forth (*Min Seng Daily*, 16 March 2003; *Min Seng Daily*, 22 March 2003). The English name SARS was used directly in Taiwan's official and popular discourses, signifying the alien nature of the disease. A clear line was thus drawn between the "foreign other" and the "local us." People associated with SARS were distinguished as "public enemy" (*China Times*, 18 May 2003), "flood"(*United Daily News*, 8 May 2003), "beasts" (*United Daily News*, 8 May 2003), "rats" (*United Daily News*, 11 April 2003), "land mine" (*United Daily News*, 17 May 2003), "gods of the plague" (*Min Seng Daily*,

27 March 2003), and so on. Due to the disease's foreign connection, words with fear-loaded appeal such as "virus airplane," "dangerous airplane," and "you are flying with patients of scary pneumonia" (e.g. *Min Seng Daily*, 21 March 2003) were used quite often in news headlines during the initial stage of the outbreak. Rumors and descriptions of unconfirmed suspected cases were also common in the stories. The following report is typical of such panic-arousing news writing at the time:

> ...A woman who had doubts about whether or not she was infected with SARS went to see the doctor at the Hospital of the National Taiwan University Medical School. Many electronic media reporters were waiting outside the hospital. Knowing that a SARS suspect-case patient was around, some patients tried to leave the hospital immediately.... (*Min Seng Daily*, 20 March 2003).

News coverage such as the above increased when the Taipei Municipal Hoping Hospital was hurriedly sealed off on 25 April, followed by the closing of other hospitals around Taiwan. As most of the SARS cases resulted from hospital transmission, tracing infected cases was placed as top priority in news coverage. Therefore, Hoping Hospital and other affected hospitals were labelled as "fatal castles" (e.g. *United Daily News*, 16 May 2003), and Ms. Tsao, the person said to have started the chain of transmissions[1] in the hospitals, was described as a "super spreader." Headlines such as "where does she live" (*China Times*, 25 March 2003) and "the fall of Hoping Hospital, epidemic out of control" (*China Times*, 24 March 2003) were highlighted. Instead of discussing what caused the disease, SARS patients were described as having to take responsibility for the outbreak.

The fears over probable-case SARS patients and the quarantine fermented became a violation of the human rights of these people. There were

---

[1] Early in April 2003, a woman from Taipei named Tsao became infected by SARS, probably as a result of being in the same rail car as an infected individual from the Amoy Gardens housing project in Hong Kong (where dozens of people had come down with the disease). Ms. Tsao went to Hoping Hospital to see a doctor, and although the hospital was on the lookout for possible cases and immediately transferred her to a better equipped teaching hospital, in the brief time that she had spent in Hoping — less than one hour — her presence set off a chain reaction with explosive results. Starting on 15 April, virtually every day there were new cases of medical staff and patients at Hoping showing high fever, and with the hospital failing to take timely measures to more strictly isolate affected persons, the virus spread quickly and could not be contained (Lee, 2003).

reports mentioning the public's panic if the aforementioned Ms. Tsao happened to be in their neighbourhood (*China Times*, 25 April 2003). Ms. Tsao and her family were afraid of returning home from the hospital because they would be discriminated by their neighbours (*China Times*, 3 May 2003). Similar descriptions were also found in public attitudes toward the quarantined people and their families (*United Daily News*, 3 May 2003; *Min Seng Daily*, 21 June 2003). Businessmen working in China were asked by their families not to return home to Taiwan (*United Daily News*, 7 May 2003). School children in quarantined families were either told not to attend classes or were isolated in the classroom corners (*United Daily News*, 2 April 2003). A "time bomb" metaphor was used to describe the SARS-related people.

The foreign connection of SARS in the news discourse seemed to work in two ways. Firstly, it functioned to maintain a psychological distance between the safe local Taiwanese and the dangerous others; in this case, people from or those who had travelled to China or Hong Kong. By labelling SARS as a foreign or imported product, the locals were reassured of their immunity to the disease. Secondly, the foreign connection of SARS justified who was to blame for the spread of the disease. Although such a stigmatising process was not contingent on people's access to social and economic power, as indicated by Link and Phelan (2001), it unfortunately occurred in the context of long-term political confrontation between Taiwan and the People's Republic of China.

Such a stigmatising process during SARS was observed during the early years of the AIDS epidemic in Taiwan. When the first AIDS case was found in December 1984, the patient's identity as "an American physician visiting Taiwan" was emphasised (*Min Seng Daily, United Daily News, China Times*, 8 March 1985). Even when the first local AIDS case was reported, the press still stressed the foreign connection by stating that the patient had lived abroad for a long time and that half of his sex partners were foreigners. Therefore, he may have contracted AIDS from those foreigners (*United Daily News, China Times, Min Seng Daily*, 30 August 1985). A metaphor of the decadent West was salient in the news discourse. Like the aforementioned government's careless statement that Taiwan still maintained a spotless record of three zeros of SARS, health officials and local medical sources had in the mid 1980s reassured the general public that "Taiwan was not a high-risk area for AIDS" (*Min Seng Daily*, 13 March 1985).

Constructing the criminal other

SARS-related people were sometimes represented not only as being horrifying, but also as criminals endangering public safety. Nevertheless, the criminalising process was not static, and it depended greatly on how agents in the popular discourse participated and interpreted the labelling of the criminal other, as mentioned previously (Davies and Harré, 1990). The news media obviously were the dominant agents in the discourse.

To begin with, the SARS epidemic in Taiwan was never a simple public health issue. Much of the controversy centred upon the power struggle between the ruling central government and the opposition-led Taipei City Government. The controversy was magnified by the aforementioned chain of transmission beginning at Hoping Hospital in which both governments blamed each other (Hsu, 2004a). In addition, the connection between SARS and China was often highlighted in the official discourse. Taiwan's President Chen Shui-bian commented that "China not only concealed the fact of its SARS epidemic, but is also on record for concealing the spread of foot-and-mouth disease" (*China Times*, 7 May 2003). Taiwan's Vice President Annette Lu[2] even described SARS as an Armageddon originating from human greed, for "there were people (i.e. Taiwanese businessmen) who were not easily satisfied with what they had in Taiwan, and thus went to China to earn more money" (*United Daily News*, 8 April 2003). While the remarks of these two top political figures were tolerated in the popular discourse, the following instance exemplified the dynamic nature of the stigmatising process. In one SARS-prevention advertisement,[3] the Department of Health decided to use the Chinese-espionage metaphor, but this immediately raised strong criticisms from the public, opposition legislators, and of course the news media (*Min Seng Daily*, *United Daily News*, *China Times*, 1 April 2003). The advertisement was soon replaced. This shows that there is still a threshold as to how far the labelling of the criminal other could go in the discourse.

---

[2] In fact, Annette Lu tends to be a controversial public speaker. When she was a special guest to endorse the occasion of the 2003 *World AIDS Day Fair*, she had commented that AIDS was a punishment from heaven, and her discriminatory remarks have also generated much coverage and heated discussions in the media (Hsu, 2004b).

[3] The advertisement slogan reads, "Both SARS and spies come from China, but the number of SARS patients is much less than that of the Chinese spies in Taiwan."

Stigmatising Chinese as the criminal other did not seem to be well received, but treating SARS probable-case and quarantined people as crime suspects within the island of Taiwan was predominant in the news discourse (*China Times*, 3 May 2003; *United Daily News*, 7 May 2003). These people, rather than the coronavirus that causes SARS, were described as "lethal murderers" (*Min Seng Daily*, 20 March 2003). *China Times* (2 May 2003) even ran a huge front-page headline, "I apologize to society" for the interview conducted with Ms. Tsao, the patient said to cause the chain of transmission in hospitals. The story was full of self-blaming expressions, such as "I feel so ashamed" and "it's all my fault." This seems like a typical open trial ritual in which a confession of a committed crime or repentance for sins (Foucault, 1979) plays an important part in justifying its reporting.

Similar examples were found for the other SARS probable-case patients in the chain of transmission (*United Daily News*, 15 May 2003; *China Times*, 21 May 2003). The news media even legitimised their own voyeurism of spying over those who were quarantined (*United Daily News*, 26 April 2003), as can be seen in the following article:

> At 7:00 am, two elderly were unmasked, taking walks at their doorway. At 8:30 am, a teacher surnamed Wang was also unmasked, driving away from home... Two reporters from our newspaper thus followed her by riding motorcycles...A nephew of a quarantined woman walked to a restaurant 200 meters from home, unmasked...At 12:20 pm, he wore a mask to ride his motorcycle, but took it off upon entering a convenience store. He wore it again after leaving the store... (*United Daily News*, 3 April 2003).

By serving as an "observer" of the quarantined people in their neighbourhood, the reporter linked the "unmasked" behaviour of these people to something that may jeopardise social security and public health. Unfortunately, such tabloid reporting style was used by the mainstream media to attract readership or increase ratings at that time.

In addition to criticisms from the public and certain legislators, the journalistic standard of balanced reporting by quoting from different sources served as a crucial agent to alter the criminalising process. For example, some SARS reports provided narratives from the probable-case patients or the quarantined people who described themselves as "being in a prison" (*Min Seng Daily*, 27 April 2003) or even "being worse than prisoners" (*United Daily News*, 7 May 2003). Discourse like these thus brought in an empathetic and positive tone for the "imprisoned" quarantined people. This may reduce public discrimination against the probable-case patients and the quarantined to some extent. In other words, the news media had a dual purpose in representing SARS-related groups or individuals.

The foregoing criminalising process as observed in the SARS news discourse, again seemed to resemble the HIV/AIDS discourse in Taiwan in the early 1990s. As in many cultures, AIDS was introduced to Taiwan as a foreign or an imported product in the early 1980s. Occasionally, stories translated from the Western news agencies regarding the exotic nature of the disease could be found in the local press (Hsu *et al.*, 2004). Beginning in the early 1990s, Taiwanese health authorities had considered foreign labourers and sex workers to be of the highest risk in passing the AIDS virus to the "innocent" locals (*United Daily News*, 27 October 1991). The foreign connection to AIDS thus switched from blaming the Westerners to blaming South Asians and Southeast Asians, sometimes including mainland Chinese. Asian countries, particularly Thailand, were seen as the origin of the modern plague, as well as its victims (Hsu *et al.*, 2004). A recurring news pattern about foreign workers who were HIV positive could be found. They purportedly came from the geographical areas where AIDS was rampant and the Taiwanese government would soon repatriate them home (*United Daily News*, 10 July 1991; *China Times, Min Seng Daily, United Daily News*, 16 October 1991). The time bomb metaphor was also found in the AIDS discourse to describe people hiring illegal foreign workers, because such an act could be "dangerous" (*China Times, Min Seng Daily, United Daily News*, 16 October 1991). In other words, foreign workers and sex workers were stigmatised not only as being scary, but as criminals endangering the local public in the HIV/AIDS discourse. Criminal labelling of foreign workers and sex workers related to HIV/AIDS had even appeared much harder to change than that associated with SARS.

Selfish other

Goffman (1963) identified a type of stigma as blemishes of individual character, i.e. certain groups or individuals are not stigmatised because of their social status or identities, but mainly due to their personalities or behaviours. For example, when homosexuality was still perceived to be correctable in Taiwan in the mid 1980s, warnings from health and expert sources about the danger of man-to-man sex, accompanied by confessions from regretful gay patients, were typical ideological apparatuses used in the news discourse (*Min Seng Daily, China Times*, 28 February 1986). Gay men were also portrayed as leading an "abnormal" or "irresponsible" sex life (*Min Seng Daily*, 24, 25 July 1987), and this portrayal was justified by an increasing death toll of HIV/AIDS.

Compared with the process of marginalising gay men in the HIV/AIDS discourse described above, individuals being stigmatised as possessing blemishes of individual character in the SARS news discourse, were mostly SARS-related people from the educated elitist groups. These people were blamed for their selfish misconduct, because they were expected to behave better than ordinary people. The following two instances best illustrate this point.

In the first instance, a student from Chien-Kuo Senior High School, the most prestigious boys' high school in Taiwan, was quarantined at home due to his mother's hospitalisation as a SARS probable-case patient. Nevertheless, he did not follow the quarantine orders and still went for his tutorial lessons at a big private institution, or what was termed as "cram school" in downtown Taipei. This caused the entire cram school student body to be placed under compulsory home quarantine. The student was then described as "selfish," "hurting the innocent," and "losing a moral conscience" in the news discourse (*United Daily News*, 4 May 2003; *China Times*, 5 May 2003). Those descriptions were mostly related to his personality or behaviour rather than to his membership in a devalued racial, ethnic, or religious group.

Another instance has to do with a researcher affiliated with Academia Sinica, the most prominent academic institute in Taiwan, as mentioned earlier in the study. This highly educated researcher was subjected to home quarantine for 10 days due to his immediate past travel in Hong Kong. Ignoring the quarantine measures, he went to his office and then flew to

Australia and the U.S. Once this case was known to the public, he was condemned as "an intellectual without moral conscience," "an educated person endangering the society and the public," "a loner," "a person with a weird personality," "destroying social order," and so on (*United Daily News, China Times*, 22 May 2003). The following story exemplifies how the researcher's image as a selfish other was created in the news discourse:

> [He] entered Academia Sinica by breaking in... He is used to going abroad without notifying his institute. He often has conflicts with his colleagues. He even wrote a paper about the negative aspects of his institute and published it abroad. Because of what he did (i.e. disobeying the quarantine orders), many of his colleagues need to be separated by home quarantine now. His behaviour has damaged the public trust for intellectuals...(*China Times*, 22 May 2003).

Criticisms of the quarantined people such as the above, which was represented in the news media, tended to focus on the lack of responsibility as intellectuals who are expected by society to be more discreet and responsible in the eyes of the general society.

Re-positioned others: Healthcare workers

The power struggle and the dynamics of positioning within it can be best observed in the othering process of the healthcare workers (HCWs) during the SARS epidemic, particularly in the news discourse dealing with the notorious instance of the shutdown of Hoping Hospital.

As mentioned before, SARS cases in Taiwan had been associated primarily with healthcare settings. Therefore, HCWs had been represented as a specific high-risk group for contracting and spreading the virus. The initial cluster of SARS cases related to HCWs at the Hoping Hospital included two nurses, a doctor, an administrator, a radiology technician, a nursing student, and another laundry worker. On the basis of epidemiologic links among the cases, 61 HCWs were identified and quarantined. By 23 April, widespread SARS transmission within the hospital was recognised, which resulted in the containment of the hospital on 24 April. Medical staff, patients and visitors were all put under quarantine (Lee *et al.*, 2003b).

The shutdown of Hoping Hospital apparently shocked many of the unprepared hospital staff. Police began maintaining security around the hospital to ensure no one enters or leaves illegally. As shown on live television newscasts, several hospital staff supposedly under quarantine tried to escape. Some staff members held banners saying it was unfair for them to be kept with SARS patients. An unidentified female hospital employee yelled, "We are normal. Why should we be quarantined? Why should we take care of SARS patients?" (*Min Seng Daily*, 26 April 2003). The staff also issued a written statement saying that because SARS patients were being kept there, everyone was at risk of eventually contracting the disease.

Scenes of the loudly protesting HCWs were even broadcasted on TV in many other countries. Both the Cabinet and the Taipei City Government claimed that they would punish those medical personnel and institutions that did not follow the quarantine orders. Taipei Mayor Ma Ying-jeou then urged medical staff at the Hoping Hospital to abide by those orders. "Fighting SARS is like fighting a real war," Ma said. "If there is any opposition, it will be regarded as defiance on the front line" (*United Daily News*, 25 April 2003). The Taipei City Government ordered police to arrest two medical staff members of Hoping Hospital who were still evading the compulsory quarantine for all the hospital's staff. HCWs suddenly became public enemies due to their irresponsible and selfish behaviours. Goffman's stigma categorisation of blemishes of individual character can be identified here.

Nevertheless, HCWs knew how to re-position themselves in response to the othering process initiated by the health authorities and the media. Some HCWs wrote letters to news media editors, demanding that the government redefine HCWs' roles. They argued that they too were victims of SARS (*China Times*, 28 April 2003). Disappointed and angry at the news coverage of the chain of SARS transmission at Hoping Hospital, some HCWs even wrote e-mails about the "truth" at Hoping, asking e-mail recipients to forward the content to as many people as possible. On 1 May, a head nurse surnamed Chen died from SARS. By paying tribute to Chen, Taipei Mayor Ma said, "She died a brave fighter in the battle against SARS. I hope her efforts will lead us to the final victory against the epidemic" (*Min Seng Daily*, 2 May 2003).

Mayor Ma's praises were meant to tone down the furor heated up over the labelling of HCWs. Indeed, positive commentaries and stories on HCWs in relation to the SARS outbreak started to surface in the news discourse, but HCWs were mostly encouraged to follow Nurse Chen's dedication in fighting against SARS (*United Daily News*, 2–4 May 2003). As expected, the framing of the heroic social identity on them was not well taken by HCWs, who claimed that they were only ordinary people with emotions and fears (*United Daily News*, 10 May 2003). In response to them being positioned as heroes or heroines, HCWs started to resign *en masse* (*China Times*, 19 May 2003). The Cabinet decided to use the "stick and carrot" tactic by giving a tougher line on those who quit, but providing rewards for HCWs who stayed on to care for the SARS patients (*China Times*, 20 May 2003). By constantly voicing out the inhuman demands imposed upon them, HCWs were finally represented in the news as regaining the understanding and empathy from the general public. The health authorities, instead of HCWs, then became the target to be criticised for using military and heroic metaphors to define HCWs' role identities.

Efforts to change the stigma associated with the disease were also made by AIDS advocacy groups in the previous decade, particularly after 1993 when gay rights activists became more involved in AIDS non-governmental organisations (Wang, 1999). Although representations of gay men have undergone changes in which more diversified perspectives can be seen in the popular and official discourses, the old blame on gay men for HIV/AIDS transmission did not disappear even after greater attention had been paid to the heterosexual others. In other words, the kind of repositioning of social identity found in the HCWs is indeed unique to the SARS discourse. A new type of othering role was first labelled on HCWs, who then tried to resist communal sanctions by emphasising their ordinariness. Such labelling was merely temporary because HCWs were soon able to resume their original role of part of the us groups. The othering process with regard to HCWs was mainly due to their proximity to the infectious disease and not to their misconduct or disadvantaged social status, as outlined by Goffman (1963). HCWs also knew how to utilise various communication and social resources to reposition themselves. Unfortunately, these two features were not found in the stigmatised groups or individuals discussed in the next section.

Everlasting others

At the early stage of the SARS outbreak, there was a prevailing fear of becoming the next mass transportation victim to be infected by SARS, as had previously happened to passengers on trains and inter-city buses. People felt constantly threatened when taking mass transportation, shopping, or working. Various socially disadvantaged groups were then labelled as carriers of the virus. For example, the news media constructed the homeless as an obstacle in the battle against SARS (*United Daily News*, 4 May 2003; *China Times*, 1 May 2003). Foreign caregivers in hospitals, foreign domestic maids and illegal immigrants were targeted as "walking carriers" or "moving carriers" that "invisibly" transmitted the disease to the general public (Yang, 2003).

Like South Asians and Southeast Asians represented in the Taiwanese HIV/AIDS discourse, certain social groups were stigmatised as endangering the so-called healthy us in the SARS discourse, regardless of the scientific evidence necessary for labelling them so. Therefore, residents in low-income communities, the homeless, foreign blue-collar workers, etc. were perceived as high-risk groups in transmitting SARS to the mainstream population.

For example, the existing stigma associated with the homeless was found to reappear in the news discourse. The homeless were filthy, sick, sleeping everywhere, and thus posed a threat to public health (*China Times*, 4 May 2003). They were also chased from time to time by the police on the streets (*United Daily News*, 5 May 2003). Such images were well integrated into the SARS outbreak when the homeless were described as using hospitals as their "day-time residence" (*United Daily News*, 24 April 2003). They were like a "malignant tumor" in the society (*China Times*, 3 May 2003). A time bomb metaphor was used again to signify the homeless as potential carriers of the infectious disease (*United Daily News*, 30 April 2003).

As most of the homeless were said to "wander around" in Taipei's Wanhua District (when the nearby Hoping Hospital was closed down) and when several elderly persons were found to be dead or infected in the Huachang Public Housing Project within the district, an urging for more strict measures to be placed upon the homeless was dominant in the news discourse. The homeless were then represented as hard to control, but still needed to be located by the police from time to time (*United Daily News*, 20,

30 May 2003). This marginalising process resembled those attempts made in the HIV/AIDS discourse to represent gay behaviour as occurring in geographical isolation such as bathhouses, certain parks, by certain riversides, etc. (*United Daily News*, 5 May, 10 July, 6 August 1988; *Min Seng Daily*, 19 July 1988).

Hospital blue-collar workers were also stigmatised as super spreaders of the SARS virus in the news discourse. A laundry worker employed at the Hoping Hospital was labelled as the "index patient." He was said to have still "remained on duty and interacted frequently with patients, staff, and visitors. He had sleeping quarters in the hospital's basement and spent off-duty time socialising in the emergency department" (Lee *et al.*, 2003b). Some media reports even mistakenly described him as coming from mainland China (*China Times*, 26 April 2003), a "scapegoating" tactic of connecting the disease to foreignness. Similar examples were found in the news coverage of SARS infection in other hospitals (*China Times*, 8 June 2003; *United Daily News*, 10 June 2003).

People from socially-disadvantaged or marginal groups were placed in distinct categories so as to accomplish some degree of separation of us from them, an important component of stigmatisation stated by Link and Phelan (2001). Those blue-collar hospital workers used to be invisible in the mainstream discourse before the SARS outbreak. Nevertheless, once they became visible in the news discourse, unlike HCWs mentioned previously, stigmatisation on the basis of class or social status was applied to define their identities. These socially-disadvantaged groups were thus deprived of their right to work. Some of them were even dismissed by the hospitals. Moreover, as they were not full-time employees, they were not considered for social welfare and compensation from the hospitals.

Discussion and Conclusion

The study has analysed the discourse on SARS in Taiwan's mainstream news media. Specifically, we have examined how others have been constructed in the news texts, informing the public about the epidemic and prevention of the infectious disease.

From the preceding analysis of the SARS news texts, we have found several patterns highlighted in the othering processes of the discourse. These processes are dynamic and the formation of the us groups depended on how others were constructed.

We have observed that various groups of others were found or created in the SARS news discourse. Due to a fear of contagion constructed among the imagined us general public, individuals or groups who were probable-case patients or their families who had travelled in other SARS-affected regions such as China and Hong Kong, or political authorities of the affected regions or the regions themselves, became the targets for blaming. Nevertheless, the othering processes of these different individuals or groups varied, depending on the existing social stratification or political ideology involved. SARS-related persons regarded as professionals, such as HCWs, researchers or students from prestigious institutions, namely, the new groups of others created in the SARS discourse, were represented merely as being selfish, a type of blemished character as categorised by Goffman (1963) for their disobedience of the quarantine orders. The labelling of these groups soon dissolved once the outbreak was controlled.

The connection of the disease to foreignness, as found in the HIV/AIDS discourse, surfaced again in the SARS news discourse. Due to the origin of SARS and the political tension across the Taiwan Strait, mainland Chinese and the Chinese government were stigmatised as being responsible for the epidemic. Although groups labelled as others in both SARS and HIV/AIDS discourses vary by their foreign connection, they are still considered the old groups. This type of othering tends to occur whenever or wherever there emerges a frightening infectious disease in society.

Another type of the old others can be found in socially-disadvantaged groups such as the homeless or blue-collar workers. They are generally invisible in the mainstream discourse. However, when the SARS outbreak became a national crisis, as had happened in other health or security-risk related events before, these groups were made visible as another target to be blamed. They were then further discriminated by being excluded from the available resources that other victims of the disease are entitled to. Foreign blue-collar workers, mostly from Southeast Asia, even appeared to be tribally stigmatised due to their perceived image of third-worldness, as represented in the mainstream Taiwanese discourse.

It should be noted that while most of the stigmatised groups in the discourse on SARS tended to be positioned by the social, cultural, and political forces at that time, only HCWs were able to empower themselves by utilising media resources and were then able to reposition themselves to be part of the us groups.

To sum up, the roles that the news media have played in shaping our understanding of the infectious diseases cannot be overlooked. News media can serve both positive and negative functions in surveillance and social integration. The accuracy and the amount of information we receive and our perceptions of risk shaped by the media may contribute to individual and public choices for action and prevention in an increasingly complex world (Singer and Endreny, 1993). In our study, the use of characterisations in the discourse on the disease may help produce varied differences between people in relation to the disease. Those who ran a higher risk of the infectious disease, be it SARS or HIV/AIDS, were characterised either as belonging to "at-risk groups" or as "victims." Some of these differences actually highlighted social categories that are already firmly established.

Implications of the results from the study are at least threefold: Firstly, they help us understand further how the agents of policy-making have influenced the othering processes in the discourse of emerging infectious diseases. Secondly, patterns drawn from the study could shed light on the role of the news media in times of health risk management and on the intertwining relationships between the media and the social, cultural, and political forces. Most importantly, a better understanding of the othering processes would tell us much more than we already know about the conditions under which the stigma is related to in real life situations. Such knowledge should form the basis for multifaceted interventions that represent our best hope for producing real change in stigma-related processes.

References

Albert E. (1986) Illness and Deviance: The Response of the Press to AIDS, in DA Feldman & TM Johnson (eds.), *The Social Dimensions of AIDS: Method and Theory*, pp. 163–178, Praeger, New York.

Archer D. (1985) Social deviance, in G Lindzey & E Aronson (eds.), *Handbook of Social Psychology*, 3rd ed, vol. 2, pp. 743–804, Random House, New York.

Bardhan N. (August 1996) *Frame of Blame: Semiosis of Newstrack's Representation of AIDS in India*. Paper presented at the Qualitative Studies Div, Assoc Edu Jour Mass Comm Ann Convention, Anaheim, California.

Center for Disease Control, Taiwan. (2003) *Memoir of Severe Acute Respiratory Syndrome Control in Taiwan*, Center for Disease Control, Taiwan, Taipei.

Center for Disease Control, Taiwan. (2004). SARS probable cases in Taiwan: One year after the outbreak, 1 July, 2004 in IJ Su (ed.), *SARS in Taiwan: One Year after the Outbreak*, Center for Disease Control, Taiwan & Taiwan Urbani Foundation, Taipei.

Chen C, Chien Y, Yang H. (2003) Epidemiology and control of Severe Acute Respiratory Syndrome (SARS) outbreak in Taiwan, in T Koh, A Plant & EH Lee (eds.), *The New Global Threat: Severe Acute Respiratory Syndrome and Its Impacts*, pp. 301–13, World Scientific, Singapore.

Chen K *et al.*, (2004). The public health response to the SARS in Taiwan, 2003, in IJ Su (ed.), *SARS in Taiwan: One Year after the Outbreak*, pp. 1–4, Center for Disease Control, Taiwan & Taiwan Urbani Foundation, Taipei.

Chu H, Chang Y, Chang L, Lin F, Chang C. (2003) A survey report on the social trends during SARS epidemic, in M Lai (ed.), *SARS in Spring, 2003: A Review of the Science, Society and Culture of SARS Epidemic,* pp. 149–94, Linking Publisher, Taipei.

Crocker J, Major B, Steele C. (1998) Social stigma, in DT Gilbert, ST Fiske & G Lindzey (eds.), *The Handbook of Social Psychology*, 4th ed., pp. 504–53, The McGraw-Hill, New York.

Davies B, Harré R. (1990) Positioning: The discursive production of selves. *J Theory Soc Behav* **20**(1): 43–63.

Foucault M. (1979) *Discipline and Punish: The Birth of the Prison*, Vintage Books, New York.

Freimuth VS, Greenberg RH, DeWitt J, Romano RM. (1984) Covering Cancer: Newspapers and the Public Interest. *J Comm* **34**(1): 62–73.

Goffman E. (1963) *Stigma: Notes on the Management of Spoiled Identity*. Prentice-Hall, Englewood Cliffs, Nj.

Hsu M. (2004a) *Reporting an Emerging Epidemic in Taiwan: Journalists' Experiences of SARS Coverage*. Paper presented at the 54th Ann Conf Int Comm Assoc, New Orleans.

Hsu M. (2004b) *HIV/AIDS Media Campaigns and Their Effectiveness in Taiwan*. Paper presented at the 2004 Bi–Ann Conf Int Assoc Media and Comm Research, Porto Alegre, Brazil.

Hsu M, Lin W, Wu T. (2004) Representations of "us" and "others" in the AIDS news discourse: A taiwanese experience, in E Micollier (ed.), *Sexual Cultures in East Asia: The Social Construction of Sexuality and Sexual Risk in a Time of AIDS*, pp. 183–222, Routledge-Curzon, UK.

Koh T, Plant A, Lee EH. (2003) WHO: At the forefront of combating SARS, in T Koh, A Plant & EH Lee (eds.), *The New Global Threat: Severe Acute Respiratory Syndrome and Its Impacts*, pp. 3–13, World Scientific, Singapore.

Lee ML *et al.*, (2003a) Use of quarantine to prevent transmission of Severe Acute Respiratory Syndrome — Taiwan. *MMWR* **52**(29): 680–3.

Lee ML *et al.*, (2003b) Severe Acute Respiratory Syndrome — Taiwan, 2003. *MMWR* **52**(20): 461–6.

Lin Y. (2003) Qualitative Analyses of SARS News reports by the domestic press: The cases of huachang public housing complex quarantine and the alleged SOS letter in a bottle from mackay memorial hospital. *Thought Words J Hum Soc Sci* **41**(4): 71–110.

Lin Y, Chen B. (2003) Representation of an Audience Reactions to Foreign Laborers in the SARS news. Paper presented at the Nov 2003 Conf on Globalization and News Reports, Taipei.

Link BG, Phelan JC. (2001) Conceptualizing stigma. *Ann Rev Soc* **27**: 363–85.

Liu C. (2004) *From Invisible to Visible: Representation of Others in SARS News Coverage.* Unpublished Masters Thesis. National Chengchi University, Taiwan.

Lu S. (January 2004) *Media Advocacy and Social Mobilization during SARS Epidemic.* Paper presented at the Conf SARS and Sustainable Development. Taipei.

Simpkins JD, Brenner DJ. (1984) Mass Media Communication and Health, in B Dervin & MJ Voigt (eds.), *Prog Commun Sci*, pp. 275–97, Ablex, Norwood, Nj.

Singer E, Endreny PM. (1993) *Reporting on Risk: How the Mass Media Portray Accidents, Diseases, Disasters and Other Hazards.* Russell Sage Foundation, New York.

Wallack L. (1990) Mass media and health promotion: Promise, problem, and challenge, in C Atkin & L Wallack (eds.), *Mass Communication and Public Health*, pp. 41–50, Sage, Newbury Park, Ca.

Wang Y. (1999) *A History of Gay Rights Movements in Taiwan.* Cheerful Sunshine Publishers, Taipei.

Watney S. (1987) *Policing Desire: Pornography, AIDS and the Media*, Methuen, London.

Weiss CH. (1974) What America's leaders read. *Pub Opin Q*, **38**: 1–21.

Yang F. (2003) Class Anxiety — "Chinese Pneumonia" — the WHO as Battlefield, in *Infectious: SARS in the World Media* (On-line). Available from http://www.opendemocracy.net/themes/article-8-1309.jsp#21

Yang S. (2003) *From Medial to Heroic Discourse: Political Power and Media Manipulation in the SARS News Events.* Paper presented at the Nov 2003 Conf on Globalization and News Reports, Taipei.

## 18

Risk Perception and Coping Responses in a SARS Outbreak in Malaysia

Chan Chee Khoon

Aspects of Risk in Public Health

Public health scientists and practitioners are much concerned with *risk analysis* and *risk communication*. *Risk analysis* and *risk estimation* are of course mainstays of the epidemiology profession; together with *risk communication*, they provide essential elements of health education and health promotion.

Much of health education and health promotion is furthermore predicated on the assumption of "rational" health behaviour of individuals, an assumption that has come under increasing scrutiny with the realisation that

> " *fully' informing individuals about health and health risk does not necessarily lead to a change in health behaviour. The natural reluctance of individuals to incorporate new health information into their existing cognitive processes means that new information will be at best only slowly incorporated"* (Whitehead and Russell, 2004).

> *"there has been a change in the perception of risk by society. We have moved to a 'risk perception society' where what is important is not whether*

351

the number or nature of risks have increased [or decreased] in their serious-
ness, but that people believe that this is so and act accordingly... 'expert'
assessment of the probability of harm appears to have become less important
than the popular perception of risk, with opinion regularly becoming the
basis on which behaviour is based" (McInnes, 2005)

For instance, the cumulative experience from the tobacco control campaign suggests that *risk perception* is an altogether more subjective and complicated matter which may be susceptible to diverse influences and life circumstances not fully captured by a natural reluctance to assimilate health information.[1]

This paper explores the theme of *risk perception* and what influences it in an emergent infectious outbreak, Severe Acute Respiratory Syndrome (SARS), which swept through East and Southeast Asia in 2002 and 2003. In particular, we will explore from the perspectives of diverse actors, their perception of risk in the unfolding SARS epidemic on the assumption that their risk perception is expressed in their coping responses, and may be furthermore modulated by the institutional dynamics within groups, agencies or enterprises.

Risk Analysis and Risk Perception in a SARS Outbreak

Speaking at a public forum in Penang on 17 April 2003, cardiologist Dr Ong Hean Teik and his Penang Medical Practitioner Society colleagues urged the Malaysian public not to over-react[2] to the Severe Acute

---

[1]It is not coincidental that tobacco advertisements, often linked to high-risk recreational activities such as skydiving, downhill skiing, rock climbing, Formula-1 motor racing, etc evidently seek to modify risk perception and to reinforce the (subliminal) message: *danger is cool, it's stylish, exciting... the Surgeon-General says smoking is dangerous for your health... so what? Life's dangerous... Danger is the Spice of Life...*

[2]Evidently, the hospital industry was not immune to over-reaction either, as when an unnamed private hospital in Kuala Lumpur imposed a 10-day quarantine without pay on two operating theater nurses after they flew back from New Zealand in April 2003 with a one-hour transit stop at Singapore's Changi airport. Deputy Director-General of Health Dr Ismail Merican deplored such excessive measures, all the more from healthcare professionals, and further noted that *"the main implication (of the quarantine) is that you will be generating a fear of reporting as healthcare staff may be afraid to report that they have been to affected countries for fear of a pay cut"* (*The Star*, 18 May 2003). This was a necessary corrective in the wake of an earlier statement by the Deputy Labor Minister Dr Abdul Latiff Ahmad who had declared that workers subjected to SARS quarantine should use their annual leave for their period of confinement, and *"if the employees have used up their annual leave, they can still apply for unpaid leave"* (*The Star*, 29 April 2003).

Respiratory Syndrome (SARS) epidemic, stressing the low case fatality ratio which at the time was crudely estimated at 4 to 5% of clinically diagnosed SARS cases (*The Star*, 19 April 2003).

Shortly after, Roy Anderson and his colleagues at Imperial College (London), at the Chinese University of Hong Kong and the University of Hong Kong re-calculated the numbers based on 1,425 cases in Hong Kong (∼ one-quarter of the cumulative total of cases worldwide at the time). They estimated a case fatality ratio of 13.2% (6.8%, non-parametric estimate) for cases below 60 years of age, and 43.3% (55%, non-parametric estimate) for those aged 60 and above (Donnelly *et al.*, 2003).

In the 1918–1919 flu pandemic which killed 30–40 million people world-wide (Johnson and Mueller, 2002), case fatality ratios were not reliably known, but have been variously cited at ∼ 1% in the US,[3] between 1 and 2% in Switzerland,[4] and the global average probably did not exceed 5%. This was in the chaotic aftermath of the horrific bloodletting between the world's imperial powers (Kolata, 1999).

A case fatality ratio[5] for SARS ranging from 7 to 55% among different age groups, in the more affluent regions of Southeast Asia and mainland China, Hong Kong, Taiwan, and suburban Toronto, in less tumultuous times, is not much cause for comfort.

Thankfully, SARS in the event was less contagious (or produced fewer symptomatic cases) when compared with flu epidemics. By the end of June 2003, the chains of transmission had been broken in the SARS-affected countries, and the much-feared scenario of uncontrolled community spread to the peri-urban and rural hinterlands (areas with weaker institutional capacity) fortunately did not materialise.

Remarkably, this rapid control was achieved in the absence of reliable diagnostics, vaccines, or efficacious therapies, notwithstanding the

---

[3]Interview with CJ Peters: SARS — The New Viral Threat (*WebMD*, 7 April 2003) http://my.webmd.com/content/article/63/71969.htm (*accessed on 1 May 2003*)

[4]Calculated from data reported in Ammon. 2002.

[5]The *case fatality ratio*, for a number of reasons, is an unstable parameter when an epidemic is rapidly evolving. It is of course an artifact of case definition criteria, at the time (early May 2003), WHO's criteria for *suspected* and *probable* SARS cases which would very likely change when more reliable laboratory tests for SARS infection became available. When used in combination with revised clinical criteria, the designated suspected and probable SARS cases may well be re-assigned to different categories, and case fatality ratios would correspondingly be revised in line with the new defining criteria.

unprecedented research collaboration (World Health Organization, 2003) which led to the rapid isolation and identification of the microbial agent involved, SARS coronavirus (Peiris et al. 2003), and the sequencing of its genome (Ruan et al., 2003).[6]

WHO gave much credit to institutional responses such as isolation, contact tracing, ring fencing, and quarantines (i.e. centuries-old techniques) for rapidly bringing the pandemic under control.[7]

Less mentioned were the individual coping responses and risk avoidance behaviours (reduced travel to SARS-affected areas, avoidance of restaurants and crowded locations, delays or cancellations of elective medical and surgical procedures, outpatients diverting to non-hospital primary care settings) and the possible contributions of seasonality effects or cross-reacting immunity from related endemic micro-organisms (Ng et al., 2003). Most importantly, the economic and financial stakes involved ensured that SARS would not be a "neglected disease".

SARS and "Collateral Damage"

Among clinicians and pathologists, there is some convergence towards the view that the lung pathology seen in SARS patients (*diffuse alveolar damage*) may in part be due to immune overreaction (*cytokine dysregulation and hyperinduction of inflammatory response*) provoked by the SARS coronavirus (Ksiazek et al., 2003; Wenzel and Edmond, 2003; Oba, 2003).

By analogy, some have lamented loudly about a societal or individual "overreaction" in the risk avoidance responses to the outbreak, with the resultant "collateral damage" on East Asian national economies disproportionate to the seriousness or severity of the epidemic of 2002–2003.

In Singapore for instance, 206 probable cases of SARS were diagnosed between March 2003 and June 2003, of whom 32 died. Malaysia, which

---

[6]These early exchanges however very soon gave way to a mutual wariness at the point when intellectual property claims were filed for the pathogen's sequences and other patentable findings with commercial potential. (see: Gold. 2003; *Lancet editorial*, 25 September 2004).

[7]Gro Harlem Brundtland, Director-General, World Health Organization "... *SARS can be contained despite the absence of robust diagnostic tests, a vaccine, or any specific treatment. When awareness, commitment, and determination are high, even such traditional control tools as isolation, contact tracing, and quarantine can be sufficiently powerful to break the chain of transmission ...*" (WHO website, accessed on 5 July 2003).

recorded five probable cases and two deaths from SARS, nonetheless suffered comparable economic losses largely visited on the travel and tourism, entertainment and hospitality, as well as the health services industries. Two months into the epidemic, average hotel occupancy rates in Singapore had fallen to 20–30% (vs. 75% for February 2003, 74% for the whole of 2002); by late April 2003, tourist arrivals were down by 67%, and retail sales down by 10–50% (Lim *et al.*, 2003), with many small traders folding. Singapore's projected GDP was forecasted to shrink at least 1% ($875 million) as a direct consequence of the SARS epidemic. Aside from tourism-related services (hotel, restaurant, retail, airlines, cruise, travel agencies, and taxi services) which together account for 5% of Singapore's GDP (2002), the health services industry also experienced markedly reduced hospital admissions from its local and regional clienteles.

In Malaysia, where tourism accounts for 7% of GDP and ranks second after manufactured exports for foreign exchange earnings, revenue losses were projected to approach $1 billion. By the end of April 2003, airlines were reporting 50–60% cancellations of bookings (Malaysian Airlines alone reportedly suffered a revenue loss of RM131 million ($34.5 million) due to the cancellation of over 700 flights to SARS-affected destinations). As a result, air-travel arrivals fell by more than 40%, and hotel occupancy rates dropped to 30–35% (Ariff, 2003). As was the case in Singapore, patient admissions into Malaysian hospitals also fell markedly. The Association of Private Hospitals of Malaysia (APHM) surveyed its 48 member hospitals in May 2003. Of the 37 hospitals that responded, 42% reported a drop of 5–10% for inpatient numbers month-on-month (comparing April 2003 with May 2003); 31% reported a decline of 15–20%; 22% reported a decline of 30%, and 2.5% reported a decline of more than 40%. Overall, patient admissions for the respondent hospitals (all with 50 beds or more) fell by 5–40% in May 2003 (Bakar, 2003; Business Times, 2003).

Faced with this novel disquieting outbreak, there were loud laments that the economic fallout was disproportionate to the seriousness or severity of the epidemic. This "collateral damage" inflicted on national economies overshadowed the direct human cost (lives lost, temporary or long-lasting infirmity, family and personal tragedies), when furthermore contrasted against the persistent, devastating, but all too often invisible plagues in the poorer countries of the South: HIV/AIDS, tuberculosis, malaria, water-borne diseases, hunger and malnutrition, which collectively (and often acting in concert) cause more than 12 million avoidable deaths annually.

Clearly, *risk perception* has consequences for the *risk avoidance* and *coping responses* of individuals and communities, quite apart from the institutional responses of state agencies in the form of isolation, contact tracing, ring fencing and quarantines, and various surveillance and epidemic control measures imposed on members of society. A more nuanced management of emergent infectious outbreaks therefore has to be sensitive not only to the characteristics of the emergent pathogens (lethality and other nonfatal sequelae; modes of transmission and sequestrability of the outbreak) and the social ecology of its emergence and spread, but also has to take into account the differentiated risk perception, risk avoidance, and the coping behaviours of diverse at-risk parties. These include the general public, travellers and intending travellers (including migrants), family members and close contacts of patients and other at-risk individuals, healthcare institutions and enterprises, healthcare staff (including diagnostic, research and other support staff), other governmental agencies, travel and hospitality industries and their staff, politicians, local (national) as well as the international disease control agencies.

In the rest of this paper, we will explore from the perspectives of diverse actors the theme of *risk perception* and what influences it, using an integrative framework which draws upon the social, biological and ecological dimensions and their interactions.

The Social Ecology of SARS in Malaysia and Singapore

The social ecology of SARS in Malaysia includes the politically influential tourism sector and its ancillary industries, with foreign exchange earnings second only to manufacturing exports, and accounting for 7% of GDP in recent years.

With the notable presence of corporations such as the Malaysian Airlines System (MAS), Faber Group Bhd, Pernas International Holdings Bhd, World Resorts Bhd, YTL Corp Bhd, Landmarks Bhd, and Sunway City Bhd in this services sector, it was unlikely that SARS would be a "neglected disease". The Malaysian Institute of Economic Research (MIER) had furthermore projected that the GDP growth for 2003 could fall from 5.7%

to 3.7% (Ariff, 2003) (subsequently revised upwards to 4.3% in July 2003), which helps explain the strenuous efforts by the authorities to keep Malaysia off the WHO list of SARS-affected countries where local transmission had been detected.

Throughout the outbreak, the local travel and hospitality industry desperately urged its nervous patrons not to "over-react" to the SARS epidemic. They may have been right about overly active survival instincts, but one would be reasonably wary about them as impartial arbiters of "appropriate" risk perception in the local context. The same individuals (and their political representatives) however urged caution upon those who contemplated travel outside the country to SARS-affected destinations such as China, Hong Kong, Taiwan, Singapore, and Toronto (*Malaysiakini.com*, 17 March 2003).

Tourism can evidently be a risk deflator under certain circumstances. In a letter to editors of the Malaysian newspapers dated 28 March 2003, Aseh Che Mat, Secretary General of the Home Ministry (which decides on the annually renewable publishing permits of Malaysian newspapers) made clear the government's preferences in information management:

> as you already know, SARS cases have received wide coverage in mainstream newspapers of different languages, including specific cases of deaths... The government is concerned that such comprehensive and widely-publicised reports will lead to undesirable implications, including striking fear among the people and jeopardising tourist arrival... Therefore, the ministry seeks the cooperation of editors to adjust the reports on the SARS, by not focusing on death cases [as this] could adversely affect the confidence of the public and tourists... (*Malaysiakini.com*, 1 April 2003)

whilst in Penang (an important regional tourist destination), State Executive Councilor for Culture, Arts & Tourism *Kee Phaik Cheen* similarly urged

> that the media should not highlight SARS stories as this would keep tourists away (*New Straits Times*, 23 March 2003).

Ms Kee had furthermore invested much effort in promoting Penang as a regional center for *medical tourism*, and she would have been keenly aware that this service sub-sector was doubly vulnerable to emergent outbreaks such as SARS, where *nosocomial transmissions* are implicated.[8]

Meanwhile, her federal counterpart Abdul Kadir Sheikh Fadzir, Minister of Culture, Arts & Tourism declared at a meeting on 23 May 2003 of ASEAN national tourism organisations:

> ASEAN countries need to find a meaningful way to cooperate. We should remove travel restrictions and cut red tape. Our tourism industry is being held ransom by these events. Hence we need to simplify existing travel procedures. We should consider travel within ASEAN as part of domestic travel ... *(Malaysiakini.com, 23 May 2003)*

In contrast, Singapore's approach to epidemic management was evidently based on the following premises:

- credibility as one of those intangibles which have enormous economic value (and costs, when it is undermined)
- bite the bullet, absorb the short-term costs
- be highly transparent, in order to curb uncontrolled, damaging rumours
- use organised, timely deployment of institutional resources
- enact tough measures infringing on individual liberties for the "greater good" (and lest we succumb to temptations to invoke "Asian values", let

---

[8]Singapore, which probably had the most detailed records of the unfolding outbreak among the SARS-affected countries, reported that as of April 30, 2003, 76% of the island state's probable SARS cases had acquired their infections in a healthcare setting, in particular in the public hospitals which took on much of the burden of handling the SARS epidemic; the remaining SARS cases either had household, multiple, or unknown exposures (*Morbidity and Mortality Weekly Report,* 9 March 2003). Likewise, in Malaysia, among the eighteen designated hospitals with special isolation wards for SARS patients, not a single private hospital was to be found. Indeed, when two foreigners insisted on being admitted into a private hospital for SARS observation, the Association of Private Hospitals of Malaysia (APHM) responded by persuading the Health Ministry to invoke emergency quarantine powers *"if a patient refused to be admitted into a public hospital.... the district health officer concerned can issue a quarantine order making it compulsory for a patient to be admitted into a dedicated [i.e. government] hospital...The [private] hospital had to admit them [at the time] because there were no guidelines outlining what private hospitals could do if they had to handle such a case. Now they know what to do,"* according to APHM president Dr Ridzwan Bakar (*The Star,* 7 April 2003). Weighing on their minds, evidently, beyond the expense of maintaining a SARS isolation ward, was the further worry that a hospital's fee-paying clientele would avoid a "SARS-tainted" hospital. One wonders how the private hospitals would cope if the hospital sector in Malaysia were ever to be completely privatised.

us note the following distinctly communitarian sentiments expressed by a prominent occidental):

today we emphasize individual rights over community needs more than we did 50 to 75 years ago. Restraining the rights and freedoms of individuals is a far greater sin than allowing the infection of others. The restraints placed on Typhoid Mary might not be acceptable today, when some would prefer to give her unlimited rein to infect others, with litigation their only recourse. In the triumph of individual rights, the public health perspective has had an uphill struggle in recent pandemics ... We typically [reconsider control measures] only after an outbreak. Perhaps we should have further debate on the social context for constraints and persuasion to contain the spread of infectious agents (Lederberg, 1997).

The Singapore government, well known for its unflinching pragmatism in matters of individual (human) rights, let alone "animal rights", was resolutely readying itself with simulation exercises in anticipation of avian flu outbreaks:

Singapore will gas and burn thousands of healthy chickens next week as part of a simulated bird flu outbreak exercise, a senior official said yesterday. There is no bird flu in Singapore but the city-state is desperate to avoid a local outbreak of the illness, which has prompted the slaughter of tens of millions of chickens across Asia and killed 19 humans. Health officials will cull the 5,000 chickens at an isolated poultry farm Wednesday by gassing and then incinerating them, said Dr Ngiam Tong Tau, Chief Executive Officer of the Agri-Food and Veterinary Authority. Police officers will be stationed around the farm to prevent unauthorised entry and civil defence officials will decontaminate personnel before they leave, Ngiam said. Doctors will also be on hand to screen workers and simulate dispensing anti-viral drugs, he added. Singapore's Deputy

Prime Minister Lee Hsien Loong has said the government would rather "overreact rather than under-react" to the bird flu threat. The city-state can ill-afford a repeat of last year's ordeal with the Severe Acute Respiratory Syndrome (SARS), which killed 33 people here and did massive damage to the nation's economy (*The Star*, 13 February 2004).

Ten days earlier, Mr Lee's Thai counterpart, Prime Minister Thaksin Shinawatra had publicly "lambasted WHO for suggesting the flu [virus] could mutate and spread to pigs and then even more easily to humans. Ethically speaking, researchers should only discuss low possibilities of such cross-strain spreads in labs, not in public," Thaksin told reporters (*The Star*, 3 February 2004) (see also footnote[9]).

Singapore, unlike Thailand, is not a leading exporter of chicken and poultry products to the world market. Nonetheless, the Singapore government has no lesser stakes invested in the travel and tourism sector (most prominently, the national air carrier Singapore Airlines), while *Temasek*, the government's investment and asset holding company, accounted for 21% of the market capitalisation of the Singapore stock exchange at that time (Financial Times, *14 February 2004*).[10]

What might explain these contrasting approaches? The answer probably lies somewhere between "Singapore exceptionalism" and the "relative autonomy of the technocratic state".

At the WHO Global Conference on SARS (2003) in Kuala Lumpur, Dick Thompson, WHO's risk communication officer re-iterated the wisdom distilled from the management of epidemic outbreaks past and present:

> People are at their best when collectively facing a difficult situation straight-on. Things get much more unstable when people begin

---

[9]In the aftermath of the Indian Ocean tsunami of 26 December 2004 which claimed more than 5200 lives (and another 4500 missing) in Thailand, it emerged that the possibility of a tidal wave hitting Thailand's most popular tourist beaches was downplayed out of concern for the country's burgeoning tourist industry (Bangkok Post, 7 January 2005).

[10]The Malaysian government's investment and asset holding company *Khazanah* has similarly large stakes (34% of market capitalisation) in the Kuala Lumpur stock exchange. (*Special Report: Reshaping Khazanah*, www.theedgedaily.com, 18 May 2004).

to feel 'handled,' misled, not levelled with. That's when they are likeliest to panic or go into denial, likeliest to ignore instructions or develop paranoid hypotheses. Make it clear what you know and what you don't know.

The Singapore government has repeatedly and publicly proclaimed the crucial importance (and competitive advantage) of *credibility* in governance and in public management, all the more emphatically as it fights to retain its carefully nurtured pre-eminence as a regional financial and business centre. This evidently extends to disease control and epidemic management, some aspects of which have been described as draconian and convenient for reinforcing social and political control in an already authoritarian polity (*chapters by Liu, and Ong, Yeoh and Teo in this volume*).

In any case, the Singapore government's blend of transparency and considered coercive measures seems to have found favour not just within international disease control agencies such as the WHO, but has also won acceptance among many of its own citizens and residents. This came across in the preliminary findings of Stella Quah (National University of Singapore's Department of Sociology) and her research collaborators at the University of Hong Kong, reported thus in the *Economic and Political Weekly*[11]:

> in spite of many similarities between the two cities, the citizens [of Hong Kong and Singapore] expressed quite different views...in their acceptance of measures undertaken by their respective governments to deal with SARS. Initial findings showed that, intriguingly, there is a discrepancy between the perception of the risk of catching SARS and the acceptance of the quarantine measures. Hong Kong residents appeared to perceive a greater risk of getting SARS; yet they were more against measures such as the quarantine than their Singaporean counterparts. Of the Singaporeans surveyed, 91% accepted being put under quarantine even in the event they had no contact with any SARS patients, compared to 72% of the Hong Kong group (Xiang & Wong, 2003).

---

[11] The Hong Kong group of course may have been quite astute in recognising that the higher prevalence of SARS in Hong Kong at that time put the uninfected quarantinees there at greater risk of nosocomial transmissions as well as residential infectious risk (such as at Amoy Gardens where there was evidence of environmental, aerosol spread).

Normalising Death and Disease

Amartya Sen once observed that if poverty itself were contagious, it would speedily dispel the nonchalance and indifference of the privileged and sequestered. He was speaking of poverty, but his dismay is equally pertinent to our troubling capacity for selective anaesthesia, for "normalising" human health disasters, especially when they occur among marginalised communities with limited "voice". Most glaringly, there were the 3.1 million AIDS deaths in 2004 (2.3 million of them in Sub-Saharan Africa — Aids Epidemic Update, December 2004), more than one million malaria deaths annually in poorer countries, and similarly high fatalities from tuberculosis, waterborne diseases (most importantly, diarrhoea), malnutrition, and other preventable diseases of poverty often acting in concert.

By contrast, the continent-wide uproar in Europe over "mad cow disease" (bovine spongiform encephalopathy, BSE) and its putative human version, variant Creutzfeld-Jakob disease (vCJD), which has recorded less than 200 deaths in the 15 years since the disease was first recognised in the late 1980s, seems grossly out of proportion.

SARS, by these yardsticks, would similarly not count as a major direct threat to global public health, notwithstanding the immense economic losses inflicted on East and SE Asian economies. Yet, precisely because of this latter consideration, SARS assuredly would not be a "neglected disease".[12]

Six weeks after issuing a global alert on SARS, the World Health Organization announced that:

> the Severe Acute Respiratory Syndrome (SARS) outbreak is beginning to come under control. Its medical officer for global alert and response Dr Mark Salter said that although the outbreak was not

---

[12]Neglected diseases, as highlighted by *Médecins Sans Frontières (MSF)*: of the 1,393 new drugs approved between 1975 and 1999, only 16 (or just over 1%) were specifically developed for tropical diseases (such as malaria, sleeping sickness, Chagas' disease, kala azar) and tuberculosis, diseases that account for 11.4% of the global disease burden. For 13 out of those 16 drugs, two were modifications of existing medicines, two were produced for the US military, and five came from veterinary research. Only 4 were developed by commercial pharmaceutical companies specifically for tropical diseases in humans. These tropical diseases mainly affect poorer communities in countries of the South, which do not constitute a valuable enough market to stimulate adequate R&D by the multinational pharmaceutical companies. (Trouiller *et al.*, 2002; Cohen, 2002; Kremer & Glannerster, 2001).

over, the disease had reached the "normalisation" phase... Since
the WHO had issued recommendations on effective control measures, the disease had been successfully controlled in several places...
In Western Europe, individual imported SARS cases have been
immediately isolated and the disease has been stopped there and
then... it was only in countries which had suffered from infections before the disease was identified that SARS was still spreading
(*The Star*, 26 April 2003).

Many infectious outbreaks become less virulent as the epidemic ages,
as host and pathogen co-evolve, as human coping behaviours impinge on
the pathogen's mechanics of transmission, and possibly on the genetics of
its virulence. Less frequently, they may transiently become more virulent
(Ewald, 1994).

Virulence aside, it would be sad if life-threatening infections became less
fearsome the more its spread was confined to marginalised communities,
where cases may emerge, transmit disease, and die (or recover) without
attracting much attention, where there was limited institutional capacity to
carry out the field epidemiology, meticulous contact tracing, ring-fencing
and quarantines which can be the mainstays against an out-of-control
community spread.

In this connection, the British Broadcasting Corporation (BBC) noted
that with privatisation and the collapse of the pioneering primary healthcare
system in China,

millions of Chinese [have] lost access to free medical care because of
[the] country's economic reforms... most people must [now] pay
in cash when they see a doctor... As 90% of patients suffering from
the atypical form of pneumonia [SARS] recover relatively quickly,
thousands of people [may be] attempting to heal themselves, or
letting chronic [or acute] disease go untreated [while] authorities
[remain] unaware of the spread of disease... It is a cheap solution for
patients unable to foot the cost of medical treatment. But it means
that authorities cannot [identify and] quarantine SARS carriers, and
thus control the disease (Williams, 15 April 2003).

By late June 2003, the chains of transmission had been broken in most of the SARS-affected countries and the much-feared scenario of uncontrolled community spread into the peri-urban and rural hinterlands (areas with weaker institutional capacity) fortunately did not materialise in countries like China.

SARS was evidently not as contagious as earlier feared, and the lower population density in rural China and lesser possibilities for nosocomial spread may have further combined with *ad hoc* community initiatives, drawing upon the institutional memories of China's barefoot doctor system to successfully deal with the limited leakage (or backflow?) from affected urban metropolises (rough and ready at times including arbitrary blockades and vigilante style sequestrations).

Concluding Remarks: Emerging Diseases, Emerging Markets

In the event of its re-emergence, effective and cheap solutions, however, may not be on the horizon given the unseemly rush to patent the SARS coronavirus genomic sequences by Canadian, US, Hong Kong, Singaporean, Chinese, and other institutions wary about each other's intentions and seemingly unable to resist the potential profits from diagnostic tests, vaccines, and medical treatments (Gold, 2003).

Further progress in SARS research may now have to contend with the secrecy dictated by commercial imperatives (Matthijis, 2004), in contrast to the early co-operative efforts and exchanges between otherwise highly competitive laboratories which identified the etiological agent in record time, and led to its sequencing within three weeks (Peiris *et al.*, 2003; Ruan *et al.*, 2003).

Dr Julie Gerberding, Director of the US Centers for Disease Control and Prevention (CDC) characterised it as "defensive patenting" on the part of the National Institutes of Health, to keep the prerogatives within the public sector domain (*Nature,* 2003).

Those who are mindful of the Bayh–Dole Act (1980) and the Stevenson–Wydler Act (1980) in the US and how they paved the way for publicly funded scientist-entrepreneurs to launch the biotechnology revolution, may be wary of this as a leaky safeguard with predictable consequences for global healthcare equity, in a market-driven setting (Keusch and Nugent, 2001).

Patents on life forms are anathema to some including myself, but if we have to live with patents in biotechnology, it might be better if patentable findings from publicly funded research, conducted in an international collaborative effort and which are of global public health importance, should be vested in an international agency such as the World Health Organization.[13]

In conclusion, we have thus argued that the perception of risk associated with the SARS infectious outbreak was disproportionate to the (direct) threat it posed to global population health. This inflated perception of risk, driven more by economic rather than epidemiological considerations, ensured that SARS would not be a "neglected" disease. Indeed, SARS was an attractive candidate for patentable research aimed at diagnostic tests, vaccines and therapies, precisely because of the perceived market potential for these commodities. As such, it underscores the irrationality and inequity

---

[13]On 3 September 1999, US activists Ralph Nader, James Love, and Robert Weissman wrote to Harold Varmus, Director of the US National Institutes of Health "to ask that you enter into an agreement with the World Health Organization (WHO), giving the WHO the right to use health care patents that the US government has rights to under 35 USC Sec 202 (c)(4) of the Bayh-Dole Act or under 37 CFR 404.7, for government-owned inventions. Under the regulations concerning government-owned inventions, the US government has an *"irrevocable, royalty-free right of the Government of the United States to practice and have practiced the invention on behalf of the United States and on behalf of any foreign government or international organisation pursuant to any existing or future treaty or agreement with the United States. 37CFR404.7(a)(2)(i)"*. With respect to government's rights in inventions funded by the US government through grants and contracts to Universities and small businesses under the Bayh-Dole Act, the US government has worldwide rights to practice or have practiced inventions on its behalf (37CFR401.14), and it may require that foreign governments or international organisations have the right to use inventions, under 37CFR401.5(d). As you must know, the US government has rights to a large portfolio of health care inventions that were invented with public funds. These include inventions in many HIV/AIDS drugs, such as government-owned inventions on ddI, ddC and FddA, and university and contractor inventions such as d4T, 3TC and Ritonavir, as well as drugs to treat malaria and many other illnesses. The private pharmaceutical companies that have obtained exclusive rights to market these products charge prices that are excessive, and too expensive for many patients, including persons in the United States and Europe. Most seriously, the hardships are particularly difficult in developing countries, where countries do not have high enough national incomes to pay for expensive medicine". Dr Varmus, in his reply dated October 19, 1999, stated that "Congress enacted the Bayh-Dole Act and the Stevenson-Wydler Technology Innovation Act (with later amendments, including the Federal Technology Transfer Act of 1986) to encourage the transfer of basic research findings to the marketplace. The primary purpose of these laws is economic development: specifically, to provide appropriate and necessary incentives [through exclusive licenses] to the private sector to invest in federally funded discoveries and to enhance US global competitiveness". A subsequent request dated 28 March 2001 and addressed to US Secretary of Health and Human Services Tommy Thompson was similarly denied.

which often arises from market-driven priorities in biomedical research and product development. Furthermore, this episode also hints at the promise and possibilities from a needs-driven scientific endeavour, utilising the coordinated talents and resources available worldwide, in contrast to the pitiful constraints of demand-driven commodified knowledge.

Acknowledgements

Helpful suggestions and references from TG Yap, HL Chee, KL Phua, J Cardosa and MP Pollack are gratefully acknowledged, but opinions expressed in this article do not necessarily reflect their views. The author was also supported by a Nippon Foundation API senior fellowship (2004–2005) for his research on health systems in transition, and health and social policies in East and SE Asia.

References

AIDS Epidemic Update. (2004) Geneva: UNAIDS/WHO.

Ammon CE. (2002) Spanish Flu Epidemic in 1918 in Geneva, Switzerland in *Eurosurveillance Monthly 7(12): 190–192*. Available at http://www.eurosurveillance.org/em/v07n12/0712-226.asp, Accessed 30 May 2005.

Ariff M. (2003) *Managing SARS' Economic Fallout*. (Unpublished memorandum, dated 3 May 2003) Malaysian Institute of Economic Research.

Bakar R. (2003) Association of Private Hospitals of Malaysia, presentation at the 2003 Malaysian Health Conference panel on *The SARS Outbreak: Counting the Costs*, 23–4 June 2003, Kuala Lumpur.

Bangkok Post. (2005) *Is Anyone to Blame for Lack of Warning?* Available at http://www.bangkokpost.com/News/07Jan2005_news42.php, Accessed 7 January 2005.

Business Times. *APHM members post drop in May patient admissions*. (23 June 2003).

Cohen R. (2002) Neglected diseases and the health burden in poor countries. *Multinational Monitor*. June 2002.

Donnelly CA, Ghani AC, Leung GM, *et al.* (2003) Epidemiological determinants of spread of causal agent of severe acute respiratory syndrome in Hong Kong. *Lancet* **361**(9371): 1761–1766.

Ewald P. (1994) *Evolution of Infectious Disease*. Oxford University Press, New York.

Financial Times, *14 February 2004*.

Gold ER. (2003) SARS Genome patent: Symptom or disease? *Lancet* **361**: 2002–2003.

Johnson NP, Mueller J. (2002) Updating the accounts: Global mortality of the 1918–1920 "Spanish" Influenza Pandemic. *Bull Hist Med* **76**(1): 105–115.

Kremer M, Glannerster R. (2001) Creating a market for vaccines. *New York Times*, 1 June 2001.

Keusch GT, Nugent RA. (2001) The Role of Intellectual Property and Licensing in Promoting Research in International Health: Perspectives from a Public Sector Biomedical Research Agency. Commission on Macroeconomics and Health (Working Paper No. WG2:7) World Health Organization, Geneva.

Kolata G. (1999) Flu: The Story of the Great Influenza Pandemic of 1918 and the Search for the Virus That Caused It. Farrar Straus & Giroux, New York.

Ksiazek TG, Erdman D, Goldsmith CS, *et al.* (2003) A novel coronavirus associated with severe acute respiratory syndrome. *New Engl J Med* **348**: 1953–1966.

Lederberg J. (1997) Infectious disease as an evolutionary paradigm. *Emerging Infect Dis* **3**(4): 417–423.

Lim TK, Chua BL, Ho T. (2003) Impact of the Severe Acute Respiratory Syndrome (SARS) on the Singapore Economy. *Economic Survey of Singapore, First Quarter 2003,* pp. 45–50, Ministry of Trade and Industry, Singapore.

Malaysiakini.com. (2003) Avoid countries affected by deadly pneumonia: Chua. Published on 17 March 2003, Accessed 24 April 2005.

Malaysiakini.com. (2003). Government orders press not to report SARS deaths. Published on 1 April 2003, Accessed 1 August 2003.

Malaysiakini.com. (2003) Malaysia urges Asean to lift travel restrictions to save tourism from SARS. Published on 23 May 2003, Accessed 23 May 2005.

Matthijs G. (2004) Patenting genes may slow down innovation, and delay availability of cheaper genetic tests (Editorial) *Br Med J* **329**: 1358–1360.

Nature. (2003) Editorial. Gene patents and the public good. *Nature* **423**(6937): 207.

McInnes C. (2005) *Health, Security and the Risk Society.* The Nuffield Trust, London.

Ng TW, Turinici G, Danchin A. (2003) A double epidemic model for the SARS propagation. *BMC Infect Dis* **3**: 19.

Oba Y. (2003) The use of corticosteroids in SARS. *NEJM* **348**: 2034–2035 (Correspondence, and Reply by Lee and Sung).

Peiris JSM, Lai ST, Poon LLM, *et al.* (2003) Coronavirus as a possible cause of severe acute respiratory syndrome. *Lancet* **361**: 1319–1325.

Ruan RJ, Lin WC, Ling AE, *et al.* (2003) Comparative full-length genome sequence analysis of 14 SARS coronavirus isolates and common mutations associated with putative origins of infection. *Lancet* **361**: 1779–1785.

The Edge Daily. *Special Report: Reshaping Khazanah,* published on 18 May 2004. Available at www.theedgedaily.com, accessed 11 August 2004.

The Lancet. (2004) Editorial: Keep genome data freely accessible. *Lancet* **364**(9440): 1099–1100.

Trouiller P, Olliaro P, Torreele E, Orbinski J, Laing R, Ford N. (2002) Drug development for neglected diseases: A deficient market and a public health policy failure. *Lancet* **359**: 2188–2194.

Wenzel RP, Edmond MB. (2003) Managing SARS amidst uncertainty. *NEJM* **348**: 1947–1948.

Whitehead D, Russell G. (2004) How effective are health education programs — Resistance, reactance, rationality and risk? Recommendations for effective practice. *Intl J Nursing Studies* **41**(2): 163–172.

Williams, H. (2003) *China's high-cost health care.* Available at British Broadcasting Corporation website published on 15 April 2003. *http://news.bbc.co.uk/2/hi/asia-pacific/2949525.stm*, Accessed 22 April 2003.

World Health Organization. (2003) A multicentre collaboration to investigate the cause of severe acute respiratory syndrome. *Lancet* **361**: 1730–1733.

Xiang B, Wong T. (2003) SARS: Public health and social science perspectives. *Economic and Political Weekly* 2480–2483.

## 19

A Defining Moment, Defining a Moment: Making SARS History in Singapore

Liew Kai Khiun

> Maybe because this person's sense of the world, that it will change for the better with struggle, maybe a person who has this neo-Hegelian positivist sense of constant historical progress towards happiness and perfection or something, who feels very powerful because he feels connected to these forces, moving uphill all the time... maybe that person can't, um, incorporate sickness into his sense of how things are supposed to go. Maybe vomit...and sores and disease...really frighten him, maybe...he isn't so good with death.

—:Taken from a play by Tony Kushner. *Angels in America; A gay fantasia on national themes* (Kushner, 1992: 25)

> I have no doubt that we will survive SARS, just what are the casualties, what is the pain that we will inflict among ourselves...But at the same time, we are now used to a high standard of life. This is a PAP (People's Action Party) Central District meeting in the Marina Mandarin Hotel! When I met the PAP branches in the 1970s, we sat down on hard benches! So that puts a great deal of pressure to

perform. Having reached this standard of living, can we progress without great pain and suffering? So I worry.

—:Former Senior Minister of Singapore Lee Kuan Yew on his opinion of the SARS epidemic (Petir, 2003: 8)

Introduction: Incorporating Sickness into Historical Progress

Although coming from radically different political orientations, both Kushner and Lee understood in their own ways the cruel impermanence of the flesh. To them, modernity and development have created comfort zones that have conjured illusionary notions of immortality and optimism. Emergent diseases like AIDS and SARS harshly reveal the frailties of the human body that has been supposedly shielded by both biomedical advances and economic affluence. Once relegated to unfortunate souls in both antiquity and the present Third World, infectious diseases demand new sets of mythos and ethos especially for the developed societies that are trying to come to grips with their wraths. As such, they tend to become selectively rationalised, historicised, politicised and memorialised.

In the larger context of Singapore's past, from its establishment as a British trading colony in 1819, the three-month duration of the SARS (Severe Acute Respiratory Syndrome) epidemic, costing ~30 lives, can be considered a footnote. Even within the historical realm of infectious diseases in the island, the presence of SARS is insignificant compared with routine occurrences of more malevolent scourges of cholera, smallpox and plague consistently listed in the colonial annual medical reports. However, this infectious disease now stands alongside the tumultuous political events from the Japanese military occupation in the 1940s to the painful separation from the Malaysian Federation as historical milestones in the annals of Singapore's history. The microbe has in effect joined the list of communist insurgents, communalist agitators, Islamic terrorists, and Darwinian geopolitics and economics as the threats defined by the Singapore state to its national survival. With commemorative books, awards and medals, as well as public memorials to the fallen victims of the epidemic, SARS has been christened by the

Republic's officialdom as "a defining moment" in Singapore's history. As stated by the former Prime Minister Goh Chok Tong in his last National Day Rally,

> "During this crisis, I saw a national spirit I have never seen before. Our country bonded with stout hearts, tenacity and determination. SARS did not break Singapore. It made us stronger." (Goh, 2003)

As such, the SARS episode has become more than a microbiological phenomenon. In its brief appearance, it has been presented and re-presented especially to reinforce the founding myths and legitimacy of the PAP government that steered the vulnerable state above the cruel waves of history to make history. The historicisation of SARS in this respect is located here within several layers. This would be discussed in the context of the relegation of the legacy of infectious diseases in the collective and institutional memories of the republic, prior to its outbreak and its elevation to that of an unprecedented crisis that tested the will of the younger leadership. As the pandemic receded, the script was again edited to congratulate the people and their national leaders in bonding together to brave through a natural calamity. In the process, SARS became a memorialised epidemic, similar to a war that acted as a national rite of passage that enshrined its combatants from ordinary health workers to government ministers as all sacrificing national heroes. It may be argued here that the lionisation of SARS in the official historical annals is a unique case when infectious diseases and epidemics are being crafted as tools of political mobilisation, and more importantly, the attempts of a new generation of leaders to entrench themselves historically alongside the towering images of their founding fathers.

Sickness and Historical Progress

Infectious diseases have been an important element in shaping the course of civilisation, by shaping the social discourses as well as the demographics of societies. In his study of epidemics in early Islamic societies, Lawrence Conrad (1992) explained that the ideological underpinnings of a social system, whether in the form of political loyalties, myth or religion, serve to rationalise the physical world in terms of the priorities, agendas and claims of the society generating these structures. They comprise an ongoing discourse of how that society views its sense of origins, identities, purposes and future. As such, threats of the gravest and most disruptive kind are posed by challenges that falsify the assumptions and claims made in these structures. Conrad (1992) points out that epidemics in particular has posed such a formidable ideological challenge, and has consistently provoked a wealth of reflection seeking to mitigate the trauma experienced.

Yet, in contrast to the more apparent political legacies from conflicts to changes of regimes, the role of diseases seems to be significantly understated. For example, compared with the literature generated by the First World War, the Spanish Influenza of 1918 which took $\sim$20 million lives around the globe remains a largely marginal subject. William McNeill, Howard Philips and David Killingray attributed its marginality to the feeling that

> "epidemic diseases...ran counter to the effort to make the past intelligible... Historians consequently played such episodes down" (Philips and Killingray, 2003).

In particular, until the recent decades, infectious diseases were perceived to be a problem that the industrialised countries have transcended with improvements brought about by progress among economic and scientific fields. Rapid advances in Western biomedical sciences have been posited as the main attribute in the belief that man has finally conquered nature in the global elimination of infectious diseases. The emergent and re-emerging diseases not only in the Third World, but at the doorstep of the most advanced economies has however shattered this progressivist myth that all societies would eventually be affluent enough to use the advanced technologies and acquire modern health portraits (Lewontin and Levins, 2003). These myths of development are given an additional dimension among the newly industrialised societies in East and Southeast Asia. In their drive towards miraculous growth rates, it is often assumed that these economies have left behind the legacy of abject Third World misery of wars, poverty and pestilence. Their sense of triumphalism however tumbled with the 1997 economic crisis, which coincided with the first outbreak of the avian flu in Hong Kong. Yet, it was the SARS pandemic in 2003 that shattered their illusionary beliefs of immunity from supposedly ancient scourges associated with Third World under-development.

Compared with other pandemics, SARS with a worldwide death toll of nearly a thousand people over several months would hardly be significant in the broader historical context. It was however instrumental in placing the political structures represented by the public health systems of the countries affected under intense scrutiny and pressure. Although SARS affected many countries, the epicentres were in the four primarily ethnic Chinese societies of Taiwan, Hong Kong, China and Singapore. From the routine issues of distribution of medical resources and the efficiency and affordability of healthcare services, public health became charged issues of political legitimacy. In trying to contain SARS, governments found themselves under the spotlight for transparency and accountability of state institutions in disseminating information on the epidemic, and the public acceptance of them.

Remembering Health and Diseases in Colonial Singapore

The reactions from the Singaporean public and officialdom to SARS seem to suggest a deeper amnesia of the island's historical experience with diseases and epidemics. Up to the 1970s, while the island was generally healthy, infectious diseases were also familiar, as were the infrastructures that contain them. As an emerging and transitory colonial port city in the 19th century, Singapore had been familiar with epidemics arising from local conditions as well as imported infections. British colonial annual medical reports reflected high mortality figures with death rates exceeding births from a range of diseases, mainly malaria, tuberculosis and pneumonia among the migrant populations from India and China. In addition, afflictions such as venereal diseases and opium addiction had also become endemic. Escaping the poverty and strife of their homes, it could be claimed that many of these migrants were already in a poor state of health upon arrival in Singapore to seek better prospects.

It was also a combination of overcrowding caused by urban congestion, coupled with the inability of a fledgling municipal sanitation and public health infrastructure to keep up with the burgeoning population, that exacerbated the situation. Nonetheless, the colonial administration did place significant attention on port health, establishing a systematic maritime health screening process and a large-scale offshore quarantine facility at St John's Island. This facility was used to enforce legislation requiring compulsory examination and notifications of vessels arriving from infected ports and passengers suspected of carrying the viruses of communicable diseases. In the 1920s, the colonial regime also supported the League of Nations's (the predecessor of the United Nations) decision to set up an epidemiological station for monitoring and disseminating information on epidemics around the world.

However, the colonial authorities were both unwilling and unable to effect widespread changes in public health policies. They saw the role and legitimacy as that of a guardianship by a small European elite over an indigenous society and entrepôt economy, and was keen to maintain the status quo of the colony as a trading port, and subsequently as a strategic naval bastion. The authorities thus favoured conservative health policies which could be enforced by a modest European-led bureaucracy over more aggressive, interventionist approaches.

Eradicating Infectious Diseases in the Singapore Story

When the PAP assumed government in 1959, it was devoted to a holistic programme to improve the living standards of the people. Cleanliness, in both its metaphorical and clinical aspects, was the hallmark presented by the PAP government. Upon coming into power, the PAP Members of Parliament (MPs) were often seen embarking on tree-planting and road-sweeping public exercises in their constituencies. On a more concrete level, the state drew up a total plan to both raise local living standards and reinforce the social and cultural fabric of the population. Aside from new public housing estates to replace the decaying and congested living quarters and shophouses, associated with the breeding of diseases such as tuberculosis, the government expanded its public health infrastructure radically as an entire network of modern hospitals and polyclinics were established around the country. Accompanied by these medical centres were the preventive health measures including cleaning up polluted rivers and districts, and countless public campaigns designed to shape the social health of Singaporeans by changing personal habits such as littering, spitting, smoking and family planning. The state also meted out hefty fines on failures to maintain public sanitation standards. This included the failure of individuals to flush public toilets and households that kept stagnant water, which could provide a potential breeding ground for mosquitoes. Whole industries and powerful political lobbying groups from farmers to street hawkers, whose trades were considered unhygienic, were phased out or marginalised.

Within a generation, the long list of infectious diseases from plague to malaria in the colonial medical reports were no longer part of the vocabulary by the 1970s. Life expectancy grew and infant mortality dived, as death rates no longer exceeds birthrates. By the same period, from a colonial port city, Singapore became the "Garden City" with a global reputation for both its cleanliness and strict laws. In the area of public health and state medicine, the "Singapore Story" became one of triumphant progressivism based on the successful application of modern Western medical and public health discourses. By 1984, the focus of healthcare has shifted from preventive public health measures and the provision of primary medical facilities to catering and mounting burden of chronic geriatric health problems associated with a rapidly ageing population (PAP, 1984).

The area of public health has been a crucial area in which both the achievements and vulnerabilities of Singapore have been played up by the official discourse. In the first paragraph of Singapore elder statesman Lee Kuan Yew's foreword for the PAP's 50th Anniversary souvenir publication, he reconstructed a more distant but harsher Singapore where:

> Young Singaporeans cannot imagine what Singapore was 50 years ago. Old photographs, films audio tapes can give some impressions, but they cannot recapture the dust, dirt and smell or the squalor and filth. The Singapore River was an open sewer exuding sulphur dioxide. Singapore had just emerged from three and a half years of Japanese occupation, during which people suffered brutality, privation hunger and disease. A harsh life tempered the spirit of the people who struggled for a better tomorrow (PAP, 2004).

The invisible and irrational microbe of SARS challenged this triumph. Even with the occasional localised dengue fever and hand, foot and mouth disease outbreaks, as well as the international concerns regarding avian flu

and BSC (mad cow) disease, the Republic continued to place little investments on epidemic control. On the eve of the outbreak of SARS, the
issue of infectious diseases received little or no mention in the health and
environment section of the Annual Yearbook on the Republic in 2002. In
fact, more attention was given to preparing for any potential incidents of
bio-terrorism. During the preparations for a commemorative book on the
fight against SARS in Tan Tock Seng Hospital, the Chief Executive Officer
realised that the institution had a precedent for dealing with contagious diseases, as it was once gazetted in 1945 as a tuberculosis (TB) ward (*The Straits
Times*, 7 May 2004). Hence, when SARS first spread uncontrollably in this
hospital from a single person infected in Hong Kong, the Health Minister
was quick to declare it a national crisis tantamount to Singapore's 9–11. This
declaration meant that the epidemic demanded a response beyond that of
the Health Ministry.

"Singaporeans are Really Scared"

While a more substantial survey would be required to gauge the actual
sentiments and experiences of the populace of SARS affected countries,
it would not be inaccurate to describe the climate as one of heightened
anxiety. Like the other Asian counterparts, the country was already gripped
by fear and panic as the usually congested malls and markets were reduced
to a trickle, while its huge international airport was left receiving a handful
of arrivals and departures. This sentiment was highlighted by then Prime
Minister Goh Chok Tong who thought in retrospect that:

> For me, the most appropriate coinage for SARS was "Singaporeans
> Are Really Scared". Yes, we were really scared. Scared for our
> lives and our loved ones. Scared of taking a taxi, scared of going to
> the hospital. Scared that tourists and customers would not return,
> and we might lose our job. For the first time in our history, all
> Singaporeans felt the same fear at the same time." (*The Straits Times*,
> 17 August 2003).

In addition, the social stigma and fear of healthcare institutions developed
quickly, and hospitals and clinics were increasingly avoided by a frightened

public. These trends prompted government leaders to appeal for calm. As Lee Kuan Yew commented:

'If we start to fear and shun all human contact, and refuse to see friends or relatives, enter a lift, or taxi, or bus or MRT (trains), or go to meetings, hawker centres, restaurants, hotels, or concerts, we will become hermits. 'We will shut down Singapore. To close down everything inside Singapore, shut off the outside world, or cut off visitors from SARS-infected countries, not travel by air and completely isolate ourselves, will be madness. 'We cannot shut ourselves off from the world (*The Straits Times*, 26 April 2003).

The government had decided from the beginning of the pandemic to be transparent with their information and policies on SARS, in order to provide a more accurate picture to both the local population and international community. This was done to prevent speculation and confusion that would be counterproductive as was shown in China's case. This alone was not sufficient, as the state found itself grappling with the fears of its citizens as much as the spread of the virus, which was still confined to the local hospitals. Finding an equilibrium formula to placate unpredictable public fears would prove to be as difficult as a search for a cure or vaccine to contain the virus. The first taste of this attempt was the Education Ministry's delayed decision to suspend the school term. As mentioned by *Asia Times,*

The most dramatic example of this was the joint Health and Education ministries' decision March 25 to close nearly all the schools — not on medical grounds, they said, but because 'principals and general practitioners have reported that parents continue to be concerned about the risk to their children in schools' (*Asia Times*, 9 April 2003)

Eventually, the two-week suspension neither fulfilled the aim of safeguarding public health nor placated parents. Students happily spent their time in malls and arcades, whilst some parents were unhappy that they had to make special arrangements for childcare.

The problem with the schools was just the tip of the iceberg requiring government's efforts to ease public tensions about SARS. Without any immediate cures in sight, it had to rely solely on "medieval" concepts of basic sanitary care, self-examination and quarantine and isolation. To convince the local population and the world that it was safe to move beyond the confines of home, it had to show the public that those infected were being kept away at a safe distance, and that the conditions for the spread of the virus were reduced to a minimum. To achieve this standard, active social consent and cooperation from the population had to be secured in order to impose medical policing and treatment. Visibly shaken by the epidemic, the bulk of the population had little disagreement to curtailing their individual autonomy and subjecting themselves to the state medical surveillance. Even without formal prompting, many were already administering their own "fever tests" by taking their temperatures and faithfully washing their hands and cleaning their homes several times daily.

However, the government felt that the general population needed to appreciate the severity of the crisis. Hence, it framed the containment of SARS in militaristic terms rather than as a public health issue. SARS was a "war" in which every citizen was a soldier and the thermometer was his or her weapon. National leaders led, for example, by showing that they were also subjected to fever checks on public occasions and in their workplace, aside from demonstrating the "correct" way of washing their hands and living hygienic lifestyles. A huge part of the public education programme lay in "fighting misguided fears and ignorance" of the epidemic that would either lead to the further spread of the disease or to social disorders through misinformation (*The Straits Times*, 26 April 2003). Meanwhile, information pamphlets and booklets on SARS accompanied by thermometers were also widely distributed to households and a "SARS television channel" was also set up to propagate such educational programmes and updates on the event.

In this "war," the negligent actions of either the "less vigilant," like hospital staff who failed to wear their protective masks and gears, or the "socially irresponsible" who breached quarantine and other public health regulations amounted to treachery. Whilst the former was merely chided, the latter received the stiffest punishments for the offences, and public shaming by the state and media machinery. Shortly after the outbreak of SARS, the PAP-dominated parliament voted to strengthen and stiffen the penalties of the Infectious Diseases Act. The passing of these amendments were marked by a solemn speech by a Parliamentarian (who was also a medical practitioner) who called for stringent laws to punish those who were shown to be socially irresponsible such as the quarantine breakers. In a stern tone, he pronounced that he was in favour of more draconian measures to fight the epidemic (*The Straits Times*, 26 April 2003). Compulsory treatment at the designed SARS hospital was required for the infected, and those who had been in contact with the victims were served Home Quarantine Orders (HQOs), which confined them to their homes for a period of ten days. The highlight of the HQOs was the enforcement, measures that included constabulary police serving the legal orders to the affected, followed by the installation of a surveillance closed circuit video camera in the household.

Members of the affected households were legally required to appear in front of the camera at random times during the day to prove their presence, and to respond to phone checks from the police. Their neighbours were also encouraged to partake in the process by reporting any suspected breaches (*The Straits Times*, 4 May 2003). Repeated quarantine breakers were also swiftly dealt with, as shown by the imprisonment of an offender who was portrayed to possess a troubled criminal background (*The Straits Times*, 10 May 2003). A family suspected of contracted SARS who defied instructions and went "doctor hopping" (seeing several doctors and thereby increasing the possibility of spreading infection) were publicly chided by the Prime Minister (Singapore Government Press Release, 22 April 2003). The scrutiny of the law was also vigorously applied to ordinary citizens. Anti-social offences like littering and spitting, which were usually dealt with by a series of fines, now warranted compulsory counselling and corrective work orders and were branded anti-patriotic during the SARS period (*The Straits Times*, 3 May 2003).

During the SARS episode, there were admirable acts of courage and empathy from health workers to ordinary citizens. There was however a corresponding and pervasive climate of paranoia in society at large, witnessed in the avoidance of those working in health institutions or those returning from SARS affected countries (*The Straits Times*, 10 October 2003). The state took an active part in handling the epidemic and certain shortfalls, given that the exigencies of the situation indeed required extraordinary measures. The underlying principles and implications of its policies should not have been left unexamined. Even as the SARS epidemic was waning, a more contrived script was already emerging.

SARS and the Repertoire of Legitimating Stories

For two months, the SARS epidemic subjected Singapore residents to intense fear and uncertainty over both their own personal health and the larger economic climate. yet, as claimed in state controlled media:

> Psychologically, a nation came together, battling a common enemy. Having come through a crisis that was both deadly and swift, Singaporeans emerged stronger with more resilient systems and with sure knowledge that together, if they could beat SARS, they can overcome other challenges (Chua, 2004).

Translated into actual events, this meant that the frontline health workers involved held the fort and contained the spread of the virus in the hospital where the first case was admitted. The general population played its by part in observing clinical and hygiene standards prescribed, as well as rendering moral and financial support to the distressed. It is however debatable whether these spirited efforts have been possible without the "decisive leadership" of the government. Its draconian enforcement of quarantine regulations, co-ordination of resources, transparency of information and public education programmes earned it popular trust and international recognition. As the epidemic unfolded, the story of SARS became "a defining moment." This positively crafted script about SARS in the Republic came not only from the official mouthpieces, but was also emphasised in carefully selected professional and anecdotal analysis and comments from international and local bodies.

So convincing was Singapore's battle against SARS that it seemed to have gained common and almost uncritical acclaim among the medical experts, the international media and even historians of medicine. A health official for WHO felt that the Singapore government had done "an excellent job" and stated that he would not characterise the state's action as draconian"

(*The Straits Times,* 6 October 2003). This sentiment was shared by the otherwise critical *Asian Wall Street Journal* (28 April 2003), whose editorial expressed that

> "We've sometimes been critical of Singapore's degree of protection of civil liberties, but when public health is seriously threatened...it is difficult to find fault with a quarantine... If only Hong Kong and China would take SARS seriously."

Responding to an interview with the local media, Dr Howard Markel, director of the Centre for the History of Medicine at the University of Michigan, endorsed the quick and decisive leadership and policies embarked in Singapore and stressed that

> "We have to keep our public health 'police force' strong, even in quiet times, and we have to make sure it's international and global in perspective" (*The Straits Times,* 4 August 2003).

These accounts were reproduced in the Singaporean media which held them up to the public as an external endorsement of the Singapore government's policies.

It was also interesting that compliance with state regulations during SARS provided a certain sense of self-gratification among Singaporeans. As noted by a doctor who is also prominently involved in civil society affairs:

> "We did not see the kind of hysteria that was evident in other places, such as hospital workers climbing out of windows to escape internment in Taiwan or anti-establishment rantings against both government action and inaction in Toronto. Singaporeans just got down to it, obeyed instructions and waited for it to blow over." (*The Straits Times,* 3 August 2003)

Perhaps the most graphic example of such unquestioned heroism and sacrifice was seen in the accounts of an infected doctor and his family at the

SARS treatment facility in the Tan Tock Seng Hospital:

> Dr Leong and his family were not allowed to use the toilets. For
> safety reasons, they had to empty their bowels in a commode, which
> was then thrown into a bin and sealed for incineration. Every day
> there was a barrage of tests. To study the virus, doctors took between
> eight and 10 tubes of blood a day from each of them for nearly
> 18 days, so much so that his wife became anaemic. Said Dr Leong:
> 'She was pregnant but she said, 'Let's do it. It's for science. If we
> die, so be it. But the mark we so leave and the information we so
> give, may hopefully help someone' (*The Straits Times*, 6 October
> 2003).

SARS and the Search for a Place in History

An essential aspect of the epidemic was the provision of a crisis around
which the second and third generation of Singaporeans and their leaders
could establish their legitimacy as equals to the toughness of their first generation counterparts, personified by the elder statesman Lee Kuan Yew. A
"young Singaporean" journalist freelancer spoke of the "end of the soft generation", when the onslaught of SARS made the "younger generation sit
up and realize that economic prosperity and something as fundamental as
good health are not givens" (*The Straits Times*, 27 April 2003). The question
of the ability of the descendents of Lee's Singapore to ensure the continued
prosperity of the city-state has not only been the concern of the octogenar-
ian himself, but also an important national issue which was widely discussed.
As Lee remarked in the celebrations of his 80th birthday a few months after
the SARS epidemic:

> The people I had to lead out of the wilderness were poor, had
> known hardship, could endure great difficulties and were prepared
> to work. The present generation has grown up in comfort. They
> expect the comfort to improve. When we say 'lower your expec-
> tations', they get terribly upset, depressed'. They say 'Oh, there is
> no future'…In my time when we faced a fight, nobody talked such
> defeatist language (Petir, 2003: 55).

Four decades after Independence, the PAP government remains concerned about shaping the writing of the country's history as a means of preserving and perpetuating its founding myths and hegemony. In the preface of his widely publicised memoirs for example, Lee states that:

> I wrote this book for a younger generation of Singaporeans who took stability, growth and prosperity for granted...Those who have been through the trauma of war in 1942 and the Japanese occupation, and taken part in building a new economy for Singapore, are not so sanguine. We cannot afford to forget that public order, personal security, economic and social progress and prosperity are not the natural order of things, they depend on ceaseless effort and attention from an honest and effective government that people must elect (Lee, 2000: 11).

While Lee's contemporaries were political activists moulded by the turmoil of their era, their younger counterparts were mostly mandarins parachuted into a significantly tamer political arena by the early 1970s. Hence, it was not surprising that Lee's successors saw in SARS an opportunity to position themselves along the same lines as their lionised predecessors. As such, policies which demonstrated "strong and decisive leadership" and portrayals of the unhesitant deployment of draconian and invasive public health measures by the government were meant to connote firmness and resoluteness in the face of adversity.

In the process, the political leadership asserted itself by conveying the seriousness of SARS in apocalyptic tones. It continuously framed the SARS campaign as analogous to a real war. Thus, hospitals have turned into battlefronts with trench, conventional and unconventional campaigns being raged against the "enemy" (Chua, 2004; Ng, 2003). The otherwise ordinary thermometers distributed became the "weapon" with which every Singaporean was being armed. In this war, the "invisible enemy" of the SARS virus had to be defeated by labelling detractors who broke quarantine and hygiene regulations as traitors. Conversely, especially the health workers who held down the fort were generously awarded, and their fallen comrades remembered in vigils. In effect, the "militarisation" of SARS serves to highlight the political leadership as battle-tested commanders and generals in times of crisis.

While serving to boost the credibility and larger legitimacy of the state, the political capitalisation of SARS through its historicisation and memorialisation becomes problematic. To begin with, the presentation of a triumphalist version has undermined a more critical public assessment of the episode. While lauding praises on the draconian actions of the government, a *Straits Times* columnist thought aloud on the need to explore its wider implications on the political culture of the republic. Therefore:

> When the dust has settled on SARS, and the level of public emergency abates, these questions must be asked: Are Singaporeans comfortable living in a society with a paternalistic government which has great powers over almost all resources in the country? In the trade-off between civil liberties and public order, is there an unbreachable line in the sand, or does anything go, so long as public safety is assured (*The Straits Times*, 10 May 2003).

This question did not provoke further discussion or review in the public sphere. In examining the relationship between the demands of transparencies and authoritarian governments, Garry Rodan noted,

> In the Singapore fight against SARS the Infectious Diseases Act was also promptly amended to legalise an assortment of measures that further erode civil liberties in the city-state. Indeed, far from SARS posing a threat to the credibility of authoritarian media controls or the regime more generally in Singapore, it had quite the opposite effect (Rodan, 2004)

In addition, by continuously playing up the myths of unity and cohesion in the discourse of fighting SARS, the broader but more subtle social fissures manifested during the epidemic were downplayed. During the epidemic, acts of fear were as prevalent as the display of courage. People avoided areas in close proximity to hospitals, shunned contact with healthcare workers, stigmatised infected victims and quarantined residents even after recovery or the lifting of restrictions. The state too was perhaps complicit in creating such a climate of fear and accusation as a result of its socially divisive policies of attributing blame and suspicion. Foreign migrant workers, for example, coming to Singapore for the first time were subjected to a compulsory ten-day quarantine upon arrival, whilst tourists from the same places were exempted. There was absolute perception that class privileges were demonstrated at the causeway checkpoints to Malaysia, where it appeared that travellers in private vehicles were often exempted from temperature checks required of those travelling by public buses. There was a controversial move by the state to cull stray cats on a massive scale, against the protests of various animal welfare groups who found the policy to be overtly reactive, cruel and counterproductive.

Finally, in placing utmost emphasis and significance on SARS, the state inevitably distorted its public health priorities on the more endemic infectious diseases, particularly that of HIV/AIDS. Compared with SARS, HIV/AIDS, which has been a chronic and growing problem in Singapore, has received little attention from the government. However, officials lay the blame for this sexually transmitted disease on the alleged promiscuity of homosexuals and heterosexual working class men. It has also implemented policies of compulsory AIDS testing for pregnant women, a group which was easier to police. In explaining the difference, the government has stated that AIDS cannot be given the same publicity as SARS, since the former involves personal choices and lifestyles (Sadasivan, 2004). For a paternalistic government prone to invasive measures, this stance seems baffling. Ironically, even though AIDS has crippled nations and societies across the world, it is unable to engender the same public fears and elicit the same commitment that SARS did, and thus it failed to mould a cohesive population led by firm and decisive leaders in Singapore. To the Singapore officialdom, the fight against AIDS is merely part of routine public health administration, whereas SARS is associated with history making and defining moments.

Conclusion: From Natural Cycle to History Making

A whole literary fiction of festivals grew up around the plague; suspended laws, lifted prohibitions...bodies mingling together without respect, individuals unmasked... allowing a quite different truth to appear. But there was also a political dream of the plague, which was exactly its reverse: Not the collective festival, but strict divisions; not laws transgressed, but the penetration of regulation into even the smallest details of everyday life through the mediation of the complete hierarchy that assumed the capillary functioning of power; not masks that were put on were taken off, but the assignment to each individual of his 'true' name, his 'true' place, his 'true' body and his 'true' disease (Foucault, 1975).

Susan Sontag had observed that the economic cleavages between the First and Third world had created imagined medical dichotomies regarding the place of infectious diseases and epidemics in the construction of histories and identities. In the former, "major calamities are history making or transformative, while in the poor African or Asian countries, they are part of a cycle, and therefore something like an aspect of nature" (Sontag, 1989). SARS has revealed the interplay between history, history making and epidemics in newly industrialised economies such as Singapore. While natural discourses no longer allude to the scourges that plagued the colonial port city and ignore the more entrenched social and chronic diseases, SARS has been memorialised since it struck an unaccustomed fear in the society and a raw nerve in the government.

As the pandemic receded, eulogies, celebrations, memorials, praises, awards and exhibitions sprung up. On their own, such expressions were tributes to the courageous and the committed. On a higher political realm, in defining SARS as a "defining moment" in Singapore's history, the state has utilised the episode as a legitimising tool to entrench the PAP's hegemonic position. From just merely emergency public policies erected to combat the epidemic, SARS was in turn carefully re-scripted to demonstrate both the logic and strengths of a paternalistic and authoritarian system of governance. Accounts of praise were carefully selected in the state-dominated media, not just from citizens but also from foreign observers to illustrate the virtues of cooperation and deference to the state's leadership in containing the epidemic. Successors of the pioneering generations of leaders could claim to have undergone their rite of passage, as their predecessors had experienced anti-colonial struggles and nation-building efforts.

The construction and historicisation of the triumphant aspects of SARS to serve broader political ends, preclude placing the episode within a more critical hindsight. The painting of an unprecedented united and cohesive society by the media and government, and the selective memories of the public sideline issues of discrimination and stigma were also prominent themes during the crisis period. Heaping praises on the firm and decisive leadership deploying invasive measures stifles critical review of the actual policies or a more informed discussion of their implications for state-society relations. In arguing that "the body is not a battlefield," Sontag (1989) has warned that the framing of diseases in military metaphors becomes more dangerous and far-reaching in its consequences, since it provides a persuasive justification for authoritarian rule and implicitly suggests the necessity of state measures as being analogous to surgical removal of the offending parts of the body politic. In the process, military imagery applied to disease "overmobilises, overdescribes, and it powerfully contributes to the excommunication and stigmatising of the ill" (Sontag, 1989). When the war on SARS continued to be remembered and revered in museums and commemorations, the fighters and victims of more chronic and endemic diseases like AIDS weaken in their claims, not so much for a proper place in the annals of "The Singapore Story," but for more support and recognition.

References

Bewell A. (1999) *Romanticism and Colonial Disease*. The John Hopkins University Press, Baltimore.

Chua MH. (2004) *A Defining Moment: How Singapore Beat SARS*. Stamford Press, Singapore.

Conrad L. (1992) Epidemic diseases in formal and popular thought in early islamic society, in T. Ranger and P. Slack (eds.), *Epidemics and Ideas: Essays on the Historical Perception of Pestilence*, Cambridge University Press, Cambridge.

Foucault M. (1975) *Discipline and Punish: The Birth of the Prison*. Penguin Books, London

Kushner T. (1992) *Angels in America; A Gay Fantasia on National Themes*. Theatre Communications Group, USA

Lee KY. (2000) *The Singapore Story: From Third World to First*. Times Academic Press, Singapore.

Lewontin R, Levins R. (2003) The return of old diseases and the appearance of new ones, in M. Gandy, A. Zumla (eds.), *The Return of the White Plague*. Verso, New York.

Ministry of Information and the Arts. (2003). *Singapore 2002*.

Ng WC. (2003) *The Silent War, 1 March–31 May 2003*. Tan Tock Seng Hospital, Singapore.

People's Action Party (2004) *PAP 50; Five Decades of the People's Action Party*. People's Action Party, Singapore.

People's Action Party (2003) *Petir*. May/June 2003.

People's Action Party (2003) *Petir*. September/October.

People's Action Party (1984) *PAP;1954–84*. Singapore: People's Action Party.

Philips H, Killingray D. (eds). (2003) *The Spanish Influenza Pandemic of 1918–19; New Perspectives*. Routledge, New York, London.

Rodan G. (2004) *Transparency and Authoritarian Rule in Southeast Asia; Singapore and Malaysia*. Routledge Curzon, London.

Singapore Government Press Release. (2003) "Fighting SARS Together." Open letter by Prime Minister Goh Chok Tong. 22 April 2003.

Singapore Government Press Release. (2003) Speech by Prime Minister Goh Chok Tong at the National Day Rally on 17 August 2003.

Singapore Government Press Release. (2004) Speech by Dr Balaji Sadasivan, Senior Minister of State (Health) at the 4th Singapore Conference on Aids on 27 Nov 2004.

Sontag S. (1989) *Aids and its Metaphors*. London, Allen Lane.

20

SARS and China's Rural Migrant Labour: Roots of a Governance Crisis

David Kelly and Xiaopeng Luo

Background

In a page-one story in *People's Daily*, senior party leader Li Changchun announced that China had succeeded in fighting SARS, thanks to the heroic efforts nationwide (Xinhua, 2003).[1] The previous week had seen a large number of such statements with the names of Communist Party Secretary General Hu Jintao and Premier Wen Jiabao standing high in the media acclaim.

Hu and Wen clearly made political capital from the crisis. They ventured early into the public arena, calling for forthright policies and opposing the cover-up which they tacitly allowed to be associated with the recently ended regime of Jiang Zemin. With dramatic public appearances in SARS-affected locations, they appeared more in the mould of Western politicians than stolid, aloof Communist leaders of the past. They announced a two-fisted

---

[1] Li was a member of the Standing committee of the Politburo and in charge of "moulding the public mind."

policy of defeating the epidemic, while maintaining economic growth and stability.[2]

In raw economic terms, SARS was contained and will have little visible effect. In some instances, worst-case scenarios simply failed to be realised, as in the prediction that the electronics industry in Guangdong province, a huge earner for the nation, would be disrupted. SARS hit at the low point in the annual production cycle and its effects were thus minimised (Xinhua, 2003a; Jingji Ribao, 2003).

Clearly, the long-term implications of the SARS epidemic reach beyond economic indicators to China's underlying social and political structures. As analysts concluded earlier on, "SARS will set off a variety of forces which the government will try to control, but which are going to be increasingly difficult to contain"(Fewsmith, 2003). The crisis allowed a period of comparative freedom of discussion, particularly in the print media. This was brought to an end in July, with controls deepening and extending in the

---

[2]In a speech to the State Council on 21 May, Wen delineated six tasks to accomplish this (Xinhua 21 May 2003b"):

1. We must persist in the principle of expanding internal demand and uphold a positive financial policy. We should fully take advantage of the fact that the market in our country is huge and that there is plenty of room for economic growth, foster strengths to make up for weaknesses, and allow investment and consumption to promote economic growth. Financial departments at all levels should *increase investment in public health facilities* to ensure sufficient funds for preventing and treating atypical pneumonia.

2. We should implement a policy of giving assistance to enterprises that have been quite seriously affected by atypical pneumonia and work out a plan to help the relevant enterprises after atypical pneumonia has gone.

3. We must do a good job in foreign trade and in using foreign investments, implement a policy that encourages exports, and effectively help foreign investors solve practical difficulties and problems in production and operations.

4. We should show concern for the production and livelihood of the masses in financial difficulties, further do a good job in providing employment and social security work, help laid-off and unemployed workers find jobs, help graduates of schools of higher learning find jobs, and pay attention to providing basic means of livelihood to families in serious financial difficulties. We should support the construction of the "six small" projects in rural areas in order to allow more peasants to find jobs.

5. We must maintain normal production and living order, ensure smooth transportation and normal flow of personnel, rectify and standardise the order of the market economy, and improve safety in production.

6. We should formulate a long-term plan for reforms and development. Wen requested that state officials have confidence in struggling against SARS, take initiatives to do their work well under the special environment of combating it, and work hard in an orderly way.

intervening two years. Yet, the discussion had shone a revealing light on the nature of China's social and political system; in some cases, it confirmed earlier analysis, whilst in others, it provided data for new interpretations.

The public health system, from its basic epidemic detection and alert system to its bureaucracy and leadership, has naturally attracted intense scrutiny, not only from international organisations spearheaded by the WHO, but from observers and the general public in China as well.

SARS exposed problems in the party-state's governance in unprecedented ways. The lack of transparency or of freedom of information in the government's handling of a massive threat to public health became an inescapable issue. What may have seemed obvious to international audiences, that secrecy about an epidemic will only increase rather than contain the risk, is partly obscured in China by references to political culture, age-old traditions attributed to Confucius and others, whose writings are generally held to impart that the masses cannot be trusted to deal rationally with threats to their security. They will panic, or worse, arbitrarily switch political allegiance, and chaos will ensue. Secrecy and misreporting are therefore legitimate tools of governance (Zhou, 2000).

Many people in China subscribe to such cultural explanations for the practices of cover-up and "positively spinning" the truth, but this often confuses the issue. For one thing, the media are *not* officially cleared to "spin" to the leadership; they are charged with reporting confidentially and factually to the higher levels (*unofficial* spin cannot of course be excluded). Suppression of vital information is a political rather an a cultural issue. "The current situation is primarily the product of systemic restraints on freedom of expression that prevented PRC citizens from talking more openly about SARS when it first appeared" (CECC, 2003).

More plausibly cultural in nature was the failure of China's medical research apparatus to follow up the initial lead of some of its own researchers in identifying SARS as a coronavirus. As the authoritative journal *Science* reported, once senior medical authorities had pronounced that it was a *Chlamydia*-like bacteria rather than a virus, the research units which had successfully proven otherwise felt it was too "disrespectful" to argue for their findings in public. As the US Congressional report suggested, a public arena for dissenting science scarcely exists in China, and it is among the nation's most glaring governance gaps (Enserink, 2003).

A major reason for the immense impact of SARS was because, unlike previous crises such as the Asian financial crisis (1997, 1998), the bombing of China's embassy in Belgrade (1999), Falun Gong (2000), or the EP3 spy plane incident (2001), SARS could not credibly be laid at the feet of foreign interests. Unlike floods, earthquakes, fires and other natural disasters, it could not be isolated to a small area as well. Everyone, rich or poor, great or humble, was a possible victim. Despite its wealth, power and the best medical facilities in the country, Beijing was seemingly powerless to prevent itself from becoming the world focus of the disease.

Disturbing as this was, there were concerns about an even greater potential disaster — that of the uncontrolled spread of the epidemic to the rural areas (Zhang, 2003), which is home to the majority of the population, and due to decades of discriminatory policies, they are deprived of the medical resources available in cities such as Beijing. If urban China was threatened, what would become of the hinterland should the disease find a vector of transmission?

In fact, the floating population of "migrant workers" from the rural areas (*nongmin gong,* referred to colloquially as *mingong*) was one such vector.[3] The widely-circulated business journal *21st Century Economic Herald* focused on this threat in an important editorial published soon after the SARS crisis was officially admitted (*Economic Herald*, 2003):

> In rural regions, after the reforms in division of financial functions, the profit motive was strengthened at every level of government; many regions had a situation in which state functions were devolved downward, while ownership of assets was transferred up. This led to serious shortfalls in local governments' public funding allocations (particularly for education and public health). This was another reason for the Centre to promote village self-government. Meanwhile in the cities, due the existence of a large surplus labour force, cheap migrant labour became the engine of economic growth of the developed regions, though improvements in their level of social security

---

[3] The expression "migrant" is troublesome as the *mingong* are not free to permanently transfer their official residence to their places of work.

were relatively slow. The tension between the advantages of cheap labour and safeguarding the rights of the migrant workers became daily more obvious with swiftly rising economic standards. Without safeguards, stability is problematic; bottlenecks in the *hukou* registration system[4] and social security create problems in the administration of a highly mobile group of migrant workers.

Mingong and SARS

The *mingong* emerged as a policy focus earlier in 2003, when Premier Zhu Rongji, drew special attention to the risks they posed to stability (Bezlova, 2003) in one of his last addresses to the National People's Congress in March. The current direction of Zhu's successor, Wen Jiabao, is consistent with this. Subsequent State Council edicts have tended to reinforce this impression as well (State Council, 2003).

The search for growth based on migrant workers has been a success on a number of levels, but at the same time, it exposed the entire system to serious risks, of which SARS was but a single case. Critical Chinese sources describe this situation as "fragility" and "vulnerability." This applies less to the economy which as a whole is reasonably robust than to the political and social systems undergirding it.

The *21st Century Economic Herald* went on to say,

> The *mingong* are "suspended in mid-air," unable to settle securely in the cities, moving between village and town year after year, not seasonally, but year-round. A body suspended in mid-air is not stable: this is a law applicable not only in physics but in human society as well. When a society of over 1 billion people is unstable, their social actions may have a direct impact on the stability of the

---

[4]The *hukou* system of permanent residence registration in use since the mid 1950s, remains a basic means of controlling internal migration. A *hukou* entitles individuals to live in a city with access to social welfare (healthcare, social welfare, housing, education, housing and much else). In most cases one inherits from one's mother the status if "agricultural" or "non-agricultural" *hukou*. See "Hukou," http://en.wikipedia.org/wiki/Hukou; "Hukou Reform Targets Urban-Rural Divide" http://www.usembassy-china.org.cn/econ/hukou.html.

society as a whole. During SARS, the danger this group brings to rural society when it returns home is only the beginning. In fact, anything which impinges on the livelihood of this group, even if its onset is less sudden, even if their actions are quite unorganised, will nonetheless not only trigger unrest within this group, but also bring about wider social instability.

This was repeated in much of the subsequent media coverage (Chow, 2003; Hu, 2003). Rural China is a major concern, simply by view of the massive population directly affected (900 million rural residents out of a total population of 1.3 billion). Furthermore, far from being segregated, it is intimately linked to other social and economic sectors. Whatever the reasons, China's leadership through the 1990s focused in relative terms on boosting the interests of urban, industrialising, modernising China, on consolidating tangible evidence of the success of reform and opening. In the Maoist framework that is still second nature to many leaders, the rural hinterland was rightly and properly the source of surplus value needed as investment capital for the nation as a whole. The need for "industry to repay agriculture" was addressed only in 2005 (Kelly, 2005).

Perhaps more importantly, the rural sector was treated as intractable. The deep issues of the lack of clarity concerning land, its ownership, allocation, usage and transfer have so far defeated the attempts of reformers. A detailed account of China's dependence on rural migrant labour and some of its ramifications in the overall national system is necessary to show the interplay of political structure and governance. It is generally assumed that there is a surplus supply of labour in China, leading to an obvious international advantage with regard to labour costs. If surplus population is common to all developing countries, why is China uniquely successful?

Origins of the mingong model of economic growth

Key features of China's evolving economic system result from the unique sequence of historical events through which it came into existence. A full account of this path dependency cannot be described here,[5] but the part which is relevant is the *mingong* model. *Mingong* forms the core of the labour

---

[5] http://en.wikipedia.org/wiki/Path_dependence

force engaged in China's export processing industry, whose cheap labour as its main competitive advantage.

The economic system is officially designated a "socialist market economy with Chinese characteristics." At its core is a hierarchical arrangement of property rights such as *state, collective* and *private* ownership. Surrounding this core are three distinctive traits of the Chinese economy

(a) State ownership dominant, but never clearly defined

The state holds ownership rights over major material assets, including visible assets of the industrial, financial, communications and major service industries. As official estimates show, this has changed little even after more than 20 years of reform. Operating assets controlled by SOEs alone account for > 170 trillion (probably exclusive of most municipal land and many non-operating assets).

However, the definition of state property is far from clear. A basic issue is that the theoretically unified property is in fact partitioned. Regional governments, for instance, control many assets, especially those created through their own investment, that the central government simply cannot recover, although they do not belong to the regional governments in theory. The deliberate retention of legal ambiguity about the demarcation of ownership gives the higher echelons more flexible control.

(b) Resource allocation according to ranking of different ownership forms

Within the economy, property was segregated in various ways: central *vs* regional, state- *vs* collectively-owned, urban *vs* rural. Prior to the reforms, collective ownership, even less clearly defined, was prevalent. This "all-but-state-owned" sector arose out of the CPC's inability to create a system of state ownership as complete as that of the USSR. The collectives, which nominally owned the assets, did not have final disposal rights in reality. Before the reforms, the state granted free medical care, education, very low-cost housing and other public goods to members of the state-owned economy. Members of the collective economy missed out. There was clear discrimination according to the differences in rank. At the apex of the pyramid sat central SOEs, below which were the regional ones and then the urban collective economy. Lowest of all was the rural collective agriculture.

A private economy emerged after the reforms, but never completely shed its pariah status. This is seen today in its lack of access to bank credit. Under the double pressure of discrimination from the state economy and the competition from the private economy, most collective ownership transferred to the latter.

(c) Hierarchy in social status corresponds to hierarchy in property arrangements

Given the ownership rank of all productive units, those working in them were also implicitly endowed with different social status — again something unknown in the socialist bloc. Before the reforms, historically unprecedented migration controls were put in place in order to preserve this hierarchy. There would be no freedom of movement, or of occupation. A quasi–caste system arose. Marriage between those in higher and lower strata was discouraged; movement from a higher to a lower stratum was favoured as a form of political punishment, whilst movement vice versa spelt political advancement. Situated at the base of the tripartite pyramid of China's polity, economy and society were the peasants on collective farms. Lacking physical freedom, they resembled medieval serfs.

First of all, the logic of the reforms was to increase the economic freedom of the bottom strata, so as to produce an externality effect which would drive market reform of the higher strata. However, "marketisation" could develop only on condition that it did not threaten the rank structure of the pyramid. This pyramid and its stability mechanisms are thus intrinsic to the economy and its reform.

Post-reform economic growth has undergone three stages. While maintaining the pyramid structure, economic growth at each stage has been realised by constantly expanding the economic freedom of the peasants, and successfully creating income opportunities for the vast rural labour force.

Phase 1: Breakthrough of household responsibility contracts and economic growth driven by growth of agriculture

The first major breakthrough in reform was the household responsibility system (HRS). In this system, peasant households gained independent economic operation, but to keep the system "socialist," ownership of the land remained in the hands of local collectives. It was leased for up to 50 years to member households who paid no rent, but were taxed by the government according to the size of their holdings. Decollectivisation greatly raised the efficiency of agriculture, but success of the HRS also laid in the fact that it was not as threatening to the entire pyramid as some party leaders had feared. This was largely because there had been no privatisation; the peasantry had only acquired usage rights over their land. The term and rules of transfer of these rights were neither defined nor safeguarded. Thus, "collective ownership of land" perpetuated the centre's control over the peasantry. Local cadres could make use of their power over land allocation and transfers to obtain personal advantage.

The major contribution of the HRS was to thoroughly eliminate material bottlenecks to the country's economic growth, and secondly to set free the rural labour power. The HRS allowed 900 million peasants to allocate their time without interference, and become a prime force driving the market economy. This was because the facts of pre-HRS surplus of labour had been concealed by the low efficiency of collectivised agriculture, while, the bulk of this surplus emerged post HRS. Making use of this rural labour surplus became an unavoidable issue for the policymakers of the time. Quite clearly, this surplus could not be used without adopting market methods and the reformist leadership made conscious use of this in pushing for market reforms.

Phase 2: Economic growth driven by development of rural industry

High rates of growth in agriculture drove the first wave of post–reform economic growth. The second wave came from rapid growth of rural industry. This was the result of combining cheap rural labour with industrial capital in the countryside. The countryside rather than the cities was imperative since it would destabilise the pyramid if the peasants came into the cities. A slogan of the time was*li tu bu li xiang* (leaving the land but not the county) let peasants start industries where they were, even though in terms of economic location and environmental protection it was far from rational, even though China's degree of urbanisation was far lower than that other countries at the same income level.

Phase 3: Economic growth driven by peasants leaving the village in search of work (mingong driven growth)

"Leaving the land but not the county" was limited in the successful coastal regions by local labour supplies and in the hinterland by local economic backwardness. Hence, in order to expand the employment of the rural labour force, peasants had to be allowed to move in search of work. While state-owned industrial capital was swelling in the midst of high-speed growth due to the need to protect the stability of the pyramid, it refrained from employing peasants even though the latter were willing to accept lower wages than urban residents. Peasants found work in other places thanks mainly to the expansion of private capital.

The combination of private capital and cheap rural labour in the developed coastal regions and cities came about through two circumstances. Firstly, foreign capital expanded the processing industries on China's coastal regions. In the early 21st century, processing industries (including local and foreign-invested) employ a total of some 20 million *mingong* directly, and an even greater number indirectly. In Guangdong alone, where export processing became most developed, *mingong* from other regions number some 12–14 million. Secondly, China's urban service industries developed rapidly. Pre-reformation, this sector was seriously retarded however, as urban residents' incomes rose and the operating environment for privately-owned business improved, many more urban jobs opened up for migrants. In the major cities, there are now some 100 million workers from the countryside, of whom over a half work in the service sector, and without whom the economy would come to a standstill.

Why mingong labour costs less than the reproduction cost of urban labour

Mingong constitute a form of wage labour unique to China. Although allowed to travel in search of jobs, they are unable to change their status as peasants in the collective economic system. This status limits their freedom to migrate. And, in particular limits their claim to rights equal to those of formal urban residents. Hence, the *mingong* are primarily the products of institutionalised discrimination towards people born in the countryside. One becomes a *mingong* simply because one's mother has rural residence status. The core discrimination is not allowing them to enjoy rights equal to those of regular urban residents, even when they have found urban jobs.[6]

The incomes of China's *mingong* are inadequate for them to set up households and have families in the city; their wages are lower than the reproduction cost of urban workers (Wen, 2003). Official economists argue that the low income levels are entirely the outcome of the action of market forces, but this is questionable. Arguably, it is the outcome of the dual action of discriminatory [internal] migrant policies and limited market forces.

Migration is limited above all by the cities. Acclaimed development economist Arthur Lewis famously described how marginal productivity in agriculture tends to zero under conditions of surplus labour (Ranis, 2004). Below a given income level, the supply of labour for the industrial (Lewis "modern") sector is unlimited. Hence, expanding the industrial sector does not cause wage rates to rise with increasing employment. If social and political factors played no roles, the modern sector, which occupies the position of buyers' advantage, could opt to pay just a little above the rural wage rate to make maximum profits.

In the classical Lewis' model, social and political factors are assumed such that the actual minimum wage the modern sector can offer must be adequate in maintaining a basic existence in the city for the workers and their families, implying the freedom to migrate there. If the state, by restricting this freedom for peasants, allows the modern sector to ignore the minimum requirements of a normal existence in the city for workers and their families, wages are brought closer to the theoretical minimum.

Rural land ownership arrangements thus impact on the opportunity costs of rural surplus labour. Collectively owned land is mainly equally allocated to rural households through the HRS. In the HRS period, agricultural productivity rose swiftly, urban demand for rural products increased at the same time and the overlap of these two advantages through the equal allocation of land meant that peasant incomes rose universally. Rural-urban income differentials diminished. The Lewis model generally assumes private ownership of land. As noted, land in China is equally allocated and cannot be

---

[6]If they can amass enough wealth, mingong can use this to buy a formal urban hukou. This is a big difference between the situation pre- and post-reform. While some rural entrepreneurs have realised this dream, relying on their ability and good fortune, for the overwhelming majority it is impossible.

privatised. This greatly increased the opportunity costs of labour in the early period, producing a much smaller pressure to urban migration than if the land were privatised. Given the same productivity and relative prices, if land were privatised, there would be mergers of holdings and some of the labour force would be squeezed out. The HRS prevented this and this raised incomes for the labour force in the beginning, thus raising the "conservation wage." Rapid growth of township and village enterprises (TVEs) in this period intensified this situation.

The good situation however did not last long; as rural products reached surplus and the growth of TVEs lost steam, urban–rural income differences began to widen again. Rural labour experienced extreme pressure to go out in search of employment:

(1) Due to equal allocation of land, operational size of farms was not only small, but the degree of self-sufficiency was very high. When prices of farm products fell, the extent of the drop in cash income from agriculture was much greater than in prices. What mainly led to it was peasants' self-sufficient production, heavily dependent on such modern inputs as improved varieties, chemical fertiliser, etc. A fall in the price paid for the sales of farm products does little to relieve the peasants' need for cash.

(2) The burden of taxes and fees in the countryside grew heavier and heavier. Their payment had to be made in cash rather than in kind; moreover, it had to be proportional to the area of land held. Hit both by excessive farm products and excessive taxes, land itself became a burden to many smaller or weaker households. In order to maintain basic livelihood in the countryside, income from other sources became more and more important.

Had the pace of urbanisation been raised higher at that point, concentration of rural land may have increased. The operational scale of households staying in the village there would have been greater. The degree of self-sufficiency would have been reduced and cash incomes correspondingly raised. This can be explained with a simple economic model. Assume a closed economy, with 80% of the population on the land, which is evenly allocated, and the degree of self-sufficiency is 80%. Without artificial barriers to migration to the cities, half the rural households would do so, the operational scale of rural land would double, the degree of self-sufficiency will decrease to 40%, and cash incomes would increase accordingly.

Thus, even if relative prices of agricultural products fell, peasants would still have no need to go out to work in order to maintain agricultural reproduction. On the other hand, if households are never allowed to migrate to the cities, when relative prices of agricultural products fall, in order to maintain agricultural reproduction, some members of all households will have to be *mingong*. The supply of *mingong* will be several times greater than if there were no limits to urbanisation. Over the past decade, China has come closer and closer to the latter situation. Maintaining basic production and life of many rural families has become increasingly reliant on *mingong* income. This leads to many *mingong* having to compete for jobs in the cities, lowering the value of their labour far below the levels seen in the Lewis model.

Conversely, when income from growing grain and the prospects for safeguarding household contracts over plots of land were both increased in the period immediately following SARS, there was an immediate reaction from the migrant workers, leading to a surprising "shortage" of migrant labour especially since the summer of 2004.

Specific features of the economic growth model based on unlimited supply of cheap migrant labour

1. Rapidly increased dependency on expansion of exports

Among the key features of economic growth based on unlimited supply of cheap migrant labour is a high level of dependency on export expansion. To a degree unprecedented in such a large country, China opened its doors to accommodate international capital which had now discovered the country's immense cost advantage. What was unique about China's labour market was that very low wages could buy very high quality labour.

Few other developing countries restrict peasant migration to the cities where better quality workers and their families would have long moved into the modern sector. Accepting lower levels of pay than the minimum required for the reproduction of labour in the cities is virtually ruled out for them. In the case of the Chinese, workers of this quality are forced to join the ranks of the *mingong*. Foreign capital was thus drawn by the quality as well as the low labour cost. Given this combination, wages of *mingong* in export processing industries are definitely lower than the marginal productivity of their labour, allowing international capital to earn super-profits from the low wages of *mingong*.

Notably, the state-owned industrial capital which dominates the Chinese economy is not interested in the cheap *mingong*. On the contrary, its growth is constantly in the capital- and technology-intensive direction. Over a long period, state capital has not substituted formal workers with *mingong*, for the obvious reason that it met with opposition from the formal workers.

2. Simultaneous rapid growth of state- and privately-owned assets accompanying overall economic growth

The value of China's state-owned assets (SOAs) is estimated to be at least 40 trillion.[7] Although quite a lot of SOAs were lost in the reform process, the total has greatly increased rather than decreased. Their increase has come mainly through three channels, i.e. the natural appreciation of existing assets through the development of the market economy, assets formed by national debt directly issued by the state, and assets formed by investment in private enterprises whose funds remain predominantly state held.

SOAs grow in a fourth way by conversion of collective assets to state ownership. According to China's laws, non-agriculturally used land must be owned by the state. Hence, due to rapid economic growth, a large amount of farmland has had to be transferred to non-agricultural and for the most part, commercial use. In the last decade, at least 15 m hectares have been converted from collective to state ownership. While the rights to usage are not always held by the state, they are state-owned as assets. By such conversion of land-ownership, the state has added no less than 2 trillion to the value of its assets. Rather than being in any way adequately compensated, the peasants who lost their land have been left with a great disaster.[8]

---

[7] If national territory and other state-owned natural resources are included in the calculation together with assets formed by investment.

[8] Private wealth has also grown immensely. In terms of its material form, the growth is mostly in housing and such materials of living. About half of private wealth probably comes under this heading, while the other half is mainly in the form of deposits in state-owned banks, and state bonds. It can be seen from this that while the regime has abandoned the dogmas of the planned economy, they have not forgotten Marx's teaching that ownership of the means of production determines everything. Of course, how much of the wealth nominally owned by the state is actually controlled by it is an entirely separate question, which we shall discuss separately.

3. The distribution of wealth is highly imbalanced

A third feature of the *mingong* labour model is a great imbalance in the urban/rural and inter-regional distribution of newly created wealth. One reason is that the *mingong* play a direct part in creating this wealth in the coastal regions, but are not allowed to stay there on an equal footing. The speed of development of cities in China in recent years has stunned the world, but little room is left for the *mingong* in their plans, despite the fact that more and more of them are moving to the cities with their entire households, and the cities are increasingly more dependant on the services they provide. The Chinese government up to the present has found the idea of slums unacceptable and has used every means to prevent them from developing. Although they cannot prevent it, the process is greatly distorted by government intervention.

4. Extreme inequitable allocation of financial resources

The financial crisis in the rural hinterland stemmed from the appropriation of regional government resources by the central government. While the central government finances were enhanced, the regions' expenditure commitments were not. The budgetary pressures of the regions, particularly in the rural hinterland, became ever heavier. Still more disastrous was that level after level of regional government followed the lead of the centre in increasing their income raising powers, and passing more and more expenditure commitments down to lower levels of regional government. Inevitably, responsibility for every kind of public expenditure was placed on the peasants. The deterioration of rural finance and the unlimited supply of cheap *mingong* workers became linked in a vicious cycle. With the withering of many county-level economies, reduced employment opportunities and lower wage levels stimulated further supplies of *mingong,* lowering even further the value of their labour.

The current leaders, recognising the gravity of the rural financial crisis, have opted to increase financial transfers to the countryside. However, given the present financial system, merely increasing central government transfer payments to the countryside will not solve the problem, not to mention that the transfer payments it is able to make are extremely limited.

China's financial system has a fundamental shortcoming, which is the basic cause of the extremely unfair distribution of financial resources. Following the swift increase in the scale of the *mingong*, the problem of unfair distribution of financial resources grew in intensity and prominence. A key World Bank report on Chinese financial expenditures points out that China transgresses international practice by passing the commitment to provide social security, something usually shouldered by the central governments, to the regions (Wong and Bhattalasi, 2002). In areas such as public health and education where the spillover effects are the greatest, the central government assumes too little responsibility. The problem is the central government can arbitrarily saddle regional governments with expenditure responsibilities which should be its own. The regional governments lack even the autonomy to adjust their own institutional structures in response to the economic development needs of their own regions. The result is that backward regional economies are simply forced to undertake responsibilities totally out of keeping with their economic capacity. For example, it is an insuperable task for governments in the hinterland to undertake provision of social security for their residents.

Conclusion

"Serve the people" is a venerable Maoist catchcry which was echoed in the inaugural statements of new leaders Hu Jintao and Wen Jiabao in early 2004. However, in the reform era, it was easy to provide a subtext that serving the people meant serving the most developed sector and this could be measured in numerical indices of economic growth such as GDP. SARS may have played a catalytic role in this evolving situation, since it delivered a message to virtually every politically conscious person in the nation that things were not well.

One dominant theme of the critical media during SARS was that the cover-up not only cost lives and threatened national wellbeing, it was also a betrayal of the fundamental social contract and revealed the self-serving mindset of the political elite. The question was openly asked whether the dismissal of the Minister for Health and the Mayor of Beijing was meaningful, if government persisted in ignoring the basic duty of care owed to its citizens.

Domestic initiatives to rectify the lack of public goods provision in regional China have undoubtedly increased, but their efficacy still hangs in the balance. Skilled observers such as Beijing University economist Yao Yang point to an overall organisational vacuum at the grassroots. Here, the unspoken subtext is that beyond simple and regionally tightly confined producer cooperatives, the state is most unwilling to give effective organisational autonomy to the peasantry (Yao, 2005; Zhang, 2005).

Attempts to remedy the social services available to *mingong* have been a feature of public policy since 2003, driven more by the "dearth of migrant labour" and the incoming regime's publicly announced emphasis on "serving the people", than by SARS itself. Public health has sector-wide weaknesses (Blumenthal and Hsiao, 2005) which reach their apogee in the countryside.

As we have seen, the rural-urban dichotomy has been placed in sharp relief by the epidemic. Some of the governance issues were spelled out succinctly by the 21st *Century Economic Herald* editorial cited earlier. The state's capacity to move to a clearer basic for land allocation, usage and transfer is an underlying factor; there are great pressures for it to do so, but the hidden agenda is systemic vested interests which undermines any such initiatives.

These institutional problems may be thought of as wave-like perturbations taking place on the rigid frame set by the unitary system which lingers from the ancient imperial tradition. It tends to defeat strong impulses toward a federalist constitution of the kind that clarifies regional governance and keeps it accountable. In China, the reform period saw a reassertion of this principle, which led to transfers of assets up to higher levels and a resulting depletion of resources of resources at the local level. It also dampens the development of citizen capabilities and identities capable of driving bottom-up social movements which might ameliorate the situation.

SARS may well have proven catalytic in resolving this issue in the medium to long term. China's leadership is likely to be more open to domestic and international NGOs who have strong capacities in assisting this change. China's incentives to prove itself a good global citizen were visibly strengthened by the SARS crisis, albeit in the most traumatic way. The nationalist sentiment that foreigners are intent on humbling China will linger, but the public mood was shifted by the very visible dependency of the central leadership on the goodwill and favourable assessment of the WHO.

Although this undoubtedly deserves close scrutiny from analysts, too much could easily be made of it. Political theatre is part of the skillset of a Chinese or any other political leader. More importantly, the Communist Party traditionally organises a great deal of skill and effort into "foreigner handling." The population's patriotic sentiments are easily aroused and the Party will do this at times to suit its convenience.

However, the events of Spring 2003 showed that the public opinion is simply not amenable to the level of control and manipulation that was once the case. Despite repeated purges, periodicals, particularly in the business sector such as *Southern Weekend, 21st Century Economic Herald, Caijing* and so forth, kept challenging the line. The question arises as to how deep the resources of the establishment would prove in a war of attrition. The public reached a level of disgust with a servile media that has little if any precedence.

References

Bezlova A. (2003) Migrant workers get attention at last. *Asia Times Online*, 8 March. Available at http://atimes.com/atimes/China/EC08Ad02.html

Blumenthal D, Hsiao W. (2005) Privatization and its discontents — the evolving Chinese health care system. *New Engl J Med* **353**: 11 (15 September), 1165-117.

CECC. (2003) Information Control and Self-Censorship in the PRC and the Spread of SARS. US Congressional-Executive Commission on China. Available at http://www.cecc.gov/pages/news/prcControl_SARS.php?PHPSESSID=66f476bbd4879e09c289285f16ae6445.

Chow C-y. (2003) SARS Outbreak Cuts Into Rural Income, *South China Morning Post*, 28 July, Foshan Labour and Security Information Net, Research Report no. 3 on 'SARS and employment'. Available at http://www.fsld.gov.cn/LbNews/2003/06/200306014.htm

Economic Herald. (2003) Nurture Citizen Awareness, Promote a Transformation of Governance. 21 *Century Economic Herald*, 15 May 2003, pp.1. Available at http://www.nanfangdaily.com.cn/jj/20030515. Translation by David Kelly available at http://newton.uor.edu/Departments&Programs/AsianStudiesDept/kelley.pdf

Enserink M. (2003) China's missed chance. *Science* **301**: 294–296. Available at http://www.sciencemag.org/cgi/content/full/301/5631/294

Fewsmith J. (2003) China's Response to SARS. *Chinese Leadership Monitor*. Available at http://www.chinaleadershipmonitor.org/20033/jf.html

Gu X, Kelly D. (forthcoming 2005) Balancing economic and social development: China's new policy initiatives in combating social injustice, in Samir Radwan (ed.) *The Changing Role of the State: Visions and Experiences*, Cairo: Economic Research Forum.

Hu F. (2003) SARS and the *Mingong* Exodus (Madian Village, Hunan). 27 June. Available at http://www.sannong.gov.cn/fxyc/ldlzy/200306270081.htm

Iyengar J. (2003) Beijing Unveils Land Reform Policy. *Asian Times Online,* 11 March. Available at http://www.atimes.com/atimes/China/EC11Ad01.html

Kelly D (ed). (2005) *Mysteries of the Chinese Economy*, Special Issue of *The Chinese Economy* **38** (4, 5 and 6).

Kelly D. (2005) Industry repays agriculture: new public policy. *East Asian Institute Bulletin* **7**(1): 5.

Qin H. (2005) Command vs. Planned Economy: 'Dispensability' of the Economic Systems of Central and Eastern Europe and of Pre-Reform China, in Kelly (ed.) *Mysteries of the Chinese Economy,* special issue of *The Chinese Economy* **38**(4).

Qin H. (2005) Justice in the economics of market transition, in Kelly (ed.) *Mysteries of the Chinese Economy,* special issue of *The Chinese Economy* **38**(5).

Qin Hui, Tax and fee reform, village autonomy and central and local finance: historical experience and realistic options, in Kelly (ed.) *Mysteries of the Chinese Economy,* special issue of *The Chinese Economy* **38**(6).

Ranis G. (2004) Arthur Lewis' Contribution to Development Thinking and Policy. 15 June. Available at http://www.rh.edu/~stodder/BE/Lewis_byRanis.htm

State Council. (2003) "Opinions on Overcoming the Impact of SARS on Increasing Peasant Incomes. 23 July. Available at http://www.ben.com.cn/BJRB/20030808/GB/BJRB%5E18333%5E1%5E08R101.htm

Wen T. (2003) Interviews on the Nongmin Gong Issue. *Dushu* **7**: 15.

Wong C, Bhattalas D. (2002) *China: National Development and Sub-National Finance: A Review of Provincial Expenditures.* World Bank Report No. 22951-CHA, 9 April.

Xinhua. (18 June 2003) Farmers' Right to Transfer Land Must Be Respected.

Xinhua. (21 May 2003a) SARS Slows China's Consumer Spending.

Xinhua. (21 May 2003) Wen Jiabao's Important Speech at State Council 2nd Plenary Session.

Xinhua. (29 July 2003) Li Changchun: PRC Success in SARS Fight Due to Heroic Efforts.

Xinhua. (29 July 2003) Economic Impact of SARS, Recovery Plans.

Yao Y. (2005) "Shi xin yimin zhenzheng rongru hexie shehui" [Genuinely Blend New Migrants into a Harmonious Society]. Available at http://news.sohu.com/20050527/n225731395.shtml

Zhang X. (2005) Nongmingong shehui baozhang zhengce zhixing zhong cunzai de wenti [Problems in Implementing Social Security for Migrant Workers]. *Zhongguo Shehui Kexueyuan Yuanbao* [Chinese Academy of Social Sciences Gazette], 29 September 2005. Available at http://www.cass.net.cn/webnew/file/2005092944278.html

Zhang X. (2003) *SARS fengbao zhong de Zhongguo jingji* [China's Economy in the SARS Upheaval], Beijing: Zhongguo Jingji Chubanshe, **2003**: 83–104.

Zhou H. (2000) Speech Governance Donors' Roundtable, DFID Office, Beijing, Friday 3 (privately circulated document). 13 June 2000. Zhou is Director, Constitutional and Administrative Law Research Department, Institute of Law, CASS.

SECTION 6

DRAWING LESSONS FROM THE PAST TO RESPOND TO FUTURE CHALLENGES

21

Avian Flu: One More Infection Challenge from Asia

Adrian C Sleigh, Rachel Safman and Phua Kai Hong

The preceding chapters have raised many issues that are applicable to the emergence in Asia of another infectious disease of potentially pandemic proportion, avian influenza (bird flu). In this chapter we will examine the available information on this nascent threat and evaluate these data in light of some of the themes raised in earlier chapters.

Influenza Pandemics

Since the start of the 20th century, there have been three significant influenza pandemics occurring in 1918, 1957 and 1968, respectively. Although the origins and dynamics of these three events are somewhat different, they are collectively an important and worrying indicator of what might lie ahead when the next virulent strain of influenza begins spreading in human populations (WHO, 2005; Kitler *et al.*, 2002)

The 1918 pandemic, which was the largest and most deadly of the three, began almost simultaneously in France, the USA and Sierra Leone, locations related to World War I troop movements among the continents. It did not originate in Spain but was widely reported from there when the population of Madrid was affected; henceforth, the pandemic acquired the name of the Spanish Flu. It also appeared in US pigs as the first report of symptomatic

411

swine flu, but we still do not know if the pigs acquired the infection from humans, or *vice versa*. The virus spread around the world in less than six months and left at least 40 million dead, killing more in that short time span than the Great War of 1914–1918. Between one third and half of the entire world population was infected and 99% of the deaths were among those aged less than 65 years, in stark contrast to the usual age groups of infants and elderly affected by influenza mortality. Many deaths were in the 20–45 year age group, and most were quick deaths from the effects of devastating viral pneumonia and not from secondary bacterial infection. The very high death rate, the frequent viral pneumonia, and the lethal impact on young healthy adults made the 1918 virus unique among influenza pandemics. The healthcare services and burial services were overwhelmed by the toll. There was no effective treatment and many countries closed schools, banned public gatherings and imposed quarantines. This may have delayed the arrival of the infection in Australia and perhaps slowed the epidemic a little elsewhere.

The 1957 pandemic was far less lethal than the pandemic of 1918, yet resulted in three million excess deaths with some deaths prevented through the use of antibiotics to treat secondary pneumonia. The pandemic was first detected in Hong Kong and from there spread to all parts of the world in less than six months. All age groups were affected, and many infants and the elderly died. Young adults also died more often than expected for seasonal influenza (Simonsen *et al.*, 1998). Public health interventions such as banning public gatherings and closing schools may have slowed its spread somewhat, and helped over-stretched healthcare systems manage the consequences.

Likewise, fatalities during the 1968 pandemic, which was also first detected in Hong Kong, were fewer than in the first pandemic of the century. Although the virus spread rapidly, it had less serious clinical effects and thus placed less stress on the healthcare services than the two previous pandemics. The excess death toll was estimated to number about one million and fatalities among young adults again exceeded the expected rates (Simonsen *et al.*, 1998). It has been surmised that the 1968 disease was less severe because this strain of the virus was similar to the previous pandemic strain, and therefore those infected during the earlier pandemic already had partial immunity.

Influenza Viruses

It is worth giving some attention to the virological characteristics of the influenza strains thought to have given rise to these three great pandemics. Influenza viruses belong to three major groups known as types A, B and C (Kitler *et al.*, 2002). Only the first two are of public health significance, the third is uncommon and causes few symptoms in infected persons.

Type B influenza is a human virus which circulates continuously and is responsible for considerable respiratory diseases. Over time, it steadily changes its antigenic structure by mutation, a process known as antigenic drift; it causes periodic outbreaks of influenza, especially among children, and is of sufficient concern to be included in human influenza vaccines.

Type A influenza is primarily a harmless enzootic infection which remains a widespread, antigenically stable and ancient component of the ecology of migratory aquatic birds. When the virus spreads to other birds or mammals, it frequently causes disease. Strains adapted to humans are of enormous public health significance because they undergo constant and rapid antigenic drift (changes in surface molecules), resulting in seasonal epidemics among humans every year in all parts of the world. Type A influenza is typically thought to pose a particular risk to children and the aged, largely as a result of secondary bacterial pneumonia. However, on occasions when the virus undergoes major antigenic shifts, which it does with some regularity, it causes global pandemics with all age groups affected. This is the result of the lack of immunity to the new strain throughout the population. It is the type A influenza virus, specifically three subtypes of the virus known as H1N1, H2N2 and H3N2, respectively, which caused the global pandemics in 1918, 1957 and 1968.

It should be noted that these three subtypes of type A influenza virus are the only subtypes known to have adapted for sustained transmission among humans, though several sub-types have been found to infect other mammals (notably, horses, pigs, seals, and recently dogs). Human subtypes can infect pigs, and they also have receptors for several other bird strains, including H5N1. It is thought that co-infection of pigs or people with two strains of type A influenza, one of which is adapted to human transmission, may have given rise to the novel strains of the virus which were responsible for the last two global pandemics (WHO, 2005; Kitler *et al.*, 2002; Hatta and Kawaoka,

2002). We know that the pandemics of 1957 and 1968 were caused by new type A viruses that were genetic combinations of avian strains and human strains which were then circulating. However, the 1918 pandemic may have arisen by a different mechanism. In 2005, it was reported that the 1918 virus, recovered and reconstructed from the tissues of its victims, appeared to be a human adaption of an entirely avian strain of the H1N1 sub-type. This 1918 virus was far more lethal in animal studies than any other influenza virus and it had several similarities to the avian strain of H5N1 that is the focus of worldwide concern today (Taubenberger *et al.,* 2005; Tumpey *et al.,* 2005).

Avian Influenza

Avian influenza was first noted as a serious disease of chickens in Italy in 1878 (WHO, 2005). It was called fowl plague and since the 1950s it has been attributed to type A influenza viruses. We now know that all known sub-types of type A viruses have a natural reservoir in wild waterfowl, especially ducks, as well as in gulls and shorebirds. These birds usually do not become ill but they carry the viruses over long distances as they migrate, contaminating water with their virus-loaded excreta along their journey. If domestic poultry become infected with avian influenza virus, the infection usually causes mild symptoms which may not be noticable. Occasionally, the virus is highly pathogenic, then the entire flock rapidly becomes ill and almost all the birds die. The highly pathogenic forms have always belonged to H5 or H7 subtypes, although these subtypes are not always lethal to poultry. Only the H5, H7 and H9 subtypes of avian influenza have ever crossed species to infect humans.

The first confirmed outbreak of highly pathogenic avian influenza was reported in Italy in 1959 (WHO, 2005). Before the current H5N1 appeared, there had been 24 documented outbreaks worldwide, 11 with H5 subtypes and the others with H7 subtypes. Most of these 24 highly pathogenic avian influenza outbreaks were confined to a few farms. Fourteen have occurred in the last 10 years. Until recently, the control strategy has been to cull infected flocks and to compartmentalise geographic areas as 'affected' or "unaffected", completely quarantining the former. The economic losses of such culling and quarantine are enormous and sentiment is shifting towards judicious use of poultry H5N1 vaccine. However, vaccination may impede export potential as importers may insist on the proof that H5N1 is not present in the flocks, which is difficult to provide if they are vaccinated. The use of sentinel unvaccinated birds may help but each country is making its own decision on the utility and economic benefit of vaccination (Normile, 2004). Furthermore, studies of long-term use of poultry vaccines for avian influenza in Mexico suggest that the virus may be induced to evolve more rapidly, diverging from the original strain to which the vaccine was directed (Lee *et al.*, 2004).

The recent regional epizootic of H5N1 infection is rewriting the book on highly pathogenic avian influenza. Never before has this disease arisen on such a large geographical scale and never before has it crossed over to humans and killed them. Rarely has it appeared in lethal form among wild bird populations that naturally harbour all the benign forms of avian influenza, and never before has avian influenza caused such huge economic losses.

It first appeared in Hong Kong in 1997, killing chickens and six out of 18 persons known to have been infected (Tam, 2002). This was the first time that an avian influenza had ever been known to kill people, with most of the victims having been exposed to pet or market chickens. Facing the threat of an emerging pandemic, a costly and painful decision was taken. The Hong Kong government decided to slaughter 1.5 million chickens, ducks and geese over three days that comprised the entire population of farm and market poultry in Hong Kong. Live bird markets were cleaned and re-opened with terrestrial and aquatic birds separated; H5N1 disappeared, only to reappear briefly in January 2003, killing two more people who had probably been infected in mainland China (Hatta and Kawaoka, 2002). In February 2003, it disappeared again from Hong Kong just as SARS broke out and spread to several other cities across the world (Abraham, 2004).

Before H5N1 reappeared in 2003, Hong Kong encountered another strain of avian influenza, also infecting humans for the first time. That was H9N2, but the two little girls who were infected eventually recovered. China then reported that H9N2 had been detected in five mainland Chinese the previous year. Avian influenza was reaching humans in ways never noted before and this caused great concern (WHO, 2005; Ferguson *et al.*, 2004).

As SARS emerged in Hong Kong in February 2003, another strain of highly pathogenic avian influenza broke out in poultry flocks in Holland, causing massive economic losses to the poultry industry in that country when 30 million birds were culled (Bosman *et al.*, 2004). It was a strain of the H7N7 subtype and it also reached the human population, causing one death. However, as expected with other avian strains of influenza, only mild disease was reported in more than 80 other people known to have been infected.

In late 2003 and again in early 2004, the lethal H5N1 strain reappeared among domestic poultry in Asia. However, this time it was much more widespread, more persistent, and even more deadly to humans. It erupted in several countries almost simultaneously, killing domestic chickens and ducks and ominously producing 11 human cases and nine deaths in Vietnam. It first appeared in Korea and Japan, but was soon reported among poultry through-out Vietnam and Thailand, in parts of Laos and Cambodia, in Indonesia and in more than half the provinces of China (WHO, 2005, Aldhous, 2005).

Throughout 2004 and 2005, the confirmed human death toll due to H5N1 infection has grown in Indochina, and then in 2005 and 2006, humans began to die in Indonesia, China and Turkey. By August 23, 2006, WHO reported that a total of 141 people had died from the infection, more than half of the 241 human cases detected, and the toll was advancing steadily. This high case-fatality rate suggests H5N1 is the most lethal strain of influenza to ever infect people, but needs to be confirmed by large population serological surveys to measure the true infection rate. Indonesia (46 deaths), Vietnam (42 deaths), Thailand (16 deaths) have suf-fered the most so far. There have been small clusters of probable human-to-human transmission, involving very close contact between relatives and dying loved ones, but no evidence of subsequent self-sustaining transmission among humans. In marked contrast to the experience with SARS, health-care workers have been infrequently infected by H5N1, further evidence that human transmissibility has not yet evolved.

Although H5N1 has not taken off in the human population, it has extended its host range to a variety of mammals, including 147 captive tigers presumed to have been fed infected chicken carcases in a Thai zoo. It has primarily affected small farms where free-range chickens, pigs, other domestic animals and people are in close contact. The humans at risk of lethal infection have so far been the subsistence farmers and their families rather than poultry workers or market traders (WHO, 2005; Aldhous, 2005). These are a very numerous and dispersed group of people in Asia, difficult to protect and surveil, yet constituting the human frontline for any possible evolution of a lethal pandemic influenza. The reason why infection has clustered among some poor farming families while usually sparing poultry workers or those involved in culling infected flocks remains unknown.

In the latter part of 2005, the frontline expanded as the highly pathogenic H5N1 virus reached birds in the Russian Federation, Kazakhstan, Mongolia, Romania, Croatia, Turkey and Ukraine. In late 2005 and early 2006, human cases and deaths appeared among poor farmers in Turkey and Iraq, and the infection reached birds in Azerbaijan, Bulgaria, Greece, Italy and Nigeria. Later in 2006, the bird-infected area extended even further in South Asia, Africa, the Middle East and Western Europe. An outbreak of highly pathogenic avian influenza on such a large geographical scale is unprecedented (WHO, 2005). H5N1 has persisted and steadily spread despite massive culling of infected flocks, with more than 200 million birds killed, vaccination of poultry in some zones, and quarantine of poultry and markets in all affected areas.

Ecological and Social Influences on Emergence of Infections

This volume opened with two chapters discussing the role of ecological and social factors on both a macro and micro scale in creating environments, within which specific pathogens could flourish. Clearly, this lens is applicable to our study of avian influenza. This lethal respiratory infection, like SARS, its most proximate historical antecedent among emergent infections, seems to have gained a foothold in human populations through the convergence of live animal markets, crowded human populations and over-stretched healthcare systems.

It is almost certainly more than coincidental that the virulent strain of avian influenza now causing alarm among international public health officials first made its appearance in Hong Kong in 1997 (Tam, 2002). Since the human influenza pandemic of 1957, if not earlier, every global influenza epidemic has had its origins in Hong Kong or Southern China where animal husbandry and marketing practices put large human populations in close contact with domestic and captured wild animals, making this area a natural jumping off point for viral pathogens adapting to move across species (WHO, 2005; Kitler *et al.*, 2002).

However, as the recent epidemiology of avian influenza has demonstrated, the movement of highly mutable pathogens from animal species to humans is not an isolated feature of the Southern Chinese environment. Since its initial appearance in Hong Kong and Southern China, this highly infectious, pathogenic variety of the H5N1 virus has made separate or serial appearances throughout many countries in Southeast Asia, which share the Chinese tradition of tightly integrating poultry farming into residential settlements, and then reached other areas at the European end of Asia that also share this characteristic. One might however ask why this century-old practice might suddenly have taken on such a lethal character. While no definitive conclusion has yet emerged, the answer may lie in the substantial growth in the size and density of human populations in the Southeast Asian region, which has turned once sparsely populated regions into increasingly urban landscapes. The shortcoming of this explanation, however, is that the affected individuals in Thailand, Vietnam and Indonesia have overwhelmingly been rural dwellers, whose residential environments are not inherently much more densely settled than were the towns and villages of earlier times.

An alternative explanation which also has its roots in human population growth, but traces its epidemiological effects through an indirect path, focuses on the advent of industrial poultry farming which has become widespread in the Southeast Asian region only in the past two decades. Building on Bradley's notion (see Chap. 3) that diseases thrive in landscapes which present ideal environments for pathogen evolution and transmission on a micro- as well as macro-scale, we might posit that these large poultry farms may have served as incubators for mutant strains of the virus. These variants may then have reached human populations, as the virus was disseminated from the ecologically homogenous environment of the mass poultry farms to the comparatively heterogeneous environment of home poultry producers (WHO, 2005; Aldhous, 2005). This could easily happen in the economic and social patchwork of rural Southeast Asia, where free-range chickens, pigs, other domestic animals and people are in close contact. In this setting, H5N1 could co-infect a person or animal already infected with another type A strain which is transmissible among humans, enabling H5N1 to genetically acquire transmissibility attributes from the other virus. H5N1 could also eventually adapt to humans after many attempts to cross the species barrier.

Mobility of People ... and Diseases

The size and geographic dispersion of the small poultry producers, who have thus far comprised the bulk of those affected by avian influenza and who constitute the human frontline for any possible evolution of a lethal pandemic influenza, draw attention to a second theme introduced in this volume, i.e., the mobility of human populations and the ability of relatively small numbers of migrants to dramatically affect the risk environment of much larger sedentary populations. This idea was both conceptually and empirically treated in the chapters by Becker and Glass, Wilder-Smith, Goh and Chew, and Lyttleton and Yang.

To date, the most alarming statistics related to the proliferation of avian influenza have been connected to the surveillance of both domesticated and wild bird populations, among whom the H5N1 virus has been found to be widespread and capable of travelling vast distances. This is demonstrated by the appearance of the disease among wild birds and poultry flocks of Central Asia, extending as far as Russia and eventually reaching Europe. From the standpoint of disease control, should the virus mutate in such a way as to make human to human transmission a common occurrence (a precondition for the virus becoming a serious threat to human health), it would not be the migration of waterfowl but rather the ever more vibrant and rapid streams of human migration that would be an issue (WHO, 2005; Ferguson, 2004; Grais *et al.,* 2003). The last three influenza pandemics spread around the world within 6 months and we can expect the next one to move even faster.

As the recent efforts to combat SARS (detailed from different perspectives in the chapters by Goh and Chew, Hsu and Liu, Chan, Liew, and Kelly and Luo) have demonstrated, national governments, including those heavily reliant on trade and tourism for their economic survival, have been willing to close their borders down or at least tighten surveillance of those moving across borders and even those within their interior, as in the case of

Singapore. Yet, as these narratives also make clear, the consistency of these controls and the feasibility of maintaining them over an extended period of time is limited. However, this would be required if the influenza pandemic persisted for many months or recurred in waves, as was the case in 1918–1919, or more recently with the H5N1 virus (re-) emergence in Hong Kong and Southern China.

We have already seen substantial gaps in the efforts of national governments to arrest the spread of avian flu in the Southeast Asian region and now in Europe. In Thailand, for example, the efficacy of widespread culls of domesticated poultry were undercut by the refusal of farmers to surrender their prize fighting cocks for which the proffered compensation was but only a fraction of the birds' true value. In Vietnam and Indonesia, containment efforts were compromised by the inability of the public health authorities to effectively communicate to their people the severity of the epidemic and the imperative of surrendering even small numbers of birds. Further difficulty arose in Thailand when potential control strategies were constrained by European markets that would not accept exports of chicken meat unless the birds had remained both healthy and unvaccinated. The importers thought that vaccination could disguise low grade H5N1 infection and although cooked chicken is safe, risk averse consumers needed reassurance that the birds were clean. The huge trade in chicken exports from Thailand to Europe has been threatened by all these events.

Influenza Containment: Cause for Hope and Concern

While much of the preceding discussion paints the prospect of an impending bird flu epidemic in a very bleak light, the forecast suggested by this book's contents is not entirely pessimistic. Indeed, contained within these chapters are studies which suggest long-term optimism for infection control. Among them is the study by Zhao *et al.*, which documents the phenomenal success which the city of Shanghai has enjoyed in increasing life expectancy and in controlling the spread of infectious diseases. The reports by Becker and Glass, and Li *et al.* in various ways illustrate the phenomenal advances which have been made in our ability to model the spread of lethal pathogens and design interventions to contain their spread. Clearly, the foundations of such research have already been laid and it is certainly needed for influenza control.

Every year, in all parts of the world, human influenza outbreaks occur on an annual basis as new virus variants arise due to antigenic drift. The infection is transmitted between people by both the airborne droplet nuclei and large respiratory droplet routes. Outbreaks often follow large gatherings, school openings or institutional recruitments. Those infected can infect others a day or two before developing symptoms, facilitating rapid virus transmission in the population. Many local health authorities track these outbreaks in their own areas and sometimes more than one strain occurs at the same time. A local outbreak involves a specific type B or type A strain, and each year the main circulating strains change. The clinical symptoms depend on the age, and the immune and health status of the host, and on the virus strain causing the infection. The disease is often quite disabling, causing high rates of absenteeism from work.

Globally, the WHO maintains a long-standing influenza surveillance network which now involves 110 laboratories in 82 countries (Kitler *et al.*, 2002). This network complements various surveillance systems for animals, which are supported by the Food and Agricultural Organization (FAO) and by the World Organisation for Animal Health (OIE). The WHO network types and tracks all human viral isolates and produces a recommendation twice a year regarding the two A strains and the B strain to include in the next vaccine. This vaccine is produced and offered to high risk groups just before the beginning of the usual transmission season, which varies from place to place. Each year, substantial morbidity occurs due to influenza, especially for children and the elderly. Among the latter, an excess mortality occurs during the influenza transmission season. This mortality can be reduced by the timely use of vaccines for preventive purposes and by the use of anti-viral drugs once infection occurs.

During both the 1957 and 1968 pandemics, specific vaccines were developed within a few months but they were not available in sufficient quantities to influence the global spread (WHO, 2005). Experimental human vaccines for H5N1 are underway but the obstacles are significant. The H5N1 virus kills the usual culture medium of embryonated chicken eggs and must be reverse engineered to enable this system to work. This introduces safety and intellectual property issues that are difficult to resolve. In the Asian region, only Japan and Australia have substantial vaccine production capacity. At present, the routine vaccines have two strains of type A influenza and one strain of type B. If a pandemic arises, the vaccine can be manufactured with just one strain and this should expand production substantially. It is a worthy goal to develop capacity to produce enough vaccine for mass global distribution. However, it remains to be seen whether this is possible and whether it can make a difference, even if the vaccine can be developed in time.

It is worth recalling that in 1976, the US government prepared a vaccine for H1N1 that had infected a few military recruits in Fort Dix, New Jersey. The first patient died and the virus appeared to be a variant of the swine version of H1N1, raising the alarm that the 1918 pandemic was about to recur. The vaccine was eventually given to 45 million people before it was realised that the pandemic had not happened (WHO, 2005; Drexler 2002). Unfortunately, there were many cases of a serious neurological disorder, an ascending polyneuritis (Guillain–Barre syndrome), that appeared to be related to the vaccine. This is a sobering reminder of what surprises may lurk ahead for any strategy involving mass use of a novel vaccine for influenza. The swine flu experience of 1976 revealed the need to be sure that a pandemic is really happening before taking drastic control measures; the criteria should include appearance of clusters of human-transmitted cases in more than one location. Furthermore, there is a need to be willing to compensate those adversely affected by such intrusive control strategies, and to communicate the risks and benefits effectively.

Anti-viral drugs were not available for any previous pandemic, but they will be available for some people during future pandemics. The older and cheaper M2 inhibitor drugs, amantadine and rimantadine, are not useful for H5N1 because resistance develops quickly (WHO, 2005). Current plans for managing future pandemics include stockpiling and the use of newer antiviral drugs oseltamivir and zanamirvir, neuraminidase inhibitors that prevent the virus from detaching from one cell to infect another, and that are known to be effective in treating or preventing H5N1 infection in humans. These drugs are in short supply, so their use must be judicious while world production is being increased. At present, it is envisaged that they could be useful in three settings. First, to treat those sporadically infected, as is now occurring in Vietnam and Thailand. Second, to treat those known or thought to have been exposed. This second use includes an early response to large human clusters that could herald the onset of human-to-human transmission of a strain that has acquired pandemic potential. The third use is to treat infections once a pandemic starts, and to protect frontline workers (who may be difficult to define) as the pandemic progresses. This third use will require large stockpiles and inevitably will reflect who has the power and resources to produce and acquire them.

Given the possibilities with both vaccines and drugs, and the much boosted surveillance capacity for influenza in animal and human populations, we can anticipate that the next pandemic will be the first to be subjected to some specific bio-technical control strategies. We must however expect that this control may have unpredictable and even some adverse effects.

Potential Impact of Avian Influenza

The economic impact of H5N1 avian influenza has already been significant. Direct economic losses for the entire East Asian region in the first 18 months of the current outbreak have been estimated at about US$10 to 15 billion, mostly in the agricultural sector (Vietnam News Agency, 22 July, 2005). Indonesia alone has confirmed that more than 9.5 million domestic fowl have died since the outbreak in early 2004. Thailand recently culled 2.7 million ducks to prevent further spread of the disease. The Thai government has proposed a US$125 million package to compensate farmers and to import frozen poultry to reduce the impact of the poultry destruction (Promed Mail, 12 Feb, 2005). The costs will increase significantly in the coming years with no end to the outbreak in sight. In addition, the effect on certain segments of society, especially on the agricultural industry, could have lingering socio-economic outcomes.

The potential for infectious diseases to spread across geographical and national boundaries are a growing concern, especially with global travel aiding transmission. The impact of diseases is also made more significant with the inter-connectivity of economies. This is especially true in East Asia, which relies heavily on trade with partners within the region and also with Europe and America. A human pandemic caused by avian influenza originating in East Asia will spread quickly throughout the region, devastating populations and ruining economies. Other countries will probably attempt to prevent spread by reducing trade and travel, although this may be a futile exercise because it is almost impossible to differentiate influenza from other upper respiratory illnesses. Nevertheless, the economic effects on the region will be significant if countries are unprepared.

While the social and economic impacts of infectious diseases are important, the direct medical costs of infectious diseases are also equally significant and should be of concern to health policy makers. Using Singapore as an example of a metropolitan Asian city, an influenza pandemic with case fatality rates of 2% (similar to conservative estimates of the rates for the 1918 pandemic), could cause more than 25,000 deaths at a direct cost to the economy of more than US$28 billion, excluding intangible costs such as loss of trade. At case fatality rates of 5%, Singapore with a four million population will experience at least 50,000 deaths at a direct economic cost of US$50 billion (Lee et al., 2006).

The impact on critical services including healthcare are also important, since a pandemic can lead to a large utilisation of hospital and medical services which will overwhelm current capacities of healthcare systems. Many patients with deteriorating conditions, especially those with pneumonia who would otherwise improve with good medical treatment, will be unable to receive prompt treatment due to the overwhelmed healthcare services. In addition, frontline healthcare workers may be exposed before precautions such as protective equipment can be distributed and worn. This will reduce the pool of healthcare workers and services available, resulting in more deaths due to influenza and the lack of available treatment for other illnesses.

Pandemic Preparedness

Many countries have decided on the stockpiling of neuraminidase inhibitors for use during a pandemic, either as treatment or prophylaxis against the virus. Available evidence points to neuraminidase inhibitors as the drugs of choice, due to their proven effectiveness in the treatment of different strains of influenza and good safety profiles (Turner et al., 2003; Kaiser et al., 2003). However, the costs of stockpiling are extremely high and the expected benefits are not immediately apparent, especially when the probability of a future pandemic and its degree of severity is unknown.

Any policy decision on stockpiling must weigh the cost of drugs and other measures to prevent the spread of any pandemic influenza strain, against the costs of the uncontrolled disease itself.

An important policy consideration in this case is the degree of protection a nation should build up as resistance against future infectious disease epidemics. Other than stockpiling of therapeutic agents, such investments include strengthening surveillance networks, infection control and other measures. These can be expensive measures for which the costs are immediate, but the accrued benefits are unknown and will not be apparent until the event actually occurs. The amount of investment in such strategies reflects the priority accorded by policy makers, reflecting the perceived severity of infectious disease epidemics and the risks they are willing to take. This situation is akin to having insurance coverage, where a bigger investment would be made against risks that are perceived to have higher probability and greater severity.

Hong Kong, for example, had purchased 1.7 million capsules of oseltamivir by January 2005, sufficient for 2.5% of its population (*Reuters*, 9 March, 2005). The government is now proposing to increase this amount to 20 million capsules at a cost of US$32.6 million. This would provide sufficient treatment courses for 25% of its population (one treatment course requires 10 capsules). The French government has ordered 13 million courses of the drug to date, and the United Kingdom has ordered 14.6 million courses, sufficient for 25% of its population. Vietnam, employing another preventive strategy, ordered 415 million doses of avian influenza vaccine for poultry. Instead of decimating its poultry stocks, it plans to vaccinate all poultry to prevent infection, and is offering a four US cent incentive for every bird vaccinated (China View, www.chinaview.cn, accessed July, 2005).

Following the call by the World Health Organization to form influenza preparedness networks, the European Union unveiled a continent-wide early warning system based on the newly created European Centre for Disease Control and Prevention (ECDC). The centre will monitor influenza outbreaks across Europe using a network of reference laboratories (Financial Times, May 18, 2005). However, the World Health Organization has warned that countries that are unable or unwilling to provide samples or to participate in the surveillance networks are undermining the efforts (Reuters,

11 May, 2005). This is especially a problem for countries that are unable to provide such support because of the costs involved. There is a need for international aid to provide support to these impoverished countries.

In the regional context, the call for national preparedness plans faces similar problems. Every nation would have limitations on the resources it can pour into such preparations, as it considers the perceived cost and benefits of investments against such threats. Throughout the vast and diverse range of countries in Asia, there is a significant disparity in the resources available. The varying perceptions of risk would depend on the relative proximity of any public health threat before any significant investment in preventive measures is committed. Policy decisions on preparedness will be affected by the availability of resources in a nation, as allocations for infectious disease programs are made in competition with other urgent priorities on a national basis.

However, due to the fast-growing connectivity of economies and societies in the region, any externalities such as spill-over effects that an infectious disease epidemic has on neighbouring nations would be magnified. Without a proper surveillance and early detection system in place, human-to-human transmission of avian influenza may not be detected until it has spread extensively across the region. As the fate of regional countries is thus intertwined, it would be in the interests of wealthier countries to invest in the surveillance and disease control programs in poorer countries, because the benefits would accrue to all countries concerned as an international public good. The World Health Organization had earlier called for an investment of US$100 million to support surveillance and control measures in Asia (WHO Regional Office for the Western Pacific, 6 July, 2005). It later recommended that investments are urgently needed at the national levels, potentially reaching US$1 billion over a three-year period, in addition to US$35 million to support immediate priority work at the international level over six months (WHO Geneva, 7–9 November 2005). In early 2006, it has managed to obtain a commitment of almost US$1.9 billion in its latest fund-raising efforts at the International Pledging Conference on Avian and Human Pandemic Influenza (WHO Conference, Beijing, January 17–18, 2006).

Another consideration is the possibility of regional stockpiling of anti-viral drugs. Due to the high cost of the drugs, wealthy countries are able to stockpile for a significant proportion of their populations while impoverished countries are left behind. To have effective control of this problem in the region, regional stockpiles of anti-viral drugs over and above national stockpiles should be built. These stockpiles can be deployed to areas of need to supplement existing national stocks. This will help reduce the impact of an outbreak and lessen the impact of the disease in the event that it result in a pandemic. This is because patients on treatment have a shorter infective period and prophylactic ring fencing of contacts is possible with sufficient stocks of anti-viral drugs.

Pandemic Avian Influenza

Many elements mentioned above point to the possibility of future pandemic H5N1 influenza and its dire consequences. Yet, we still have some crucial knowledge gaps that must be closed, the most important being the viral mutation or reassortment needed to develop human transmissibility and to retain high human virulence. Without this knowledge, we cannot estimate the likelihood of the H5N1 virus acquiring pandemic attributes. However, we can be certain that pandemic viruses emerge and that H5N1 is a candidate for the next pandemic that is showing abilities to evolve and adapt to many new ecological niches, and to reach humans, the first step in the pandemic journey. Based on past experience, we can expect the next pandemic to be a new H serotype and H5 qualifies on that count. We can also expect it to emerge from Asia, especially from Southern China and H5N1 qualifies again. As our surveillance systems have improved substantially, we can expect forewarning of the next pandemic, unlike previous pandemics. As we are so much more interconnected, we can expect the next pandemic to spread faster across the world than any previous pandemic. It may take just two or three months to reach most populations.

In reaction to the threat, WHO and FAO have been assisting all countries to develop plans to control avian influenza and prepare for an influenza pandemic. A good example is the plan released by Thailand, which is an important development, given the adverse health and economic impact that H5N1 is having in that country (Wibulpolprasert, 2005). The aim is to abort transmission of avian influenza within poultry flocks or from poultry to humans within two years, and to reduce the incidence of transmission within domestic poultry, fighting cocks and exotic birds within 3 years. The plan is very detailed and lays out strategies to achieve these goals. Part of the plan involves knowledge generation and engagement with the civil society because the Thais realise that governments cannot do this alone. Education of small subsistence farmers and improved farming conditions will be important elements as the plan is activated over the next year. Other countries have developed their own plans and the region will be better prepared than it has ever been, once these plans are implemented over 2005 and 2006. We cannot predict the final impact on H5N1 as this infection is being driven by many powerful forces which have not abated (Weiss and McMichael, 2004).

In this final chapter, we have reviewed the dangerous emergence in the Asian region of yet another novel infection in the aftermath of SARS. We have connected the emergence and multi-continental spread of H5N1 to themes covered by this book, noting forces that are drivers and others that appear as consequences. Existing social orders and divides are highlighted repeatedly, as are world trade, farming systems, rural poverty, education, cultural traditions and social ecology. Other recurrent issues, including migration, urbanisation and population change, also relate to the unfold-ing threat from H5N1. All these phenomena are outcomes of complex ecological and socio-economic structures undergoing rapid change, readily apparent throughout this multi-disciplinary assessment of infectious diseases and population dynamics in Asia today. Sophisticated responses to popu-lation infection threats, such as that now posed by H5N1, should take all these issues into consideration. Effective control strategies require transdis-ciplinary understanding of both the nature of the threat and of our potential to contain it. We anticipate that the contents of this book will make such approaches more possible.

References

Abraham T. (2004) *Twenty-first Century Plague: The Story of SARS.* Hong Kong University Press, Hong Kong.

Aldhous P. (2005) Vietnam's war on flu. *Nature* **433**: 102–104.

Bosman A, Mulder YM, de Leeuw JRJ, Meijer A, Du Ruy van Beest Holle M, Kamst RA, van der Veiden PG, Conyn-van Spaendonck MAE, Koopman

MPG, Ruijten MWMM. (2004) *Avian Flu Epidemic 2003: Public Health Consequences.* National Institute for Public Health and the Environment (RIVM) and the Institute for Psychotrauma, Bilthoven, The Netherlands. RIVM Report 630940001/2004.

Drexler M. (2002) *Secret Agents: The Menace of Emerging Infections.* Joseph Henry Press, National Academy of Sciences, Washington, DC.

Ferguson N, Fraser C, Donnelly CA, Ghani AC, Anderson RM. (2004) Public health risk from the avian H5N1 epidemic. *Science* **304**: 968–969.

Grais RF, Ellis JH, Glass GE. (2003) Assessing the impact of airline travel on the geographic spread of pandemic influenza. *Eur. J. Epidemiol.* **18**(11): 1065–1072.

Hatta M, Kawaoka Y. (2002) The continued pandemic threat posed by avian influenza viruses in Hong Kong. *Trends Microbiol* **10**: 340–344.

Kaiser L, Wat C, Mills T, Mahoney P, Ward P, Hayden F. (2003) Impact of oseltamivir treatment on influenza-related lower respiratory tract complications and hospitalizations. *Arch Int Med* **163**: 1667–1672.

Kitler ME, Gavinio P, Lavanchy D. (2002) Influenza and the work of the world health organization. *Vaccine* **20**: S4–S14.

Lee CW, Senne DA, Suarez DL. (2004) Effect of vaccine use in the evolution of mexican lineage H5N2 avian influenza virus. *J Virol* **78**: 8372–8381.

Lee VJ, Phua KH, Chen MI, Chow A, Ma S, Goh KT, Leo YS. (2006) Economics of neuraminidase inhibitor stockpiling for pandemic influenza, Singapore. *Emerg Infect Dis* **12**(1): 95–102.

Normile D. (2004) Vaccinating birds may help to curtail virus's spread. *Science* **306**: 398–399.

Simonsen L, Clarke MJ, Schonberger LB, Arden NH, Cox NJ, Fukuda K. (1998) Pandemic versus epidemic influenza mortality: A pattern of changing age distribution. *J Infect Dis* **178**: 53–60.

Tam JS. (2002) Influenza A (H5N1) in Hong Kong: An overview. *Vaccine* **20**: 577–581.

Taubenberger JK, Reid AH, Lourens RM, Wang R, Jin G, Fanning TG. (2005) Characterization of the 1918 influenza virus polymerase genes. *Nature* **437**: 889–893.

Tumpey TM, Basler CF, Aguilar PV, Zeng H, Solorzano A, Swayne DE, Cox NJ, Katz JM, Taubenberger JK, Palese P, Garcia-Sastre A. (2005) Characterization of the reconstructed 1918 spanish influenza pandemic virus. *Science* **310**: 77–80.

Turner D, Wailoo A, Nicholson K, Cooper N, Sutton A, Abrams K. (2003) Systematic review and economic decision modeling for the prevention and treatment of influenza A and B. *Health Technol Assessment* **7**: 1–182.

Weiss RA, McMichael AJ. (2004) Social and environmental risk factors in the emergence of infectious diseases. *Nat Med* **10**: S70–S76.

Wibulpolprasert S, Chunsuttiwat S, Ungchusak K, Kanchanchitra C, Teokul W, Prempree P (eds). (2005) *National Strategic Plan for Avian Influenza Control and Influenza Pandemic Preparedness in Thailand, 2005–2007.* Ministry of Public Health and Thai Health Promotion Foundation, Bangkok.

World Health Organization. (2005) *Avian Influenza: Assessing the Pandemic Threat.* WHO, Geneva.

World Health Organization. (2005) Avian Influenza and Human Pandemic Influenza, Summary Report of Meeting held in Geneva, Switzerland, 7–9 November 2005. WHO, Geneva.

World Health Organization. (2006) *Beijing Declaration*, International Pledging Conference on Avian and Human Pandemic Influenza, 17–18 January 2006, Beijing.

Index

Abdul Kadir Sheikh Fadzir, 358
acute respiratory infections, 137, 142, 143
  (*see also* respiratory infections)
  - almost 4 million people killed annually, 26
  - resistance to drugs, 151
Aedes aegypti, 30, 33, 45
Aedes africanus, 45
Aedes albopictus, see Asian tiger mosquito
Aedes simpsoni, 45
Africa, bush-meat consumption, 29
AIDS, *see* HIV/AIDS
AIDS Organisation
  (*see also* non-governmental organisations)
  - activities, past and present, 174–177
  - ethnographic study of, 164–165
  - networks and support groups, 174
Akha villagers (Laos), 211, 216, 217, 219, 221,
  223, 225
Al Haram mosque (Saudi Arabia), 272
An. dirus, see mosquitoes
An. minimus, see mosquitoes
Anderson, Roy, 353
animal parasites, 25
Anopheles mosquitoes, 144
antibiotic era, 23
antibiotics
  (*see also* drug resistance)
  - bacteria's resistance to commonly used drugs
    e.g. ampicillin, gentamicin etc., 151–152
  - communicable disease resistance to, 98
  - drug resistance to, 151

Aseh Che Mat, 357
Asia
  (*see also* other subject headings e.g. avian
    influenza, population etc.)
  - economy:
    'Four Tigers': Hong Kong, S. Korea,
      Singapore and Taiwan, 97, 99
    newly industrialising economies: Malaysia,
      Thailand and Indonesia, 97
  - healthcare systems, 12
  national, 99, 107
  - infectious diseases, 8; emergence and
    resurgence, 100
  - mortality
    rates lower in cities than rural areas, due to
      health advantage, 7
  - population, aging and growth declining,
    98–99
  - public health and diseases, 98–99
  - urbanisation increasing, 6–7
Asia, South, cholera pandemic (eighth)
  emerged, 24
Asian MetaCentre for Population and
  Sustainable Development Analysis, National
  University of Singapore, 3
Asian Development Bank
  - infrastructure development in Greater
    Mekong Sub-region, 210
Asian tiger mosquito, 30
Audy, J.R., *Red Mites and Typhus*, 45
avian influenza, 8, 24, 40

431

(*see also* influenza)
- control measures, 420–423:
  WHO's influenza surveillance and
      preparedness networks, 421, 424
- drugs, antiviral: oseltamivir, zanamirvir and
      neuraminidase inhibitors, 422
  human vaccines for H5N1 virus underway,
      421
  vaccines and drug production, 421–423
- economic impact on East Asia, 423–424
- first noted in Italy 1878, known as 'fowl
      plague', 414
- outbreaks
  in: Asia (2003–2004), 416
      Holland, 30 million birds culled, 416
      Hong Kong (1997), 372, 415
      Italy (1959), 414
      Singapore, 5000 chickens killed, 359
      Thailand, Prime Minister Thaksin
          Shinawatra's statement, 360
      worldwide (2005), 417
  ongoing outbreak may cause severe
      socio-economic damages, 103
- pandemic preparedness:
  Asian countries call for preparedness plan,
      426–427
  European Union continent-wide early
      warning system, 425
  stockpiling of drugs by national governments,
      424–425
- Pledging Conference on Avian and Human
      Pandemic Influenza (WHO), Beijing (Jan
      17–18, 2006), 426
- virus containment:
  causes for concern, 420
  environment conducive to virus growth,
      418–420

bat-borne virus, 31
Bayh-Dole Act (US 1980), 364
bilharzia (Africa), *see* schistosomiasis
bird flu, *see* avian influenza
blood-borne diseases, *see* diseases
Body Shop to employ AIDS sufferers, 197
Borrelia burgdorferi, see Lyme disease (borreliosis)
bovine spongiform encephalopathy (BSE), *see*
      'mad cow disease'
Brazil
- Amazon deforestation, 51
British Broadcasting Corporation

- effects of the collapse of the Chinese
      pioneering primary healthcare system, BBC
      report, 363
British Overseas Development Administration,
      61–62
bronchitis, acute, 140, 141
  in Vietnam, 135, 143
brucellosis
- Saudi Arabia endemic, 273–274
Business Coalition on AIDS Singapore (formed
      in 2000), 197

C. jejuni, see Campylobacter enteritis
California, University of (LA)
- loneliness scale and attitude scale for
      measuring social isolation and lax social
      control, used in a China's survey, 254
Campylobacter enteritis
- detected in Singapore, 288
- infection caused by *C. jejuni*, 288
cattle-borne zoonotic disease, *see* diseases
CCHF, *see* Crimean-Congo hemorrhagic fever
Cernea, Michael, 62
Chan, Roy (President, Action of AIDS)
- AIDS cases in Singapore, statement, 187
China
(*see also* Shanghai and other subject headings
      e.g. population, women etc.)
- dams, ecological and social impacts of,
      58–59, 62
- diseases
  (*see also* other countries e.g. Malaysia,
      Singapore, etc.)
  HIV/AIDS: 128, 130;
      Premier Wen Jiabao shaking hands with
          AIDS sufferers at a Beijing hospital,
          193
  SARS outbreak:
      exchange of information agreement with
          ASEAN, Japan and S. Korea, 296
      failure to identify the virus early, 391
      government policies for fighting the
          disease, 389–390
      success in containment (official
          announcement), 389
      outbreak cover-up criticised, 391
      rural-urban dichotomy in wealth linked
          to spread of disease, 403–405
  tuberculosis:

control in Gongyi, Linying, Yuzhou,
  and Zhenping counties, 233–235
costs of treatment, 238–241
high occurrence rate among off-farm
  migrants, 232
occurrences poverty-related, 232
pulmonary tuberculosis, occurrence in
  Henan province (2002–2004), 232
research method and results, 233–238
WHO's "directly observed therapy
  short-course' strategy adopted,
  232–233
- economic development:
  (*see also* rural sector and urban sector under
    China)
fast-tracked export industrialisation, 232
growth dependent on cheap migrant labour,
  401
household responsibility system, 396, 399
township and village enterprises, rapid
  growth, 400
wealth distribution highly imbalanced, 403
- local government:
village self-government promoted, 392
- migrant workers *(mingong)*:
female temporary migrants vulnerable to
  sexually transmitted diseases, 246
individual characteristics by migrant status
  among females 18 years or older,
  survey results (statistics), 256
model of economic growth, 394–396, 398
socio-economic environment conducive to
  STD/HIV risk sexual behaviour, 247
status and income of workers, 398
temporary migrants from rural to urban areas,
  245, 392
- migration:
hukou registration system, 393
phenomenal migration of the rural poor to
  the cities, 232, 245, 248
sexually transmitted disease risks, 246–247
temporary labour migration and gender
  inequality, 248–251
- population
affected by infectious diseases, 128
ageing, 130
- public health:
  effects of the collapse of the pioneering
    primary healthcare system, BBC report,
    363

system under WHO's intense scrutiny for
  transparency due to SARS, 391
- rural sector:
agricultural industry developed, 397
grave financial crisis, 403
surplus labour supply to the urban sector,
  394, 401
- Southwestern region:
population-based survey on HIV/AIDS cases
  (2003), 251–255
STATA software used for data analysis, 253;
  results, 255–264
- urban sector:
service industries boom, 398
state and private wealth, rapid growth of, 402
unlimited supply of cheap migrant labour
  from the rural sector, 394, 401
- water:
'hydraulic centralism', 60
irrigated agriculture system, 60
large dams, flood control, irrigation and water
  supply, 60
pollution, 58, 61
Cholera
in: Shanghai (1912–1949), 114
  Singapore, 370
  South Asia, eighth pandemic emerged, 24
- pandemic (seventh) extended globally, 25
Cholera, Bengal (*Vibrio cholerae* O139)
- outbreak in India and Bangladesh (1992), 288
- spread to Thailand, US and UK, 288
chronotones, 11, 40, 45, 46
(*see also* ecotones)
climate changes, global, 33, 34
(*see also* environmental changes, global)
communicable diseases, *see* diseases,
  communicable, infectious diseases
Conrad, Lawrence, 371–372
contagious diseases, *see* infectious diseases
coronavirus, *see* Severe Acute Respiratory
  Syndrome
Creutzfeldt-Jakob disease, 23, 362
Crimean-Congo hemorrhagic fever, 274
Culex mosquitoes, 30
cyclosporiasis, 27

dams, 11
and diseases, 11–12, 62–65
and politics, 66
and reservoirs, 46, 58

- Amazon deforestation due to dam construction, 51
- 'Dam and Development Forums', UN environment programme, 67
- dams in ancient period: Mesopotamia, Middle East and China, 59
- development in Europe, N. America and China (past and present), 61
- displacement of people, 63–64; psychological problems, 65
- health and socio-economic effects, adverse, 62, 64–65
- industry and environmentalists meeting co-convened by World Bank and World Conservation Union, Switzerland (1997), 67
- large dams and irrigation systems in China and India, environment transformed, 57–58
- protests against:
  Narmada river dams in India, 66
  Three Gorges dam in China, 66
- World Bank and other development banks, present role of, 61
dengue fever, 8, 9, 24, 29, 33, 64
in: Singapore, 375
Vietnam, 140, 147
diarrhoea, 64, 68, 140, 141, 142
diarrhoeal diseases killed 3 million people annually, 26
in: Shanghai, 117–118, 129
Vietnam, 135, 137, 140, 141, 142, 152
diphtheria, 27, 124
'directly observed therapy short-course' on tuberculosis control, 232–233
diseases
(*see also* infectious diseases)
- air-borne, 275
- blood-borne, 274
- cattle-borne zoonotic, 274
- food-borne from animal products, 274
- mosquito-borne, 64
- rodent-borne, 31
- vector-borne, *see* vector-borne diseases
- water-borne, 58, 356
diseases, communicable, 273–274
(*see also* infectious diseases)
- epidemiology, 41, 52
  descriptive, 41

- Hajj pilgrims to Mecca, transmission risk, 273
- resistance to common antibiotics, 98
diseases, non-communicable, 273
and ageing population, 98, 99
diseases, vaccine-preventable, 276
(*see also* immunisation)
- importation and immunisation, 73–74
- mathematical models, 74
DOTS, *see* 'directly observed therapy short-course'
drug abuse and trafficking
in Thailand, intravenous drug use and transmission of HIV/AIDS, 167
drug resistance
(*see also* antibiotics)
- bacteria to commonly used antibiotics, 151–152
- falciparum malaria to chloroquine, sulphadoxine, and pyrimethamine, 144
- microbes, 43
- pathogens, 40
- tuberculosis, 146, 151
dysentery, 140, 141, 142

'East Asian miracle', 97
ecotones, 11, 45, 46
(*see also* chronotones)
and epidemiology of emergent infections, 40
and scrub typhus in Malaysia, 45
El Nino
- dengue fever occurrences affected by the fluctuations, 33
- event (1991–92), 32
- Southern Oscillation phenomenon, 42
El Tor strain, 25
elephantiasis, 64
encephalitis,
enterovirus (71), 291
Japanese, 8, 64, 140
in: Malaysia, 101; 100 deaths (1998–99), 290
Singapore, 101
Vietnam, 140
- tick-borne, 34, 44
- viral, 33, 135
environmental changes, global
(*see also* climate changes, global)
- UN Environment Programme, 67
enzootic microbes, 25–26
Ertan Dam (China), 59, 68

European Centre for Disease Control and Prevention, 425

falciparum malaria, 47, 50, 144
- resistance to chloroquine, sulphadoxine, pyrimethamine, 144
Food and Agriculture Organization, 61, 421, 427
food-borne diseases, *see* diseases
food market, globalisation of, 29
foot and mouth disease
- UK (2002), 52
Foundation for Advancement of Media Excellence (Taiwan)
- SARS coverage, content analysis in 7 Taiwanese newspapers (March-May, 2003), 332
Fourneyron, Benoit (inventor of water turbine), 61
'fowl plague', *see* avian influenza

Ganges river valley, 57
gastroenteritis
  in Singapore, 93 cases, 288–289
gender inequality, *see* women
genetic variation, *see* pathogens
geographical information systems, 39, 41, 44,
- used for control of malaria, 46, 47
Gerberding, Julie (US Centers for Disease Control and Prevention Director), 364
GIS, *see* geographical information systems
global changes, *see* climate changes, global; environmental changes, global
globalisation linked to transmission of infectious diseases, 100
Goh, Chok Tong (Singapore, Prime Minister)
  SARS outbreak, statement on, 376
Gongyi county (China), 233
gonorrhoea
  (*see also* sexually transmitted diseases)
  in: Laos, 221
  Shanghai (1955–2003), 117, 128

Greater Mekong Sub-region,
- Asian Development Bank infrastructure development, 210
group B arboviruses, mice's resistance to, 40

H. influenzae
- bacteria found during Hajj pilgrimage in Mecca, 275
hand, food and mouth disease
- outbreaks in:
  Sarawak (1997), 291
  Singapore, 375
  Taiwan (1998), 291
Hanta viruses, 31
hantavirus pulmonary syndrome, 32
- rodent-borne hantavirus widespread in agricultural systems in S. America, 31
health and diseases, 98–99
health care
  (*see also* public health and individual countries e.g. China, Singapore etc.)
  in Thailand:
    non-governmental organisations' programmes for HIV/AIDS sufferers, home-based and a support network, 161, 169
    outreach care needed for mobile sufferers, 161, 169, 180–182
- rising costs of, 107
- systems in Asia, 99, 107
    overwhelming demand for services during flu pandemic, 106
"health impact assessment", WHO's submission, 67
Hendra virus, 31
hepatitis, 127, 129
  (*see also* viral hepatitis)
  and liver diseases and cancer, 145
  in: Vietnam, 140, 141, 144–145
- mouse, 40
- viral, *see* viral hepatitis
hepatitis A, 27, 274
  in: Shanghai, 116, 128, 129
hepatitis B, 145, 274
hepatitis C, 23, 145, 274
hepatitis, acute
  in Shanghai (1955–2003), 117
HIV/AIDS, 23, 27, 29, 34, 64, 68, 98, 356
  (*see also* migration, human and individual countries e.g. Laos, Singapore etc.)

- 2.5 million people killed annually, 26
- antiretrovirals drug, costs of, 191–192
in: China, migration and female temporary
  migrants' vulnerability, 246, 261
    Southwestern region, population-based
      survey (2003), 251–255
    Shanghai, virus spreading, 128, 130
    STATA software used for data analysis,
      253; results, 255
  Laos, Chinese migrant workers' sexual
    interaction with Akha women, 224–228
    ethnic sexual customs and HIV
      vulnerability, 222–224
    high occurrence rate in northern region,
      218
  Singapore, 370; compulsory AIDS test for
    pregnant women, 385
    Fourth Singapore AIDS Conference
      (2004), 193
  Thailand, non-governmental organisations'
    programmes for sufferers, 160–161
- risk groups identified: commercial sex
  workers, intravenous drug users and
  haemophiliacs, 166, 169
- spread of virus linked to human migration,
  207
- World AIDS Day (2003), 193
homosexuality and heterosexuality
- Fridae.com (online gay portal) based in Hong
  Kong, 200
- link to HIV/AIDS identified (1984), 165
Hong Kong
  (*see also* Severe Acute Respiratory Syndrome,
    and other countries e.g. Malaysia,
    Singapore etc.)
- flu pandemic detected (in 1957 and 1968),
  412
- SARS outbreak in Amoy Gardens (2003),
  305, 325:
  drainage system
    as a possible transmission route, 313–316
    as the virus-laden bio-aerosol source,
      316–317
  faeco-respiratory airborne route, 325
  investigation data and methods, 307–310;
    results, 310–325
  potential spread in high population density
    and built environment facilities, 305–325
  wind spread, 319
hookworm, 8

host snails, *see* vector mosquitoes
Hu, Jintao (China, President)
  government policies for fighting SARS,
    389–390
human immunodeficiency virus, *see* HIV/AIDS
human mobility and spread of diseases, *see*
  migration, human

immunisation
  (*see also* diseases, vaccine-preventable)
- Shanghai, Expanded Programme of
    Immunisation widely implemented, 124
India
- diseases:
  Bengal cholera (1992), 288
  plague, 100
- environment transformed by large dams and
    irrigation systems, 57–58
- Great Kumbh annual religious festival in
    Upper Ganges, 24
- population, 4
infectious diseases
  (*see also* specific types e.g. HIV/AIDS, SARS,
    tuberculosis etc. and sexually transmitted
    diseases)
- 30 new diseases identified, 23
- dam-associated, 58
- deaths, 26; rate in Shanghai, 118
- economic impact, 102, 104
- future pattern, 32
- importation, 73; effect of, 76, 79, 81
  interrupted transmission, 76–79
  mean outbreak size from a single importation
    (statistics), 82
  SEIR model, 75–76
  susceptible fraction, 76, 78–79, 81–86
  transmission model, 75, 88
  secondary transmission probability, 89–90
- infection:
  dam-related, 58
  water-related, 58
- information dissemination, role of the news
    media, 348
- preventive measures:
  costs of, 104–106
  stockpiling of anti-viral drugs, 104
- re-emergence and spread, 10, 24, 30
  due to globalisation, 100
- social impact of, 104, 105
influenza, 140, 141

(*see also* avian influenza)
during Hajj pilgrimage in Mecca, 275, 280
- pandemics
in: 1918–1919, 30–40 million people killed
worldwide, 353
1918, 1957 and 1968, 411–412
- outbreak in:
Shanghai, 130
Vietnam, 137, 140, 143
- overwhelming demand for health services
during pandemic, 106
- transmission among Hajj pilgrims to Mecca,
275
- viruses, types A, B and C, 413
type A subtypes (H1N1, H2N2, H3N2), 413
International Workshop on the Population
Dynamics of Infectious Diseases in Asia (Oct.
27–29, 2004), 3
interstitial pneumonitis, 291
Islam
- Hajj pilgrimage to Mecca, 271–272
great potential for zoonotic diseases, 273

Japan
- population ageing, 99
- SARS, exchange of information agreement
with ASEAN, China and S. Korea, 296

K. pneumoniae
- bacteria found during Hajj pilgrimage in
Mecca, 275
Kee, Phaik Cheen, 357
Korea, South
- SARS, exchange of information agreement
with ASEAN, China and Japan, 296
Kui villagers (Laos), 217, 221, 225–226
Kunming (China)
- land transport systems to Haiphong and
Burmese frontier developed, 209

land use and environmental change, 31–32
Landes, David, 59–60
landscape ecology, 44
landscape epidemiology, 39, 41, 44, 53
landslides, reservoir-induced, 65
Lao Cai (Vietnam), *see* Vietnam
Laos
- gonorrhoea, high level in ethnic villages, 221
- HIV/AIDS:

Chinese migrant workers' sexual interaction
with Akha women, 224–228
ethnic sexual customs and HIV vulnerability,
222–224
high occurrence rate in northern region,
217–218
- Luang Namtha province:
estimated population (in 1998), 212
Sing and Long districts:
Chinese traders and workers arrive in large
numbers, 215
ethnic diversity (statistics 2003), 212–213
government resettlement plan, 216;
displacement and relocation problems,
216
HIV risk, 211
increased migration due to ban on opium
cultivation, 216
movement of Sing and Long, 213
sexual interactions along route 17B and
Xiengkok, 219–221
- migration linked to HIV/AIDS vulnerability,
213
- trade with China, cross-border traffic
increases, 215
- Upper Mekong Region:
historical background, 208
infrastructure development to promote
transnational mobility, 208–209
migrants as a key HIV/AIDS 'risk group', 210
Tai settlers, 212
Lee, Hsien Loong (Singapore, Prime Minister)
- avian flu, Singapore "under-react" to the
threat, statement, 360
- future of Singapore politics and society,
speech, 196
Lee, Kuan Yew (Singapore, elder statesman)
- comments on Singapore: SARS outbreak,
377; young generation's high expectations,
375, 382
- memoirs, 370, 377, 383
leishmaniasis, 33, 44
- visceral, 40
leprosy, 27
Levi Strauss Co. to employ AIDS sufferers, 197
Linying county (China), 233
Lyme disease (borreliosis), 32

'mad cow disease', 23, 28, 34, 362, 376
malaria, 9, 24, 26, 68, 140, 141, 356

(*see also* specific types e.g. falciparum malaria, vivax malaria etc.)
- 1.5 million people killed annually, 26
- dam-induced, 64, 67
- deforestation increases incidence rate, 45
- Malaria Control Programme, 47
- operations of control, study of
   Brazilian Amazon (1990), 46
   Pacific coastal plain, Colombia, (2004), 46
   Yunnan province, China, (2001), 46
- outbreaks in:
   China, South, 40
   Kenya, 49
   Shanghai, 117, 118
   Singapore, 373, 375
   Uganda, 42
   UK, 48
   Vietnam, 137, 140, 144
- preventive measures, European Union project, 144
- resistance to drug, 151
Malaria Reference Laboratory (UK), 47
- MRL database, 50
Malaysia
- economy affected by SARS, 356
- SARS outbreak in 2003, statements by:
   Abdul Kari Sheikh Fadgir (Minister of Culture, Arts & Tourism), 358
   Aseh Che Mat, (Home Ministry), 357
   Kee Phaik Cheen (State Executive Councillor), 357
Mandela, Nelson, statement on AIDS, 193
Markel, Howard, 381
measles, 73, 74, 79
- epidemic resurgence after sustained interrupted transmission, 77–86
- importation rate, number per year (statistics), 77; lowering rate through global control, 86
in: Australia, 14 outbreaks (1998–2001), 75
   Shanghai, statistics (1955–2003), 117, 118, 121, 129
   US, 41 outbreaks (1997–1999), 74
Mecca (Saudi Arabia), Hajj pilgrimage to, 271–272
Mediterranean Zoonosis Control Programme, 274
meningitis
- outbreak in Shanghai, 129
meningococcal disease, 9, 30, 277–280, 279, 290

- caused by *Neisseria meningitidis* serogroup W135, 278–280, 290
- infection found among Hajj pilgrims in Mecca, 277–280
- transmitted through pilgrims returning from Mecca to: Africa, 280; Singapore, 279
microbes, 29, 35
(*see also* enzootic microbes)
- conditions to become human infections, 34
- resistance to drug, 43
migration, human
(*see also* individual countries e.g. China, Laos etc.)
- human mobility and spread of infectious diseases, 29, 40, 46–49
in: Asia, migrants in labour-importing countries 2000 (statistics), 6
   China, female migrant service and entertainment workers, 255–264
      HIV/AIDS risk, 261
   Laos, migration linked to HIV vulnerability, 213
   UK, postcode used to detect changing location, 51
   Vietnam, infectious diseases spread by internal migration, 150
- migration, gender and sexually transmitted diseases, 251
- mobility risks to HIV/AIDS/ SARS and public health, 207–208
monkey pox virus, 31
Moslem, *see* Islam
mosquitoes, 64
   Anopheles, see Anopheles mosquitoes
   Culex, see Culex mosquitoes
   vector, *see* vector mosquitoes
movement, travel and migration, *see* migration, human
Muslim, *see* Islam
Mycobacterium tuberculosis, see tuberculosis
myocarditis, 291

N. meningitidis W135, *see* meningococcal disease
Narmada river dams (India),
- social and environmental impact of, 66
National Centre for Epidemiology and Population Health, Australian National University, 3
Neisseria meningitidis, see meningococcal disease
Nematode worms, 64

Ngiam, Tong Tau, 359
NGO, *see* non-governmental organisations
Nipah virus
- identification of, 23
in: Malaysia, 31
Singapore, transmitted from Malaysia, 290
- outbreak (1998–99), 100, 101
non-governmental organisations
(*see also* AIDS Organisation)
- comparison with community-based
organisations, 172–173
- guidelines for organisational activities and
services, 170–173
- healthcare programmes for HIV/AIDS
sufferers in Thailand, 161, 162, 169,
problems of the sufferers, 180–182
- important sites for global and local
epidemiological discourses, 163
- support groups, proliferation in Upper North
of Thailand, 163
Norovirus gastroenteritis
- outbreak in Singapore, caused by imported
oysters from China, 289
North American Free Trade Agreement, 27

onchocerciasis, 33, 44
Ong, Hean Teik, 352
orf (viral disease), 274

P. falciparum, see falciparum malaria
Palovsky, E.N
"Landscape Epidemiology" work, 43–44
parapox virus, 274
parasites, animal, *see* animal parasites
paratyphoid, outbreak in Shanghai, 114
patent for
coronavirus genomic sequences sought by
Canadian, US, Hong Kong and
Singaporean institutions, 364
- public funded biomedical research to be
vested in WHO (a suggestion), 365
pathogens
- infections, 35
- movement of, 29
- presented as metapopulations, 43
- resistance to drug, 40
pertussis, 275–276
- International Consensus Group on Pertussis
Immunisation, recommendations, 276
- outbreak in Shanghai, 117

phytoplankton, vibrio-harbouring, 25
plague
in: India, 100,
Singapore, 370, 375
Plasmodium falciparum, see falciparum malaria
Plasmodium vivax, see vivax malaria
pneumonia, 64, 140, 141, 142
(*see also* viral pneumonia)
in: Saudi Arabia, during Hajj pilgrimage in
Mecca, 276
Shanghai, 130
Singapore, 290, 373
Vietnam, 135, 137, 140
poliomyelitis
in: Shanghai, decreasing, 124
population
- ageing and vulnerable to non-communicable
diseases, 98, 99
- in Asia, growth declining and ageing, 4
Japan, ageing, 99
- infectious diseases, 8
- life expectancy in Hong Kong, Japan,
Shanghai, and Taiwan, 119
- migration and labour mobility, 5
- urbanisation, percent in 1975, 2000 and 2030
(statistics), 6, 7
Porcupine Co. to employ AIDS sufferers, 197
public health
- risk analysis and risk communication, 351
- vulnerability linked to migration, 207

Quah, Stella
risk perception of SARS in Hong Kong and
Singapore, research report, 361
quarantine
- SARS (2003):
in: Singapore, strict regulations to control the
spread, 378, 385
Taiwan, widespread measures to isolate the
risk groups, 330
healthcare workers, 342–344
probable-case patients, 335–337

reproductive tract infections, *see* women
reservoirs, *see* landslides, reservoir-induced
respiratory infections, 275
(*see also* acute respiratory infections)
in Vietnam, 76% of the children treated with
antibiotics, 151
Rickettsia tsutsugamushi, 45

Rift Valley hemorrhagic fever, 64, 274
Rodan, Garry, 384
rodents
- rodent-borne hantavirus widespread in
   agricultural systems in S. America, 31
S. japonicum, see Schistosoma japonicum
S. pneumoniae
  bacteria found during Hajj pilgrimage in
   Mecca, 275
S. typhimurium DT104L, *see Salmonella* species
Sadasivan, Balaji (Singapore, Senior Minister for
   Health), 193, 194, 195, 200
Salmonella species, 29
- *S. typhimurium* DT104L detected in
   Singapore, 289
Sardar Sarovar Dam (India), 66
SARS, *see* Severe Acute Respiratory Syndrome
Saudi Arabia
- Al Haram mosque developed for pilgrims,
   272
- brucellosis, highly endemic, 273
- Rift Valley hemorrhagic fever outbreak,
   (2000–2001), 274
  imported sheep from endemic countries
   banned, 274
Schistosoma haematobium, 42
Schistosoma japonicum, 63
schistosomiasis, 33, 63, 64, 67, 68
- epidemics in Volta Lake, Ghana, 46
- known as: bilharzia in Africa, snail fever in
   Asia, water-belly in S. America, 63
Severe Acute Respiratory Syndrome, 8, 23, 24,
   28, 34, 74, 87,100, 103
(see also infectious diseases and individual
   countries)
and 'collateral damage' on East Asian
   economies, 354–355
- affected countries, WHO's list of, 357, 373
- case fatality ratio in Southeast Asia, China,
   Taiwan and Toronto, 353; Roy Anderson's
   estimate, 353
- coronavirus, 354:
  China's failure to identify the virus early, 391
  environment conducive to the virus growth,
   417
  genomic sequences, patent sought by
   Canadian, US, Hong Kong and
   Singaporean institutions, 364

transmission in high-rise buildings, case study
   of Amoy Gardens in Hong Kong, 306,
   307, 310–319
- disease under control 6 weeks after alert,
   WHO's announcement, 362
- economic impact on Canada and East Asia,
   103
- health risk to Hajj pilgrims in Mecca, 277
- outbreak in Amoy Gardens, Hong Kong
   2003, *see* Hong Kong
- vulnerability linked to migration, *see*
   migration, human
sexually transmitted diseases, 64, 98
(see also infectious diseases and individual
   countries e.g. Laos, Thailand etc.)
in China:
  epidemic growth in last 2 decades, 245
  female temporary migrants and
   casual/unprotected sex, survey of, 260
  high occurrence rate linked to migration and
   commercial sex, 246
  STD risk sexual behaviour and STDs by
   migrant status and by gender (statistics),
   258
- spread of diseases linked to:
  diversity of sexual contacts, 28
  migration and gender inequality, 251–251
- syphilis, 64, 68
Shanghai (China)
- food production and distribution control
   system, 126
- infectious diseases, 114–119, 122
  control and prevention measures:
  diseases surveillance network, 123
  drug use and prostitution eradication, 127,
   130
  Municipal Bureau of Health vaccination
   programme, 123–124
  endemics (pre-1950), 114
  incidence rates (1955–1965), 116
  notification system, 123
  health and mortality statistics (after 1950), 115
  public awareness promotion, 126
  registration of births and deaths in urban
   areas, 123
  sexually transmitted,
   gonorrhoea (1955–2003), 117, 128
   syphilis (1955–2003), 117, 128
  three-tier medical and health service network,
   122

- mortality,
  caused by major diseases, 119; age structure of
    deaths, 120
  infant mortality, 121
  rate declines, 120; statistics, 115
- population: ageing, 130 ; life expectancy
  rising, 119–120
- sex revolution since 1980's, 129
- socio-economic development, 113
- water supply, plants construction, 125
Shanghai Municipal Centre for Disease Control
  and Prevention, 113
Shinawatra, Thaksin (Thailand, Prime Minister)
- avian flu mutation, statement, 360
Singapore
- 'Action For AIDS', promotion of safe sex
  practices, 200
- avian flu outbreak, 5000 chickens killed, 359
- health and diseases during the colonial
  period, 373
- healthcare schemes: Medisave, Medishield,
  Medifund, 191
- HIV/AIDS:
  compulsory AIDS test for pregnant women,
    385
  deportation of foreign sufferers, 192, 199
  embalming dead bodies banned to reduce
    risk, 200
  female sufferers increase, 194
  incidence rates by ethnic and occupational
    groups, 189
  infection first reported in 1985, 187
  Ministry of Health's 4 education messages,
    195
  Patient Care Centre's scheme to help
    sufferers, 198, 199
  pattern of infection, 189
  preventive measures through education, 190
  restorative healthcare, 190
  Singapore Press Holdings survey, 191
  sufferers integrating in the workforce and
    their rights protected, 188
- infectious diseases, control strategy of, 287
- living standards, great improvement since
  1959, 374
- public health:
  geriatric health problems, 375
  infrastructure radically expanded, 374
  public sanitation standards maintained, 375
- SARS outbreak (2003), 17, 88, 90

cases, 296
Contact Tracing Centre, 301
containment framed in militaristic terms, 378
Crisis Management Groups, roles and
  responsibilities, 297, 299
foreign migrant workers quarantined on
  arrival, 385
Health Check System, 301
infectious disease alert and clinical database
  system, 301
Infectious Diseases Act, penalties stiffened,
  379
national crisis declared by Health Minister,
  376
pandemic, 370, 372
political aspect, 381, 384, 386–387
preventive and control strategy, 294–301
quarantine regulations set up to control the
  disease, 378, 385
residents' fear and panic, 376
risk analysis and perception, 352–354
schools closed for 2 weeks, 377
three colour-coded alert status, 297
transmission, mathematical models, 88–94
- sickness in historical progress, 370–376
Singapore AIDS Conference, Fourth (2004),
  193
Singapore National Employers' Federation
- employment guidelines for handling
  HIV/AIDS workers, 197
smallpox
- outbreak in:
  Shanghai, 114
  Singapore, 370
snail fever (Asia), *see* schistosomiasis
Sontag, Susan, 386–387
Spanish influenza of 1918, *see* influenza
Stevenson-Wydler Act (US 1980), 364
syphilis, *see* sexually transmitted diseases

Taiwan
- HIV/AIDS:
  first case discovered (1984), 337
  gay rights activists involved more in AIDS
    non-governmental organisations since
    1993, 344
  sufferers and diseased-related groups
    stigmatised in the 'othering' process,
    332–333, 347
- SARS outbreak, 16:

cases and control measures, 330
healthcare demands fell due to public fear of
    utilising the facilities, 103
high-risk groups: healthcare and foreign
    workers, and socially disadvantaged,
    342–346
news media involved in the 'othering
    process', 332–336
political aspect of, 338, 342
public panic triggered by the mass media, 330
qualitative textual analysis of new reports, 334
sufferers stigmatised in the 'othering
    processes', 332, 335, 336, 339
Taiwanese Broadcasting Fund
- national survey on SARS reported by the
    news media in Taiwan, 331
Thailand
- AIDS Organisation, ethnographic study of,
    164–165
    networks and support groups to be
        developed, 174
- avian flu outbreak, Prime Minister Thaksin
    Shinawatra's statement, 360
- HIV/AIDS:
    Chiang Mai sufferer (Porn)'s story, 159–160
    epidemic explosion in the northern region,
        13, 167–168, 170
    non-governmental organizations' healthcare
        programmes for sufferers,
    funded by the Thai Government, 173
    home-based programme and a support
        group network, 161, 169
    outreach needed for mobile sufferers, 161,
        169
    serve as important sites through which
        epidemiological discourses flow, 163
- protection of the 'general population' against
    virus transmission, 168
- sufferers defining their role, training and
    contribution as healthcare volunteers,
    177–178
- virus transmission,
    causes of growth and spreading, 166
    from urban to rural areas, 169
    migrants' vulnerability to HIV/AIDS, 160
    Southern Sipsongpanna (Laos), Tai Lue
        people's migration linked to transmission,
        212
Thompson, Dick, 360
Three Gorges Dam (China), 58, 66, 68

transmissible diseases, *see* infectious diseases
trypanosomiasis, 44
tuberculosis, 9, 24, 27, 40, 64, 68, 127, 129,
    130, 355
- Hajj pilgrimage to Mecca, a transmission risk,
    276, 280
- killed 2 million people annually, 26
- *Mycobacterium tuberculosis*, 276
- outbreaks in:
    China, 4th national survey (2000), 233
        high occurrence rate among off-farm
            migrants, 241–242
        occurrences poverty-related, 231–243
    Singapore, 373–374
    Vietnam:
        Lao Cai, 137, 146
        Northern Mountain Region, 135
- pulmonary tuberculosis, 276
    outbreak in Henan province (China), 232
- resistance to drug, 146, 151
- respiratory tuberculosis, 140
- WHO's 'directly observed therapy
    short-course', 232–233
- World Bank project, 240
- worldwide occurrences re-emerged since
    mid-1980s, 232
typhoid fever, 27

United Nations AIDS Programme, 187
United Nations Development Programme, 61
*Basic need for resettled communities in the Lao
    PDR*, document, 217
United Nations Environment Programme, 67
United States Agency for International
    Development, 61
urbanisation
    (*see also* migration, human)
    in: Asia, population shift from rural to urban
        settings increasing, 6–7
    China, rural-urban dichotomy linked to
        spread of infectious diseases, 405

Vaccination, *see* immunisation
Vaiont Dam (Italian Alps), 65
vector-borne diseases, 29, 33, 41, 42, 44, 49
- dam related, 63
vector mosquitoes (host snails), 29, 64
vectors
- resistance to insecticide, 40, 41
Vibrio cholerae 0139, *see* cholera, Bengal

Vietnam
- Lao Cai:
  health service problems, 151
  infectious endemics, causes of , 154
  research on 4 local communities, 136–138
    ethnographic fieldwork (2003–04), 139
    method of research, 140–141; findings,
    140–155
- Hmong people's migration linked to
  transmission of malaria, 144
- Northern Mountain Region:
  ethnic minorities of, 133
  mortality, leading causes of, 135
Vietnamese-Chinese conflict (1977–1983), 214
viral encephalitis, *see* encephalitis
viral hepatitis, 231, 274
viral pneumonia, 412
virus and viruses
  (*see also* influenza, and specific types, Hendra
    virus, Nipah virus etc.)
- resistance to drugs, 40
vivax malaria, 47, 48

water
  and economic development, 65
- hydraulic systems built in ancient Middle
  East, Asia and S. America, 59
  in: Asia, water-stressed regions, 66
    Brazil, water-related diseases, 58
    Shanghai, water supply system improved,
    124–125
water-belly (S. America), *see* schistosomiasis
water-borne disease, *see* diseases
Wen, Jiabao (China, Premier), 389, 393
- shaking hands with AIDS sufferers at a
  Beijing hospital, 193
West Nile virus, 30–31, 293–294
- environment conducive to the virus survival,
  30
- outbreak in:
  Mexico, state of emergency declared, 31
  United States, endemic, 31
women
  (*see also* individual countries e.g. China, Laos
    etc.)
- gender inequality and HIV/STD risk, 250

in: China, female migrants vulnerable to
  sexually transmitted diseases, 248–251,
  265–266
  individual characteristics by migrant status
    among female 18 years or older, survey
    results, 256
  Singapore, compulsory AIDS test for
    pregnant women, 385
  Vietnam, reproductive tract infection, 140,
  145
World Bank, 61, 67
- tuberculosis control project, 240
World Commission on Dams report (2000), 62,
  68
World Conservation Union, 67
World Health Organization
- assessment of national health systems, 107
- 'directly observed therapy short-course',
  232–233
- Global Conference on SARS, Kuala Lumpur
  (2003), 360
- "Health Impact Assessment" report, 67
- SARS outbreaks, WHO's recommendations
  ignored by international reaction, 101
World Organisation for Animal Health, 421

Yangtze river valley, 57
Yao, Yang, 405
yellow fever, 33, 40, 45
Yellow river, 60
youth
  in Singapore: young generation's high
    expectations, Lee Kuan Yew's comment,
    375, 382
Yuzhou county (China), 233

Zhenping county (China), 233
zoonoses,
  epidemiology of, 43
  in Saudi Arabia, 273
zooplankton, 25